AYURVEDIC SYSTEM OF PATHOLOGY
(Roga Nidānaṁ)

AYURVEDIC SYSTEM OF PATHOLOGY

(Roga Nidānaṁ)

By

KAVIRAJ RUSSICK LAL GUPTA

BKP

BHARATIYA KALA PRAKASHAN

DELHI (INDIA)

Revised Edition : 2006

Published by **C.P. Gautam**
BHARATIYA KALA PRAKASHAN
3421-A, IInd Floor Narang Colony, Tri Nagar,
Delhi-110035. Phone : 27393083, 30967505 (O), 27522129 (R)

ISBN : 81-8090-088-6

Laser Type Setting by
A-ONE GRAPHICS
JD-18C, IInd Floor, Pitampura, Delhi-110088
Phone : 55640278, Mob. : 9811167357

Printed By :
BDH Printer at Salasar Imaging Systems
Delhi, Ph. 9312245804

PREFACE

"Old fashions please me best, I am not so nice
To change true rules for odd intentions."

—Shakespere

The tendencies and prejudice of the people are half revealed or not revealed to those who have not cared to watch with some interest the numerous editions and translations of ancient books that are printed off every month. What makes these possible? Not certainly the increasing figures of population or the rising education of the people, but a reactionary feeling for encouraging the proper recognition of the genius of our sages. A revival has set in—a revival of the old faith for old institutions—especially for the old medical system. No one now puts it down as a huge sham—a pure product of fertile fancy. The people can now understand what a precions store house of medical knowledge is represented by the few old volumes that have descended to us. Even foreigners have not failed to admit, there are many things in them that were never dreamt of in the modern science of medicine. It is an established creed at present that the old system is the genuine creation of long experience and varied experiments and that it can be thus profitably made an excellent hand-maid to the modern one. When such a belief is once awakened, it is no wonder that editions and translations of a *Charaka* or a *Susruta* will spring up with a formidable rapidity. I myself have had the honour of appearing before the public as a translator of some of the oldest but noblest works of medicine and I have met with the greatest the greatest encouragement on every occasion. Relying on the same patronage of our people, I have undertaken to translate into English the Sanskrit treatise on pathology (compiled by Madhava Kar and generally known under the name of Nidāna) giving a full account of the diseases known to the ancient Hindus. It contains many truths which have been recognised by several eminent scientists of Europe and it contains many other whose importance, a remote generation can alone realise. It is moreover a great aid to European scholars as supplying history of diseases which prevailed in past times but have now completely disappeared. The mere fact that it has been the text-book on medicine of native physicians from so long a time should not fail to recommend it to the public. "Our virtues lie in the interpretation of the time." Greatness is not greatness unless approved by time and age. Time has proved that there is infinite truth in the doctrines of Nidāna. What higher testimony of its worth can there be than that a posterity separated by so many hundreds of years should still adore it and should not grudge to be guided by it. A translation of such a book can never be unwelcome. It has been already translated into Bengali. But an English translation is greatly calculated to make its use more general and I have therefore attempted to render it into English which is one day destined to be the language of the universe. The present work is not simply a literal translation of the Sanskrit text. It contains even much of the valuable information to be found in the commentary of Nidāna by Bijoy Rakshit and Sreekanta Dutta. If the translation conveys an idea of the Hindu system of pathology to those who are unacquainted with Sanskrit and if it thus tends in any way to enhance the respect for those great men whose blood still runs in our veins, I shall think my labours amply rewarded.

—K.R.L. Gupta

CONTENTS

ROGA NIDĀNAṀ

(रोग निदानम्)

ज्वरनिदानम्

दक्षापमानसंक्रुद्धरुद्रनिश्वाससम्भवः।
ज्वरोष्टऽधा पृथग् हन्द संङ्जाता गन्तुजः स्मतः॥
मिथ्याहारबिहारस्य दोषा ह्यामाशयाश्रयाः।
वहिर्निरस्य कोष्टाग्निं ज्वरदाः स्यूरसानुगाः॥
खेदावरोधः संतापः सर्व्वाङ्गग्रहणन्तथा।
युगपद् यत्र रोगे च स ज्वरो व्यपदिश्यते॥

FEVERS (*Jwara*)

Fevers are first considered because it is said that man is born and dies with fever ; because it affects the whole body, the organs of senses, and the mind; and is so severe that only man and gods can survive it, and by which various other diseases are produced.

Dakshya the father-in-law of *Shiva* did not invite him to a feast given to the gods, and spoke disrespectfully of him. His wife *Durgā* was present, and was so enraged, at the disrespect, that she considered it better to die than live under such a disgrace; and while sitting, her spirit left her body. *Nundi* the servant of *Durgā* seeing her die, went and informed *Shiva* of the event. He in grief for his loss, tore off one of his locks, and it fell into the fire, and a great devil named *Birabhadra* was produced from it. Others say that in his anger he heaved a deep sigh, and from his mouth the devil was produced. *Birabhadra* asked *Shiva* to be allowed to destroy his father-in-

श्रमोऽरतिविवर्णत्वं वैरस्यं नयनप्लवः।
इच्छाद्वेषौ मुहुश्चापि शीतवातातपादिषु॥
जृम्भाङ्गमर्द्दो गुरुता रोमहर्षोऽरुचिस्तमः।
अप्रहर्षश्च शीतञ्च भवल्युत्पत्स्यति ज्वरे॥
सामान्यतो विशेषेण जृम्भात्यर्थं समीरणात्।
पित्तान्नयनयोर्द्दाहः कफादन्नारुचिर्भवेत्॥
रुपैरन्यतराभ्या तु संसृष्टेर्द्वन्द्वजं विदुः।
सर्व्वत्र समलिङ्गञ्च सर्व्वदोषप्रकोपजे॥
वेपथुर्बिषमो वेगः कण्ठौष्ठपरिशोषणम्।
निद्रानाशः क्षवस्तम्भो गात्राणां रौक्षमेव च॥

law. This was permitted, and after polluting the sacred fire of *Dakshya,* destroying many of his guests, and tearing his hair, he wrenched his head from his body. It was during the paroxysm of grief and rage of *Shiva* for the death of *Durgā* that the breath which proceeded from his nostrils, hot, and destructive, gave origin to fevers, which attack all persons, of all ages, and in all conditions.

The *cause* of all the principal varieties of fever, with the exception of five from accidents (*āgantuka*), is using improper mixtures of food ; as eating fish and milk ; the want of seasoning in food; sleeping at improper hours; fighting with a strong man; exposure to the morning sun while fasting; eating voraciously of food of a very hot nature, when the body has been previously weakened by extreme hunger; and by fatigue, fear, grief, and watching. Fevers are also produced by poisons, drinking stagnant water, in which withered leaves have fallen; taking a full meal without any appetite, or after delivery, especially if improperly treated. In other cases the first secretion of milk in the breast, produces fever, exposure to unseasonable weather, or to sudden vicissitudes of temperature ; checked perspiration, long continued constipation ; and living in wooded, ill ventilated valleys. Other causes of fever are the

शिरोह्वग्दात्ररुग्वद्ब वैरस्यं गाढ़विट्कता।
शूलाध्माने जृम्भणञ्च भवत्यनिलजे ज्वरे।
वेगस्तीक्ष्णोतिसारश्च निद्राल्पत्वं तथा वमिः।
कण्ठौष्ठमुखनासानां पाकः स्वेदश्च जायते॥
प्रलापो वक्क्रटुता भूर्च्छादाहौ मदस्तृषा।
पीतविन्मूत्रनेत्रत्वं पैत्तिके भ्रम एव च॥
स्तमित्यं स्तिमितो वेग आलस्य मधुरास्यता।
शुक्लमूत्रपुरीषत्वं स्तम्भस्तृप्तिरथापि च।
गौरवं शीतभुतक्वे दो रोमहर्षोऽतिनिद्रता।
प्रतिश्यायोरुचिः कासः कफजेऽक्ष्णोश्च शुल्कता॥

influence of bad stars, neglected adoration of saints or gods ; visiting a new climate ; the malign influence of evil spirits, and severe local diseases, or injuries. By such causes the air, bile, and phlegm are deranged, pass into the stomach (*āmīshay*), and thus expel the internal heat. The humors stop also the chyle vessels, and derange the heate, which digests the food : in other words, whatever exposes our moral qualities, or bodily frame, to deviations from their natural and accustomed movements, produces fever ; and it requires remedies to drive back the heat, to its natural position, when the person is restored to health.

GENERAL SYMPTOMS OF FEVER.

The attack of fever commences with the person complaining of lassitude and fatigue ; he is continually yawning, and stretching ; his skin loses its natural colour, and there is a bad taste in his mouth; his eyes are watery, and he alternately wants the application of heat, and cold to thc body. Littlc, and much food distresses the person, as it is not digested; he has no appetite, the body is chilly and heavy, with dejection of mind ; and he is quarrelsome, and ready to fight with a much stronger person than himself.

तृष्णा मूर्च्छा भ्रमो दाहः स्वप्नाशः शिरोरुजा।
कण्ठास्यशोषो वमथुरोमहर्षऽरुचिस्तमः।
पर्व्वभेदश्च जृम्भा च वातपित्तज्वराकृतिः॥
स्तैमित्यं पर्व्वणाम्भोदो निद्रागौरव मेव च।
शिरोग्रहः प्रतिश्यायः कासः स्वेदाप्रवर्त्तनम्॥
सन्तापो मध्यवेगश्च बात श्लेष्मज्वराकृतिः।
लिप्ततिक्तास्यता तन्द्रा मोहः कासोऽरुचिस्तृषाः।
मुहुर्दाहो मुहुःशीतं पित्त श्लेष्मज्वरान्तिः॥

These precursory symptoms are followed by heat of the surface, cessation of perspiration, and pain affecting the whole body, but particularly the members. There is also pain in the chest, languor and drowsiness, loss of appetite, restlessness, heaviness of the abdomen with costiveness, and a copious flow of urine. These symptoms are always present in fevers ; but, when *air* is deranged, there is also much gaping ; when *bile* is affected the eyes feel hot, and when *phlegm* is deranged there is no appetite.

1*st Variety of Fever.* *Bātik-jwara* is that variety which is produced by a derangement of the air (*bāyu*).

This fever commences with shivering, there is sometimes much at other times little heat ; the throat, mouth, and lips are dry, the patient has no sleep, does not sneeze, his skin is dry, with head-ache, and pain in the chest, as well as over the body. Whatever is taken into the stomach feels heavy, and creates uneasiness ; the stools are very hard ; pain in the abdomen ; flatulence as if much food had been eaten , and he is frequently yawning.

2nd form of Fever. When Bile is deranged, producing fever, it is called (*Paittika Jwara*). This form of fever commences with a shivering fit, followed by a severe hot stage ; a frequent desire to go to stool, vomiting, a bitter taste in the mouth, and restlessness. Aphthae form in the throat, lips, mouth, and nose;

क्षणे दाहः क्षणे शीत मस्थिसन्धिशिरोरुजा।
सास्त्रावे कलुषे रक्ते निर्भुग्ने चापि लोचने॥
सरुनौ सरुजौ कर्णौ कण्ठः शूकैरिवावृतः।
तन्द्रा मोहः प्रलापश्च कासः श्वासोरुचिर्भ्रमः॥
परिदग्धा खरणार्थ। जिह्वास्त्रस्ताङ्गता परम्।
ष्ठीवनं रक्तपित्तस्य कफेनोन्मिश्रितसा च।
शिरसो लोढनं तृष्णा विद्रानाशो हृदिवाथा।
स्वेदमूत्रपुरीषाणां चिराद्दर्शनमल्पशः॥
कृशत्वं नातिगात्राणां प्रततं कण्ठकुजनम्।
कोढानां शबरक्तानां मण्डलानाञ्च दर्शनम्।

the patient perspires freely, often speaks nonsense, and has sometimes fainting fits, and attacks of giddiness. Such a patient is very listless, his body is pale, with a burning sensation over the surface, he has great thirst, the stools and urine have a yellow colour, as well as the eye, which is often also red.

3rd form of Fever. Derangement of phlegm (*Kapha*), produces a fever named *shlaishmik-jwara,* or *kapha-jwara*. This fever is ushered in by loss of appetite, and the symptoms of the hot stage is less marked than in the last form of fever. The person feels languid, and listless, with a sweet taste in his mouth. In this fever the body feels cold, as if wrapped in a wet cloth, and stools and urine are white. Such a person remains quiet and silent, does not eat ; but feels as if he had eaten too much, his body is very heavy, eyes white, with nausea attended with cough. He is very sleepy, and there is a discharge of mucus from the eyes, mouth, and nose.

4th.Bāta-paittika Jwara. This fever commences with giddiness, fainting and thirst : the body feels cold to another person, although he complains of his body being hot and burning, loss of memory, no sleep, pain in all the joints, headache, cough, throat and mouth dry, vomiting, goose-skin, no perspiration, low spirits, and yawning.

मूकत्वं स्त्रोतसां पाको गुरुत्वमुदरस्य च॥
चिरात् पाकश्च दोषाणां सन्निपातज्वराकृतिः॥
दोषि विवद्धे नष्टेऽग्नौ सर्व्वसम्पूर्णलक्षणः।
सन्निपातज्वरो साध्यः कृऽच्छसाध्य स्ततोऽन्यथा।
सप्तमे दिवसे प्राप्ते दशमे द्वादशेऽपि वा।
पुनर्घोरतरो भूत्वा प्रशमं याति हन्ति वा॥
सप्तमी द्विगुणा चैव नवम्येकादशी तथा।
एषा त्रिदोषमर्यादा मोक्षाय च वधाय च॥
सन्निपातज्वरस्यान्ते कर्णमूले सदारुणः।
शोथः सञ्जायते तेन कश्चिदेव प्रमुच्यते॥
त्रयः प्रकुपित दोषा उरःस्त्रोतोऽनुगामिनः।

5th. Bāta-shlaishmik Jwara. This form of fever is not very severe in its accession. The body feels cold, with slight shivering and pain in the bones ; the person sleeps much, has pain in the head, with much saliva in the mouth, and running at the nose, with cough, a dry skin, and body hot.

6th. Bile and Phlegm, (Pitta-shlaishmik Jwara). The mouth is clammy and sour, with much saliva, in this form of fever. Ther person is always dozing, complains of faintness, and coughs; has no appetite, thirst and is at one time hot, and at another time cold.

7th. Mixed Remittent or Synochus Fever, (Sannipāt Jwara Bikāra). In this form of fever the air, bile, and phlegm, are deranged ; and it is always dangerous. At one time the patient is hot, at other times cold, with pains in the bones, and joints ; the eyes are watery, of a dirty yellow colour, and hollow; the patient complains of ringing, and pain in the ears, with pain in the head, neck, and thorax ; is always dozing, but cannot sleep at night; has no memory, and is often delirious. Bodies seem to turn round, and sometimes he is laughing, crying, performs unnatural actions, is always coughing, has quick

आमातिवृद्ध्या ग्रथिता बुद्धीन्द्रियमनोगताः।
जनयन्ति महाघोरमभिन्यासं ज्वरं दृढ़म्।
श्रुतौ नेत्रे प्रसुप्तिः स्यान्न चेष्टां काञ्चिदीहते।
न च दष्टिर्भवेत्त्वस्य समर्था रूपदर्शने।
न घ्रानं न च संणशं शब्दं वा नैव बुध्यते।
शिरो लोढयतेऽभीक्ष्ण-माहारं नाभिनन्दति।
कुजति तुद्यते चैव परिवर्त्तनमीहते।
अल्प प्रभाषते किञ्चिदभिन्यासः स उच्यते।
प्रत्याख्यातः स भूयिष्ठः कश्चिदेवात्र सिध्यति॥
अभिघाताभिचाराभ्यामभिषङ्गाभिशापतः।

breathing, no appetite, the tongue is black like charcoal, and irregular like that of a cow, with pain. Blood, phlegm, air and bile flow from the mouth, the patient moves head about continually, with thirst, watching, and pain in the breast. The urine is secreted in small quantities, with costiveness and no perspiration ; great thirst, noises in the throat, so that there is a difficulty in comprehending what the sick person says ; with round elevations, and central depressions of a blue and red colour, over the surface of the body. The person vomits blood, mixed with phlegm, and his abdomen diminishes in size. His body does not become thin, but his belly is heavy and enlarged. This kind of fever remains long, and much care and proper medicines are required for its cure. After the first stage, should the fever continue severe, it will be generally fatal ; and at the last stage of the fever the lower part of the ear (the parotid gland) swells. This is supposed to be a fatal sign.

The 7th, 10th, 12th days, are always the days on which the fever is severe, or from these periods the symptoms diminish in severity.

In other books it is stated that the critical days are the 7th, 9th, 11th, 14th, 18th, 22nd ; from which period the desease is

आगन्तुजायते दोषैर्यथास्वं त्वं विभावयेत्।
श्यावास्यता विषकृते तथातीसार एव च।
भक्तारुचिः पिपासा च तोदश्च सह मूर्च्छया।
ओषधीगन्धजे मूर्च्छा शिरोरुग्वमथु स्तथा।।
कामजे चित्तबिभ्रंश स्तन्द्रालस्यमभोजनम्।
भयात् प्रलापः शोकाच्च भवेत् कोपाच्च वेपथुः।।
अभिचाराभिशापाभ्यां मोहस्त्यृष्णा च जायते।
भूताभिषङ्गादुहेगो हास्यरोदनकम्पनम्।।
कामशोकभयाद्वायुः क्रोधात् पित्तं त्रयो मलाः।

diminished or increased. Those who live till the 22nd day generally recover.

There are thirteen kinds of mixed fever. In three kinds one of humours, that is the air, bile, or phlegm, are morbidly increased, or diminished beyond the others. In a second form two are increased or diminished. The thirteenth variety is that in which the three humours are morbidly increased.

1. ***Bisfaraka Bātulbana.*** When the air is increased, the usual symptoms of this form of fever will be accompanied with a bad taste in the mouth, difficulty of breathing, shivering, cough, yawning, giddiness, syncope, delirium, and pain in the sides of the belly.

2. ***Pittulbana or Asukarī*** **.** The peculiar symptoms of this form are looseness, giddiness, fainting, aphthae in the mouth, red spots, and a burning sensation, over the body.

3. ***Korupono or Kaphulbana,*** is distinguished by a feeling of languor, a difficulty in speaking, sleeping much, eyes cloudy, and a sweet taste in the mouth.

4. ***Pobru Bobru. Bālapittulbana.*** When bile is increased the person feels as if he had taken narcotic medicines, complaining of thirst, dry mouth, drowsiness, flatulence, loss

भूताभिषङ्गात् कुप्यन्ति भूतसामान्यलक्षणाः॥
दोषोल्पोऽहितसम्भूतो ज्वरोत्सृष्टस्य वा पुनः।
धातुमन्यतमं प्राप्य करोति विषमज्वरम्॥
सन्ततं सततान्येद्यस्ततीयकचतुर्थकान्।
सन्ततं रसरक्तस्थः सोऽन्येदुऽः पिशिताश्रितः॥
मेदोगत स्तृतीयेऽह्नि अस्थिमज्जागतः पुनः।
कुर्य्याच्चातुर्थकं घोरमन्तकं रोगसङ्करम्॥
सप्ताहं वा दशाहं वा द्वादशाहमथापि वा।
सन्त्यत्यायोऽविसर्गी स्यात् सन्त्यतं स निगद्यते॥
अहोरात्रे सततको द्वौ कालावनुवर्त्तते।
अन्येदुष्कस्त्वहोरात्र एककालं प्रवर्त्तते॥
तृतीयकस्ततीयेऽह्नि चतुर्थेऽह्नि चतुर्थकः।
केचिद्भूताभिषङ्गोत्थं व्रुबते विषमज्वरम्॥

of appetite, cough, difficulty of breathing, giddiness, and languor.

5. ***Bato Soleso, Ulbono, or Sigrokarī.*** When the air and phlegm around the neck is stopped, fever comes on with shivering, fainting, sneezing, thirst, pains in the sides of the body and in the abdomen, and difficulty in breathing.

6. ***Petu Soleso Bono Bolu.*** Is distinguished by a burning sensation in the body with chilliness, much thirst, pain in the right side of the chest, head-ache, pain in the breast and throat, vomiting phlegm and bile, looseness, difficulty of breathing, hiccough, and drowsiness.

7. ***Bato-Peto-Soliso-Ulbono*** or ***Kutopākolo.*** In this form the three air, bile and phlegm are morbidly increased, and like thunder, fire and sword, it kills quickly. The peculiar symptoms of this form of fever are, the patient breathes slowly and imperfectly, he is motionless, his eyes are fixed, and after three days he dies.

कफपित्तात्रिकग्राही पृष्ठाद्यातकफात्मकः।
वातपित्ताच्छिरोग्राही त्रिविध स्यात्ततीयकः॥
चातुर्थको दर्शयति प्रभावं द्विबिधं ज्वरः॥
जङ्घाभ्यां श्लैष्मिकं पूर्व्वं शिरस्तोऽनिलसम्भवः।
विषमज्वर एवान्यश्चातुर्थकविपर्ययः।
मध्येऽहनि ज्वरयतीत्यादावन्त्ये च मुञ्चति॥
नित्यं मन्दज्वरो रुक्षमः शूनकस्तेन सीदति।
स्तब्धाङ्गः श्लेष्मभूयिष्ठो नरो वातवलासकी।
प्रलिम्पन्निव गात्राणि घर्म्मेण गैरवेण वा।
मन्दज्वरविलेपी च सशीतः स्यात् प्रलेपकः॥
विदग्धेऽन्नरसे देहे श्लेष्मपित्ते व्यवस्थिते।
तेनार्द्धं शीतलं देहे चार्द्धचोष्णां प्रजायते।

8. ***Songonohohoko.*** The peculiar symptoms of this variety are delirium, languor, faintness, shivering, giddiness, and paralysis of half the body. This is a very dangerous disease.

9. ***Pākolo.*** Faintness, delirium, stiffness of the neck, head-ache, cough, difficulty of breathing, giddiness, drowsiness, severe pain in the chest, hemorrhage from the mouth, and nose, and the eyes being fixed characterise this form of fever. The patient generally dies within three days.

10. ***Jammo.*** In this variety severe pain in the chest, and abscesses form in the liver, spleen and lungs ; and both the patient's stools, and the matter vomited contain blood and pus.

11. ***Korkotoko.*** Is accompanied with a burning sensation internally, the person cannot speak, his face and eyes become red, he cannot expectorate the phlegm from his throat, has severe lancinating pains in the breast, with drowsiness, difficulty of breathing, and hiccough. These symptoms increase daily ; the patient's tongue becomes black and rough, his throat

कायेे दुष्टं यदा पित्त्रं श्लेष्मा चान्त्ये व्यवस्थितः।
तेनोष्णत्वं शरीरस्य शीतत्वं हस्तपादयोः।
काये श्लेष्मा यदा दष्टः पित्तञ्चान्ते व्यवस्थितम्।
शीतत्वं तेन गात्राणां उष्णत्वं हस्तपादयोः।
त्वक्रुख्यौ श्लेष्मानिलौ शीतमादौ जनयतो ज्वरे।
तयोः प्रशान्तयोः पित्तमन्ते दाहं करोति च॥
करोत्यादौ तथा पित्तं त्वक्रुख्यं दाहमतीव च।
तस्मिन् प्रशान्ते त्वितरौ कुरुतः शीतमन्ततः॥
द्वावितौ दाहशीतादिज्वरौ संसर्गजौ स्मृतौ।
दाहपूर्व्वस्तयोः कष्टः कच्छसाध्यतमश्च स॥

becomes covered with prickles, involuntary evacuations follow; he moans much ; like the cooing of a pigeon ; his mouth, lips, and palate are dry, he sleeps much, and he cannot speak, with convulsions, or nausea and vomiting.

12. ***Boidārīko.*** In this fever there is pain in the loins, the body is cool, and during the accession the body feels cold, with diarrhoea, giddiness, languor, head-ache, drowsiness, pain in the neck and chest, cough, difficulty of breathing, and insensibility.

13. ***Abhinyāsa Jwara.*** Is characterized by dryness of the mouth, by the patient being always sleepy, and his body feels as if it belonged to another person ; he seaks very little, and with great pain, is stupid, and breathes with difficulty. His internal heat is diminished, he feels an internal burning sensation accompanied with weakness, and a dead like feeling of the skin.

8th. Accidental fever, (Āgantuka.) The causes of this order of fevers are injuries ; such as wounds, *etc.* They may also be produced by the evil designs of an enemy, or a devil ; by the passions ; by the curses of a guru, a brāhman, or a prophet ;

गुरुता हृदयोत्क्लेशः सदनं छर्द्यरोचकौ।
रसस्थे तु ज्वरे लिङ्गं दैनञ्चास्योपजायते॥
रक्तनिष्ठीवनं दाहो मोहश्छर्द्दनविभ्रमौ।
प्रलापः पीडका तृष्णा रक्तप्राप्ते ज्वरे नृनाम्॥
पिण्डिकोद्देष्टनं तृष्णा सृष्टमूत्र पुरीषता।
उष्मान्तर्द्दाहविक्षेपौ ग्लानिः स्यान्मांसगे ज्वरे।
भृशं स्वेदस्तृया मूर्च्छा प्रलापश्छर्द्दिरेव च।
दौर्गन्धयारोचकौ ग्लानिः मेंदख्ये चा सहिष्णुता॥
भेदोस्थां कूजनं श्वासो विरेकश्छर्द्दिरेव च।
विक्षेपणञ्च गात्राणाभेतदख्यिगते ज्वरे॥

by poison, or by the effects of air mixed with deleterious matter, as that proceeding from a kind of poisonous trees which are supposed to come from the east. These causes derange the air, bile, and phlegm, and thus produce fever.

Adultery, grief for parents, friends, etc. derange also the air, anger deranges bile, and devils derange both air, bile, and phlegm.

When a man wants to kill another, or to remove an obnoxious individual to another country ; or to have command of him, certain *mantras,* and directions are given in the *Tantra Shāstra* for accomplishing these. But should he err in any of the injunctions enjoined, the person himself will be attacked with the fever, and he will not have power to injure the other. In some such cases the two front teeth are extracted to prevent the person blundering in pronouncing *mantras*.

When the fever is produced by poisons the tongue is white, or black in the middle, the person has frequent stools, and fainting fits, and has no appetite, or memory, and complains of thirst, and pain over the body. By improper medicines this fever is sometimes produced with swooning, head-ache, and vomiting.

तमः प्रवेशनं हिक्का कासः शैत्तं वमिस्तथा।
अन्तर्द्दाहो महाश्वासो मर्म्मभेदश्च मज्वगे।
मरणं प्राप्नुयात्तत्र शुक्रख्यानगते ज्वरे॥
शेफसः स्तब्धता मोक्षः शुक्रस्य तु विशेषतः॥
वर्षा शरद्वसन्तेषु वातादैः प्राकृतः क्रमात्।
वैकृतोऽन्यः स दुःसाध्यः प्राकृतश्चानिलोद्भवः।
वर्षासु मारुतो दुष्टः पित्त्वश्लेष्मान्वितो ज्वरं॥
कुर्यात् पित्तञ्च शरदि तस्य चानुबलः कफः।
तत्प्रकृत्या विसर्गाच्च तत्रनानशनाद्भयम्॥
कफी वसन्ते तमपि वातपित्तं भवेदनु।
काले यथास्वं सर्व्वेषां प्रवृत्तिर्वृद्धिरेव वा।

When it is produced by the passion of love there is no memory, the person dozes, is lazy, and delirious.

When produced by the curses of a good man, or by the sorcery of another, want of memory and thirst are peculiar symptoms present ; and when an evil spirit produces it, the person alternately is sorrowful and laughing ; and at other times he cries and laughs.

9th. Intermittent fevers (Bishama Jwara). This is another form of fever, which occurs before and after attacks of other kinds of fever ; by the derangements of the humours of the body. The essential parts of the body such as chyle, blood, muscles, fat, bone, semen, and marrow, in the order now mentioned may be affected. One or more are sometimes deranged, and form so many types of fever.

These are *Santata, Satata, Anyejyuka, Tritīyaka, Chāturthaka*. The general symptoms of intermittent fever are as follows: when the paroxysm occurs at uncertain periods the patient feels first cold, then hot, and afterwards perspires.

निदानोक्तानुपशयो विपरीतीपशायिता॥
अन्तर्द्दाहोऽधिकस्तृष्णा प्रलापः श्वशनं भ्रमः।
सन्ध्यस्थिशूलमस्वेदो दोषो वर्च्चो विनिग्रहः।
अन्तर्व्वेगस्य लिङ्गानि ज्वर स्यैतानि लक्षयेत्।
सन्तापो ह्यधिको वाह्य स्तृष्णादीनाञ्च मार्द्दवम्।
बहिर्व्वेगसा लिङ्गानि सुखसाध्यत्वमेव च॥
लालाप्रसेको हृल्लासो हृदयाशुद्ध्यरोचकाः।
तन्द्रालस्याविपाकास्य वैरस्यं गुँरुगात्रता॥
क्षुन्नाशो बहुमूत्रत्वं स्तब्धता बलवान् ज्वरः।
आमज्वरस्य लिङ्गानि न दद्यात्तत्र भेषजम्॥

The following five varieties are described :

1. *Santata* continues for several days without an intermission.
2. *Satata* has two paroxysms daily.
3. *Anyejyuka* occurs daily, at the same hour.
4. *Tritīyaka* occurs on alternate days.
5. *Chāturthaka* occurs every fourth day.

The following varieties of this class of fevers are described by Ancient Medical writers.

1. ***Santata-jwara*** affects the chyle and blood ; and it continues for 7, 10, or 12 days ; followed by an interval and again occurs, and remains for several days.

2. ***Satata*** has two paroxysms daily, one in night and another during the day.

Others say there are two kinds of this fever, one of which commences with a cold fit, and another with a hot fit. The first gives much uneasiness, and is cured with difficulty.

भेषजं ह्यामदोषस्य भूयो ज्वलयति ज्वरम्॥
ज्वरवेगऽधिकस्तृष्णा प्रलापः श्वसनं भ्रमः।
मलप्रवृत्तिरुत्क्लेशः पच्यमानस्य लक्षणम्॥
क्षुत्क्षामता लघुत्वञ्च गात्राणां ज्वरमार्द्दवम्।
दोषप्रवृत्तिरष्टाहौ निरामज्वरलक्षणम्॥
बलवत् स्वल्पदोषेषु ज्वरः साध्यऽनुपद्रवः।
हेतुभिर्बह्वभि र्जातो बलिभिर्वह्वलक्षणः॥
ज्वरः प्राणान्तकृद् यश्च शीघ्रमिन्द्रियनाशनः।
ज्वरः क्षौणस्या शून्यस्य गम्भीरो दैर्घरात्रिकः॥
असाध्यो बलवान् यश्च केशसीमन्तकृत् ज्ज्वरः।

3. If the paroxysm of fever recurs at the same hour daily, it is called *Anyejyuka*.

4. When the fever returns at an interval of one day it is called *Tritīyaka*. These are the following three varieties of this fever :

a. When *phlegm* and *bile* are deranged in this fever, before the accession, pain is felt at the nape of the neck.

b. When *spirit* and *phlegm* are deranged, the patient first feels pain in the loins.

c. When *air* and *bile* are deranged, the fever is introduced with head-ache.

5. In *Chāturthaka,* the paroxysms of this fever occur every fourth day. When the paroxysm continues for two days, there is no paroxysm on the first and fourth day, the fever is that called *Chāturthaka Biparjyaya*.

This fever presents the following symptoms. It commences with shivering, dryness, and swelling. The patient has no strength, so as not to be able to walk. He evacuates much bile, air, and phlegm which are particularly affected.

गम्भीरस्तु ज्वरो ज्ञेयो ह्यन्तर्दाहेतेन तृष्णया।
आनद्धत्वेन दोषाणां श्वासकासोद्गमेन च।
आरम्भाद्विषमो यस्तु यश्च वा दैर्घरात्रिकः।
क्षीणसा चातिरुक्षस्य गम्भीरी यस्य हन्ति तम्।
विसंज्ञस्ताम्यते यस्तु शेते निपतितोऽपि वा॥
शीतार्द्दितोऽन्तरुक्षश्च ज्वरेण म्रियते नरः।
यो हृष्टरोमा रक्ताक्षो हृदि संघातशूलवान्।
वक्त्रेण चैवोच्द्दछ्रसिति तं ज्वरो हन्ति मानवम्।
हिक्काश्वासतृषायुक्तं मूढं। विभ्रान्तलोचनम्॥
सन्ततोच्छासिनं क्षीनं नरं क्षपयति ज्वरः॥
हतप्रभेन्द्रियं क्षीणमरोचकनिपीड़ितम्॥

When the body is heavy, with perspiration, and little fever and stools, it is called *Proapiko*.

When half the body is hot, and the other cold ; when what is eaten is not digested, and does harm ; the deranged bile and phlegm have produced these morbid symptoms. When the bile of the body is deranged, and phlegm of the arms and legs, the body is hot and the hands and feet cold. When the phlegm of the body is deranged, and bile of the hands and feet, the body is cold, and the hands and feet are hot.

The fever is also modified, as the essential parts are deranged. Thus the air may be deranged in the blood, flesh, bone, marrow and semen ; and the supposed danger increasing in the order above stated, until the last, the semen, when the fever is considered always fatal.

The type of the fever varies also according to the season of the year. Each of them forms two lunar months; during June and July, the rainy season (*Barshā*), air predominates, and the fevers takes on the characters of deranged air. The season called *Sharata,* autumn, or sultry months (Sept. and Oct.), the bile and the phlegm predominate ; *Basanta* or spring (Feb. March

गम्भीरतीक्ष्णवेगाप्तं ज्वरितं परिवर्ज्जयेत्॥
दाहः स्वेदो भ्रमस्तृष्णा कम्पबिड्भेदसंज्ञिता।
कूजनञ्चास्य वैगन्ध्यमाकृतिर्ज्वरमोक्षणे।
स्वेदो लघुत्वं शिरसः कण्डुः पाको मुखस्य च।
क्षबथुश्चान्नलिप्सा च ज्वरमुक्तस्य लक्षणम्॥

अतीसारनिदाम्

गुर्व्वतिस्निग्धरुक्षोष्ण द्रवस्त्यूलातिशीतलैः।
विरुद्धाध्यसनाजीर्णै विषमैश्चापि भोजनैः॥
स्नेहादौ रतियुक्तैश्च मिथ्यायुक्तैर्विषैर्भयेः।

and April), the phlegm is in excess, and is succeeded by derangement of the air and bile, followed by fever.

Āhaka-jwara*, *(Nakra* or *Nāsā-jwara.) We are subject to this peculiar form of intermittent fever. The description of it is not contained in the more ancient medical works. It is produced by a swelling of the Schniderian membrance, and is said to be caused by the air and phlegm deranging the blood of the part. It is accompanied with pain over the body, but particularly in the neck and back, and other symptoms of fever.

It is of frequent occurrence in Bengal ; attacks adults alone, between the age of 20 and 40 years of age.

DYSENTERY (*Atīsār*)

Dysentery is produced by a variety of causes ; such as exposure to cold, eating very cold articles of food in considerable quantities, eating much ghee and oily articles, very heavy or hot substances, or very thin or dry articles of food ; eating several articles of food with contrary qualities, such as milk and fish, etc., or any kind of indigestable food, causes this disease. In other cases it is produced by the food not being properly boiled or mixed, or being eaten at improper times ; or when not properly seasoned, or in unusually small or large

शोकाद्दुष्टाम्वुमद्यातिपानैः सात्म्यर्त्तुपर्य्ययैः॥
जलाभिरमणैगर्व्वेविघातैः क्रिमिदोषतः।
नृणां भवत्यतीसारो लक्षणं तस्य वक्ष्यते॥
संशम्यापां धातुरग्निं प्रवृद्धः शकृन्मिश्रो वायुनाधःप्रणुन्नः।
सरत्यतीवातिसारं तमाहुर्व्याधिं द्योरं षड्बिधं वदन्ति॥
एकैकशः सर्व्वशश्चापि दोषैः शोकेनान्यः षष्ठ आमेन चोक्तः।
हृन्नाभिपायूदरकुक्षितोद्गात्रावसादानिलसन्निरोधाः॥
विट्संज्ञ आध्मानथाविपाको भविष्य स्तस्य पुरःसराणि॥
अरुणं फेनिलं रुक्षः मल्पमल्पं मुहुर्मुहुः।
शकृदामंसरुक्शब्दं मारुतेनातिसार्य्यते॥
पित्तात् पीतं हरितं लोहितं वा तृष्णा मूर्च्छा दाहपाकोपपन्नम्।

quantities. In some cases the disease is produced by poisons, great fear, or grief ; by unwholesome drinking water; by much wine, and peculiar food which thus affects certain persons ; and by irregular or sudden changes in the seasons. Remaining long in the water while bathing, worms, deranged or constipated alvine, or other excretions, sometimes produce the disease. The symptoms are explained by the internal fire being diminished by morbid watery secretions, or phlegm generated in the intestines ; this is mixed with the faeces, and is carried off downwards by the air of the part. Hence the production of watery stools, etc. In some cases the fever cccurs first from the derangement of air, bile, and phlegm ; in other cases the dysentery precedes the fever, and sometimes both occur together. In these cases abstinence from eating the drinking is to be observed, and such medicines are to be given as prepare the food that is in the abdomen. If dysentery is present such medicines are to be used as will dry up and stop this discharge, and the physician is to decide in each case which sort of remedies are to be given, whether they should be to cure first the fever or the diarrhoea.

शुक्लं सान्द्रं सकफं श्लेष्मणा तु विस्त्रं शीतं हृष्टरोमा मनुष्यः॥
वराहस्नेहमांसाम्बु सदृशं सर्व्वरूपिणम।
कृच्छ्रताध्यमतीसारं विद्याद्दोषत्रयोद्भवम्॥
तैंस्तेंर्भावैः शोचतोऽल्पाशनस्य वाष्पोष्मावैं वह्निभावित्तजन्तोः।
कोष्ठं गत्वा क्षोभयेत्तसा रक्तं तच्चाधस्तात् काकणन्ती प्रकाशम्॥
निर्गच्छद्वै विड्विमिश्र ह्यबिड़ वा निर्गन्धं वा गन्धवद्वातिसारः।
शोकोत्पन्न दुश्चिकित्स्योऽतिमात्रं रोगो वैद्यैः कष्ट एष प्रदृष्टः।
अन्नाजीर्णात् प्रद्रुताः क्षोभयन्तः कोष्ठं दोषा धातुसङ्घान्भलांश्च।
नानावर्णैकशः सारयन्ति शूलोपेतं षष्ठमेनं वदन्ति॥

There are six varieties of this disease, as when the air, bile, and phlegm are deranged, it forms so many kinds ; when the three deranged together, when produced by grief, and when caused by mucus in the abdomen. *Dhanantwari* says, there are many other varieties as the symptoms vary from time to time.

Before this disease develops itself a sharp pain is felt in the chest, umbiliacus, and anus, and in the abdomen under the false ribs, which is succeeded by want of appetite, languor, and lassitude of the body; no air passed by the anus, the patient is costive, the abdomen swelled, and every thing taken remains undigested. When air produces the disease it commences with great pain; the dejections are of a dark yellow colour, frothy, dry and frequent, and in small quantities mixed with the indigested substances, which have been eaten, pain is felt in the anus on the expulsion of air, and the urine is scanty.

2. When bile is deranged, the dejections are expelled with an effort. They have a bad smell, are hot; and of a red yellowish colour, like the water in which flesh had been steeped. In other cases they are of a blue or red colour, and are accompained with thirst, dozing, heat of body, free perspirations and tenesmus at the time of the evacuation. There is often in such cases inflammation of the rectum with violent fever.

3. When phlegm is deranged, the person dozes, the

संसृष्टमेभिर्दोषैस्तु न्यस्तमपस्ववसीदति।
पुरीषं भृशदुर्गन्धि पिच्छिलञ्चामसंज्ञितम्॥
एतान्येव तु लिङ्गानि विपरीतानि यस्य वै।
लाघवञ्च विशेषेण तस्य पक्कं विनिर्द्दिषेत्॥
पक्कजाम्बवसङ्काशं यकृत् पिण्डनिभं तनु।
घृततैलवसामञ्जवेश वारपयोदधि॥
मांसधावनतोयाभं कृष्णां नीलारुणप्रभम्।
भेचकं स्निग्धककवरं चन्द्रकोपगतं घनम्।
कुणपं मस्तुलुङ्गाभं सुगन्धि कथित वहु।
तृष्णा दाहतमःश्वासहिक्कापार्शख्यिशूलिनम्।
संमूर्च्छारतिसंमोहयुक्तं पक्कवलीगुदम्।

dejections are white, thick, and constipated, mixed with phlegm. He has no appetite, complains of languor and lassitude with dozing, and has frequent calls to stool, which are passed without any noise.

4. When the above three humours are deranged the dejections are of different colours. The patient is very thirsty with languor, dejection of mind, and drowsiness. This kind of dysentery is fatal when children and old people are attacked, and in all cases it is difficult to cure, and will cause much vexation to the physician. The symptoms will vary according as one or other of the above forms predominate. The cause of the disease will likewise vary the symptoms.

5. When grief produces dysentery, the person has the internal fire of *pakasia* deranged by the watery vapours, which are formed by grief , and passing into *pakasia* mixes with the fire, and deranges the bright blood of the part. This blood is mixed with the dejections, often becomes putrid, and is expelled with them. In other cases it is discharged by itself. Sometimes it has a bad smell, in other cases it has not. The cure is tedious, and physicians are vexed by its obstinacy. If the dejections are frequent, the cure will be very difficult.

प्रलापयुक्तञ्च भिषग्वर्ज्जयेदतिसारणिम्।
असंवृतगुदं क्षीणं दुराधनातमुपद्रुतम्॥
गुदे पक्के गतोष्माणमतिसारकिण त्यजेत॥
श्वासशूलपिपासार्त्तक्षीणं ज्वरनिपीड़ितम।
विशेषेण नरं वृद्धमतीसारो विनाशयेत्।
पित्तकृन्ति यदात्यर्थं द्रव्याण्यश्नाति पैत्तिके।
तदोपजायतेभिक्षणां रक्तातीसार उलबण:।
वायु: प्रवृद्धोनिचितं बलाशं नुदत्यधस्तादहिताशनसा।

6. The sixth form is when it is produced by mucus, which deranges the stomach and is discharged frequently of various colours.

There are also two forms of dysentery, one being acute (*Āmaapāka*) or crude, and the other chronic (Pākātisār) or mature

ACUTE DYSENTERY (*Āmaraktātīsār*)

This from is known by the dejections sinking in water, and being very foetid. In the pāka variety the opposite symptoms to the above are most prominent, and the abdomen does not feel heavy.

The unfavourable symptoms are a stiffness of the body, dejections of a dark bluish colour, like the ripe rose-apple; in other cases the colour of the dejections is like that of the lime, of ghee, or of oil, of tallow or marrow; in other cases they are like milk or curds; or like water in which flesh had been washed; or black, blue, or yellow; or like the colour of these three mixed together in different proportions; or like the water of Madar. In other cases they are very thin, of a foetid smell, and cold; or of the colour of peacock's feathers, or that of thc rainbow, or dry and hot. Sometimes the dejections are consistent, or like the brain, or like the refuse of well washed and beaten bark (fibrous), or its decoction, and are evacuated in large quantities. When the sick person is thirsty and hot,

प्रवाहतोऽल्पं वहुशो मलाक्तं प्रवाहिकां तां प्रवदन्ति तज्ज्ञाः।
प्रवाहिका वातकृता सशूला पित्तात् सदाहा सकफा कफाच्च।
सशोणिता शोणितसम्भवाच्चताः स्नेहरुक्षप्रभवा मतास्तु।
तासामतीसारवदादिशेच्च लिङ्ग क्रमञ्चामविपक्कताञ्च।
यस्योपचारं विना मूत्रं समग्वायुश्च गच्छ्रति॥
दीप्ताग्ने र्लघुकोष्ठस्य स्थिततस्योदरामयः॥

ग्रहणीरोगनिदानम्

अतीसारे निवृत्तेऽपि मन्दाग्नेरहितासिनः।
भूयः संदूषितो वह्निर्ग्रहणीमभिदूषयेत्॥
एकैकशः सर्व्वशश्च दोषैरत्यर्थमूच्छितैः।
सा दुष्टावहुभो भुक्तमाममेव विमुञ्चति॥
पक्कं वा सरुजं पूति मुहुर्व्वद्धं मुहुर्द्रवम।

breathes through the nose, has hiccough, and pain in the side, and skin, with loss of memory, dosing and stupor, the disease will be fatal. Such a person has no inclination to do any thing, and remains stupid and complains of pain in the anus, like that of a ripe boil. He speaks incoherently and becomes insensible, with an involuntary discharges from the anus : such person will not live. When the person is very much reduced in flesh, is cold and the abdomen distended, with pain in the anus: such a person should not be attended by the practitioner, as the disease is incurable.

The physician should be able to distinguish the symptoms of *Ama*, of acute, from those of chronic dysentery. Without this he will not be able to treat the disease properly.

DIARRHOEA (*Grihinī*)

By the use of improper food the internal fire is weakened, which deranges the place where it is situated, between the stomach and place of the chyle. When any thing is eaten, which is not properly digested, and is frequently discharged, with or

ग्रहणीरोगमाहुस्तमायुर्व्वेदविदो जनाः॥
पूर्व्वरुपन्तु तस्येदं तृष्णालस्यं बलक्षयः।
विदाहोऽन्नसा पाकश्च चिरात कायस्य गौरवम्॥
कटुतिक्तकषायातिरुक्षसंदुष्टभोजनैः।
प्रमितानशनात्यध्व वेगविनिग्रहमैथुनैः॥
मारुतः कुपितो वह्निं संछाद्य कुरुते गदान्।
तस्यान्नं पच्यते दुःखं शुक्तपाकं खराङ्गता॥
कण्ठास्यशोषः क्षुतृष्णा तिमिरं कर्णयोः स्वनः।
पार्शोरुवङक्षणग्रीवारुगभीक्षणं विसूचिका॥
हृतप्रीड़कार्श्यदौर्व्वल्यं वैरसां परिकर्त्तिका।
गृद्धिः सर्व्वरसानाञ्च मनसः सदनन्तथा।
जिर्णे जीर्यति चाध्मानं भुक्त्वे स्वाख्य्यमुपैति च।
न वातगुल्महृद्रोगप्लीहापूङ्गी च मानवः॥
चिराद्दुखं ट्रवं शुष्कं तन्वामं शब्दफेनवत्।
पुनः पुनः सृजेहर्च्चं कासशासर्हितोऽनिलात्॥
कट्वजीर्णविदह्यम्लक्षाराद्यै पित्तमुल्वणम्।

without pain, sometimes, liquid, at other times consistent, sometimes it is evacuated without air, and at other times it is foetid, it forms this disease. Before it commences the patient complains of lassitude and weakness of the body, accompanied with noise in the intestines, sour and bitter eructations, and a bad taste in the mouth. When a singing of the ears, oedema in the hands and feet, with pain in the joints, vomiting, fever, thirst, loss of appetite, and a heaviness and burning sensation the the body occurs, in old cases, the prognosis should be guarded. These symptoms are varied when either the air, bile, or phlegm, or their peculiar symptoms are present.

Another form of Diarrhoea is called *Sangraha Grihinī;* from *Sangraha,* (a collection,) and *Grihinī,* (place of internal

आप्लावयद्धन्त्या नलं जलन्तप्तमिवानलम्।।
सोऽजीर्णं नीलपीताभं पीताभः सार्यते द्रवम्।
पूत्यम्लोद्गरहृततकण्ठदाहरुचितृड़र्द्दितः।।
गुर्ब्बतिस्निग्धशीतादिभोजनादतिभोजनात्।
भुक्त्वामात्रस्य च स्वप्लाद्धन्त्यग्निं कुपितः कफः।
तस्यान्नं पच्यते दूःखं हृल्लासकृर्द्दरोचकाः
आसोप्यदेहमाधुर्य्यं कासष्ठीवनपीनसा।।
हृदयं मन्यते स्त्यान मुदरः स्तिमितं गुरु।
दुष्टो मधुरउद्गार सदनं स्त्रीषहर्षणम्।
भिन्नाम श्लेष्मसंश्लिष्टं गुरुवर्च्चप्रवर्त्तनं।
अकृशस्यापि दौर्व्वला मालस्याञ्च कफात्मके।
पृथग्वातादिनिर्द्दिष्ट हेतुलिङ्गसमागमे।।
त्रिदोषं निद्दिशेदेवं तेषां वक्ष्यामि भेषजं।।
अन्त्रकूजनमालस्यं दौवल्यं सदनन्तथा।
द्रवं शीतं घनं स्निग्धं सकटिवेदनं शकृत्।
आमं वहु सपैच्छिल्यं सशब्दं मन्दवेदनम्।।
पक्षमान्मासाद्दशाहाद्वा नित्यं वापथ्य मुञ्चति।।
दिवा प्रकोपो भवति रात्रौ शान्तिं व्रजेच्च सा।
दुर्व्विज्ञेया दुश्चिकित्सा चिरकालानुवर्द्धिनौ।
सा भवेदामवातेन संग्रहग्रहणी मता।

fire;) in which there is much noise in the stomach, with laziness, weakness and lassitude. The stools are unnatural, irregular, and evacuated with noise; sometimes they are thin, and in other cases they are consistent or hard, and of a pale colour like indigested food. Some people remain ten or fifteen days, or even one month, without any fecal discharge; other patients feel well during the day, but have frequent dejections during the night. The prognosis of this form of disease is unfavourable, as it is obstinate and is cured with much difficulty.

अर्शोनिदानम्

पृयग्दोषैः समस्तैश्च शोणितैः सहजानि च।
अर्शांशि षट् प्रकराणि विद्यादगुदवलित्रये॥
दोषास्तङ्यांसमेदांसि संदुष्य विविधाकृतीन्।
मांसाङ्कुरानपानादौ कुर्व्वन्त्यर्शंसितान् जगुः॥
कषायकदुतिक्तानि रुक्षशीतलधूनि च।
प्रमिताल्पाशनं तीक्ष्णं मद्यं मैथुनसेवनम्॥
लंघनं देशकालौ च शीतौ क्यायामकर्म च।
शोको वातातपर्स्मशों हेतुर्व्वातार्शसां मतः।
कट्वम्लवणोष्णाणि व्यायाममन्यातपप्रभाः।
देशकालावशिशिरो क्रोधो गद्यमसूयनम्।
विदाही तिक्ष्ण सुषाञ्च सर्व्वं पानान्नभेषजम्।

Arsa (*Piles*)

There are six varieties of this disease according as it is produced from deranged air, bile, phlegm, the three humours deranged at the same time, diseased blood, and the last form is congenital or hereditary.

That part of the rectum called *guda* is five and a half fingers breadth in length, has three spiral turns called *Prabāhini* which accelerates or assists in expelling its contents. The second is called *Bisarjini*, or that which expells; and *Sambarini*, or sphincter. Piles are usually situated in these parts, the causes producing them are as follows: The improper mixtures, of food, excessive venery, the unnatural position of the body when long indulged in horse riding, and the want of attention to the calls of nature. By these causes the humours are deranged in the anus and produce tubercles, or piles.

When air is deranged it affords the following signs : round the anus small tumors from, which are dry, slightly painful red, and irregular like the *kadamba* fruit. The disease is accom-

पित्तोल्वणनां विज्ञेयः प्रकोपे हेतुरर्शसाम्॥
मधुरस्निग्धशितानि लवणाम्लगुरूणि च।
अव्यायाम दिवास्वप्न शय्यासनसुखे रतिः॥
प्राग्वातसेवा शीतो च देशकालावचिन्तनम्।
श्लैष्मिकानां समुद्दिष्टमेतत् कारणमर्शसाम॥
हेतु लक्षणसंसर्गाद्विद्याद्द्वन्दोल्वणानि च।
सर्व्व हेतु स्त्रिदोषाणां सहजैर्लक्षणैः समम्॥
विष्टम्भौऽन्नस्य दौर्व्वल्यं कुक्षेराटोप एव च।
कार्श्यमुद्गार वाहुल्यं स किथ्सादोऽल्पविट्कता॥
ग्रहणीदोष पाण्ड्वत्तेराशद्ध चोदरस्य च।
पूर्व्वरूपाणि निर्द्दिष्टान्यर्शसामभिवृद्धये॥
गुदाक्षुरा वह्निलाः शुष्का श्रिमचिमान्विताः॥

panied with constipation, pain in the back, loins, penis, anus, and umbiliacus, and is occasionally accompanied with pain in the breast, want of appetite, cough, and noise in breathing; sometimes the appetite is good, at other times it is much impaired. The blood is often evacuated by a small orifice from time to time. The skin, eyes, face, mouth, teeth, and nails appear dirty and yellow with unhealthy yellowish dejections and urine. Symptoms likewise appear like *Gulma* or spleen, or it even produces these diseases. In other cases the piles produce *Astila,* a kind of hysterical ball.

When bile is deranged the swelling has an erysipelatous appearance; at other times it has a blue yellow, red, or black colour, with orifices in its surface like the mouths of leeches. The blood evacuated is very thin, and there is a considerable discharge, with pain in the part, accompanied with fever, thirst, and fainting.

When phlegm is deranged the tumors are pendulous, near each other, hard, round, shining, and of a white colour, like

म्लानाः श्यावारूणास्तब्धा विषादा परुषाः खराः॥
मिथो विसदशा वक्रा स्तीक्ष्णा विस्फुटिताननाः।
विम्बीखर्ज्जूरकर्कन्दुकार्पासीफलसन्निभाः।
केचित् कदम्वपुष्पाभाः केचित् सिद्धार्थकोपमाः।
शिरः पार्श्वांश कट्यूरुवङ्गणाद्यधिकव्यथा।
क्षवथुद्गारविष्ठम्भः हृद्गुहारोचकप्रदाः।
काशश्वासाग्निवैषमा कर्णनाद भ्रमावहाः॥
तैरार्त्तो ग्रथितं स्तोकं सशब्दं सप्रवाहिकम्।
रुक्फेनापिच्छानुगतं विबद्धमुपवेश्यते।
कृष्णत्वङ्नखविण्मूत्रनेत्रवक्त्वृश्च जायते।
गुल्मप्लीहोदराष्ठीला सम्भवस्तत एव च॥
पित्तोत्तरा नीलमुखा रक्तपीतासितप्रभा।
तन्वस्त्रास्त्रविणो विस्त्रा स्तनवो मृदवः श्लथाः।
शुकजिह्वायकृत्खण्डजलौक वक्त्रसन्निभाः।
दाहपाकज्वरस्वेद-तृण्मूर्च्छारुचिमोहदाः।
सोष्मार्ग द्रवनीलोष्णपीतरक्तामवर्च्चसः।
यवमध्या हरितपीतहारिद्रत्वद्धनखादयः॥

the paps of the cow. There is no discharge, they are cold, itchy, heavy, remain stationary, and the stools are mixed with mucus, and appear like water in which flesh had been washed. In some cases the disease is accompanied with swelling of the extremities, with feverishness, loss of appetite, heaviness and pain of the head; and the skin, nails, eyes, face, urine, and faeces becomes white. In these diseases there is a great discharge of urine, the person often becomes impotent, and digestion is impaired, with vomiting. Those diseases which impair digestion, produce this disease. When the three humours are diseased, the symptoms of the three separate diseases are present.

श्लेष्मोल्वण महामूला घना मन्दरुजः सिताः।
उत्सन्नोपत्ति स्निग्धाः स्तब्धवृत्तगुरुस्थ्यिराः।
पिच्छिलाः स्तिमिताः श्ललक्ष्ण कण्ड्वढ्याः णर्शनप्रियाः।
करीरपनसाख्याभा स्तथा गोस्ता सन्निभाः।
वङ्क्षणानाहिनः पायुस्तिनाभिविकर्षिणः।
सश्वास कासहृल्लासप्रसेकारुचिपीनसाः।
मेहकृच्छ्रशिरोजाड्य शिशि ज्वरकारिणः।
क्लेव्याग्निमार्द्दवः छर्द्दिरामप्राय विकारदाः।
वसाभ सकफप्राह्य पुरीषाः सप्रवाहिकाः।
न स्त्रवन्ति न भिद्यन्ते पाण्डुस्निग्धत्वगादयः।
सर्व्वैः सर्व्वात्मकान्याहु लक्षणैः सहजानि च।
रक्तील्वणा गुदे कीलाः पित्ताकृतिसमन्विताः।
वटप्ररोहसहशा गुञ्जाविद्रुमसन्निभाः॥
तेऽत्यर्थे दुष्टसुष्याञ्च गाढविट्क प्रपीड़ताः।
स्त्रवन्ति सहसा रक्त्वं तस्य चातिप्रवर्त्तितः॥
मेकाभः पीड्यते दुःखैः शोणितक्षयसम्भवैः।

When blood produces the disease, the pain is like that of a needle thrust into the skin, and symptoms appear like those of deranged bile. The tumors resemble the hanging roots of the banian tree, or the *kunch* seeds, small red seeds with black spots, or they are like coral. When costiveness occurs it is accompanied with a free and rapid discharge of blood, which is hot, and produces the usual effects of a great and sudden loss of blood; the person with this disease remains yellow, like the yellow frog; weak, silent, and sad; his skin is dirty, and all his senses perform their office imperfectly or they are depraved. The dejections are gray, like smoke, dry and hard, and in others they are thin, yellow, and frothy.

The last form of this disease is produced by hereditary

हीनवर्णवलोत्साहो हतौजाः क्रलुषेन्द्रियः।
विट्श्याबं कठिनं रुक्षमधोवायुर्न वर्त्तते।
तनु चारुणवर्णञ्च फेनिलच्चासमृगर्शसाम्।
कट्टूयरुगुदशूलञ्च दौर्व्वल्यं यदि चाधिकम्।
तवानुवन्धो वातस्य हेतुर्यदि च रुक्षणम्॥
शिथिलं स्वेतपीतञ्च बिट्स्निग्धं गुरु शीतलम्।
यद्यर्शसां घनञ्चासृक् तन्तुमत् पाण्डुपिच्छिलम्।
गुदं सपिश्छं स्तिमितं गुरु स्निग्धञ्च कारणम्।
श्लेष्मानुबन्धो विज्ञेय स्तत्र रक्तर्शर्षां बुधैः॥
पञ्चात्माः मारुतः पित्तं कफो गुदबलीत्रयम्।
सर्व्व एवं प्रकुप्यन्ति गुदजानां समुद्भवे॥
तस्मादर्शांसि दुःखानि वहुत्याधिकराणि च।
सर्व्वदेहोपतापनि प्रायः कृच्छ्रतमानि च॥
वाह्यायान्तु बलौ जातान्येकदोषोल्वणानि च।
अर्शांसि सुखसाधानि न चिरोत्पतितानि च॥
द्वन्द्वजानि द्वितीयायां नलौ यान्याश्रितानि च।
कृच्छ्रसाध्यानि तान्याहुः परिसंवत्सराणि च।

disposition, from the taint being mixed in the semen and female blood. The tumors in this form become rough, of a white unnatural colour, with internal openings. The patient cannot eat much, his body has large veins over the surface, and his voice is low. He is impatient, is easily roused, has little appetite, is afflicted with disease of the eyes, ears, nose and head, and is always complaining of diseases of the stomach and intestines.

When piles are external they are easily cured, but when situated internally they are cured with difficulty, or are incurable. Tumors like those of piles sometimes form in the cavities of the ear, nose, mouth, vagina, and upon the penis.

सहजानि त्रिदोषानि यानि चाभ्यन्तरां बलिम्।
जायन्तेऽर्शांसि संश्रिता तान्यसाध्यानि निर्दिशेत्।
शेषत्वादत्युषस्तानि चतुष्पादः समन्विते॥
याप्यन्ते दीप्तकायाग्नेः प्रत्याखेययान्यातोऽन्यथा।
हस्ते पादे मुखे नाभ्यां गुदे वृषणयोस्तथा॥
शोथो हृतपार्श्वं शूलञ्च यस्यासाध्योऽर्शसो हि सः।
हृत्पार्श्वशूलं संमोहश्चद्रिरङ्गसा रुग्ज्वरः॥
तृष्णा गुदस्य पाकश्च निहन्युर्गुदजातुरम्।
तृष्णारोचकशूलार्त्तमतिप्रश्रुतशोणितम्॥
शोथातिसारसंयुक्तमर्शांसिक्षपयन्ति हि।
मेढ्रादिष्वपि वक्ष्यन्ते यथास्वं नाभिजानि च।
गण्डूपदासारूपाणि पिच्छिलानि मृदूनि च।

When affecting the internal ear, they produce deafness, pain, and a fetid discharge from the organ. In the eyes they cover the eyelids; and sometimes destroy the sight of the organ. When in the mouth, they are attached to the throat, lips, and palate, they impair the voice and taste, and produce other diseases of the mouth. When in the nostrils they produce difficult breathing, a fetid smell, a change of voice, pain in the head, and a considerable discharge from the nose.

The deranged humours produce the disease on the surface of the body when they form tumors of different sizes, which are called *Charmkīla*. When the air is deranged the disease is accompanied with throbbing; when phlegm, the colour or the tumor is the colour of the skin and hard. When bile and blood are deranged, producing the disease, the tumors become black and rough. Those piles which form externally are curable, as also those in the first and second convolutions of the rectum, but in the third the disease is incurable, and also after they have existed for upwards of a year.

:

अग्निमान्ध्यांजीर्णविसूचिकालसक विलम्बिकानिदानम्

मन्दस्तीक्ष्णोऽथ विषमः समश्चेति चतुर्व्विधः।
कफपित्तानिलाधिक्यात्तत्साम्याज्जाठरोऽनलः॥
विषमो वातजान् रोगान् तीक्ष्णः पित्तनिमित्तजान्।
करोत्यग्नि स्तथा मन्दो विकारान् कफ सम्भवान्॥
समासमाग्नेरसितामात्रा सम्यग्विपच्यते।
स्वल्वापि नेव मन्दाग्ने र्विषमाग्नेस्तु देहिनः॥
कदाचित् पच्यते सम्यक् कदाचिच्च न पच्यते।
मात्रातिमात्राप्यसिता सुखं यस्य विपच्यते।
तिक्ष्णाग्निरिति तं विद्यात् समाग्निः श्रेष्ठ उच्यते।
आमं विदग्धं विष्टब्धं कफपित्तानिलैस्त्रिभिः।
अजीर्णं केचिदिच्छन्ति चतुर्थं रसशेषतः।
अजीर्णं पञ्चमं केचिन्निर्द्दोषं दिनपावि च।
वदन्ति षष्ठं चाजीर्णं प्राकृतं प्रतिवासरम्॥

Ajirna, (*Indigestion*)

This disease is divided into three varieties, *Āma Ajīrna Bistabdha Ajīrna,* and *Bidagdha Ajīrna.* When digestion is good, the food is properly prepared for the use of the body, the eructations are free and without taste, and the dejections are natural, the body is light and elastic, and the person is inclined to exertion, he has a good appetite and the food is tasty, and is accompanied with thirst.

When digestion is imperfect the person's temper becomes bad, he is subject to anger, is fearful, and becomes covėtous. The food of persons with a bad and hasty temper is not properly digested. When indigestion occurs, there is a disinclination to exertion, with giddiness; the body is heavy, the colour of the skin bad, and there is no passage of air; such a person does not like his food, his understanding is impaired, and his bowels are either constipated or there are copious dejections.

अत्यम्बुपानाद्विषमाशनाच्च संधारणात् स्वप्नविपर्यवाच्च।
कालेऽपि सात्मत्यं लघु चापि भुक्त मन्नं न पाकं भजते नरस्य॥
तत्रामे गुरुतोत्क्लेदः शोथो गण्डाक्षिकुटगः।
उद्गरश्च यथा भुक्त्व मविदग्धः प्रवर्त्तते॥
विष्टब्धे शूलमाध्मानं विविधा वातवेदना।
मलवाताप्रवृत्तिय स्तम्भो मोहाङ्गपीड़नम्॥
विदग्धे भ्रमतृन्मूर्च्छाः पित्ताच्च विविधा रुजः।
उद्भारश्च सधुमाम्लः स्वेदो दाहश्च जायते॥

The unfavourable symptoms of this disease are fainting, delirium, vomiting, a copious discharge of saliva from the mouth, with languor, and giddiness.

Āma Ajīrna. In this disease the body feels heavy, with a flow of saliva and phlegm from the nose. The eyelids swell, and there are eructations of the substances eaten, some time before.

In ***Bistabdha Ajīrna,*** the air is deranged, and produces severe pain in the stomach, with flatulency. The stomach swells there are no dejections, no air escapes, and the person remains stupid, with his understanding impaired, and pain over the body.

In ***Bidagdha Ajīrna,*** the bile is deranged, the person has sour eructations, complains of thirst, is giddy and often dozes. He has a free perspiration over the body, which feels hot.

When there is want of digestion, although the individual thinks the appetite good and eats, still it does not nourish the body, but acts as a poison in destroying the person. When the food is not taken in the usual quantities, digestion is not performed, and is often followed by disease. When a person eats like an animal, without consideration, he will be affected with indigestion, which is the cause of other diseases, as cholera, drum-belly, and constipation.

रसशेषेऽन्नविद्वेषो हृदयाशुद्धिगौरवे॥
मूर्च्छा प्रलापो वमथः प्रसेकः सदनं भ्रमम्।
उपद्रवा भवन्त्येते मरणं वाप्यजीर्णतः।
अनात्मवन्तः पशुवद्भुञ्जते येऽप्रमाणतः।
रोगानीकस्य ते भूल मजीर्णं प्राप्नुवन्ति हि॥

विसूची-अलसक-विलम्विका निदानम्

अजीर्णमामं विष्टब्धं विदग्धञ्च यदीरितम्।
विसूच्यलसकौ तस्माद्भवेच्चापि विलम्विका॥
सूचीभिरिव गात्रणि तुदद् सन्तिठष्तेऽनिलः।
यस्याजीर्णेन सा वैद्यै र्विसूचीति निगद्यते।
न तां परिमिताहारा लभन्ते विदितागमाः।

Ālasaka, (drum-belly). The abdomen in this disease becomes enlarged and tight, with a rumbling noise, the air passes upwards, followed by a constipation of faeces and air; with great thirst, eructations, and pain in the stomacii.

Bilambika, or constipation, is somewhat different from drum-belly, as there is no swelling nor tightness of the abdomen; nor is the indigested food either rejected by vomiting nor by stool; but is retained in the abdomen causing much pain there, and likewise producing various diseases in different parts of the body. Constipation is always difficult to cure.

DYSPEPSIA (*Agnī Māndya*)

This disease is supposed to be produced by derangements of the internal fire. It has four varieties.

1st. When there is too little fire, it is called *Manda Agnī* ; when food is not digested, or only imperfectly. In this form, the diseases of phlegm are often present.

2nd. When the fire is too strong, as when bile is deranged, it is called *Tikhna Agnī*. In this case, little or even

मूढ़ास्तामजितात्मानो लभन्तेऽशनलोलुपाः।
मूर्च्छातिसारो वमथुः पिपासा मूलभ्रमोद्वेष्टनजृम्भदाहाः।
वैवर्ण कम्पो हृदये रुजश्च भवन्ति तस्थां शिरस्य भेदः।
कुक्षिरानह्यतेऽत्यर्थे प्रताभ्येत परिकूजति।
निरुद्धो मारुतश्चैव कुक्षावुपरि धावति।
वातवर्च्चोनिरोधश्च यख्यात्यर्थं भवेदपि।

large quantities of food are digested ; and the diseases of bile are liable to occur.

3rd. When the air is deranged the food is sometimes digested and sometimes not ; from fire being sometimes in the natural state, and at other times it is deranged. In this case the disease is called *Bishama Agnī*, when other diseases of air are present.

4th. *Bhasma Agnī*, *(Bulimia,)* when pungent, sour and dry food are taken for some time ; phlegm is diminished, and air is much increased ; the internal fire, with the deranged air, absorbs the liquid part of the body, and the food when taken is soon digested, or reduced to ashes, the person is not satisfied. This disease is accompanied with great thirst, dry cough, fainting, giddiness, burning of the body and emaciation, with severe constipation, and much perspiration.

When there is no increase or diminution of the air, bile, and phlegm, in the same person ; the fire remains in the natural state, and is called *Sama Agni*. This is not a disease, but is the most favourable state of digestion, and is the condition in which food is properly digested ; when not taken in too small, or too large quantities. The divisions of the digestive organs into the parts in which the food are received, *Amasia,* (stomach;) *Agniaria,* (the duodenum;) and in which the digested food is removed *Pakasia,* (the small intestines,) is probably from the known structure of the intestines of the inferior animals.

This disease is produced by drinking much water, and eating at unusual hours, when very little food is taken, and the calls of nature are resisted ; when the person is sleepy or is in

तस्यलसकमाचष्टे तृष्णाद्गारौ च यस्य तु॥
दुष्टन्तु भुक्त्वं कफमारुताभ्यां प्रवर्त्तते नोर्द्धमधश्च यस्य।
विलम्विकां तां भृशदुश्चिकित्सा।
माचक्षते शास्त्रविदः पुराणाः।
यत्रस्थमाम् विरुजेत्तमेव देद्यं विशेषेण विकारजातेः।
दोषिण येनावततं शरीरं तल्लक्षणैरामसमुद्भवैश्च।
यः श्यावदन्तोष्ठनखोऽल्पसंज्ञो वम्यर्द्दितोऽभ्यन्तरयातनेत्रः।
क्षामस्वरः सर्व्वविमुक्तसन्धिर्यायान्नरः सोऽपुनरागमाय।
उद्गारशुद्धिरुत्साहो वेगोत्सर्गो यथोचितः।
लघुता क्षुत्पिपासा च जीर्णाहारस्य लक्षणम्॥

a passion, or is afraid, grieved, or fatigued at the time of eating; and when he dislikes the food during the time of eating. It is also produced, when the person sleeps during the day, instead of at night, or is irregular in the time of sleeping and when at the usual time of dinner, little is eaten. By such causes the food is not digested in the proper manner. When phlegm is deranged the food tastes sweet, and is indigested when bile, the taste is sour, and the food in the stomach produces eructations ; and air when deranged causes the partially digested food to be dried up, with pain in the stomach.

CHOLERA (Bisuchika)

The person first feels pain, as from indigestion, in the abdomen followed by frequent stools and vomiting, great thirst, and pain in the abdomen, fainting, giddiness, yawning, and cramps in the legs. The colour of the body is altered, accompanied with shivering, pain in the chest, and head-ache. The unfavourable symptoms of cholera are, the lips, teeth and nails become blackish, the person insensible, with frequent vomiting. The eyes become sunken, voice feeble, and the joints loose, with great debility. Such a person may be taken out to the burnt, as he will not recover. The most fatal symptoms of cholera are, want of sleep, restlessness, shivering, no secretion of urine, and insensibility.

क्रिमिनिदानम्

क्रिमयश्च द्विधा प्रोक्ता वाह्याभ्यन्तरभेदतः।
वहिर्मलकफासृग्विट् जन्मभेदाच्चतुर्व्विधाः॥
नामतो विंशतिविधा वाह्यास्तच्च मलोद्भवाः॥
तिलप्रमाणसंख्यानवर्णाः। केशाम्बराश्रयाः॥
बहुपादाश्च सूक्ष्माश्च युका लिख्याश्च नामतः।
द्विधा ते कोठपिड़क कण्डुगण्डान् प्रकुर्व्वते॥
अजीर्णभोजी मधुराम्लनित्यो द्रवप्रियः
पिष्टगुड़ोपभोक्ता व्यायामवर्ज्जी च
दिवाशयानो विरुद्धभुक् संलभते क्रिमींस्तु॥

WORMS (*Krimi*)

There is an internal sort of worms, and another which appears upon the surface of the body. Others say that there are four kinds ; one is external and produced by filth on the surface; others are internal and are produced by phlegm, by food and by the faeces. There are twenty varieties of worms, of which has a particular name. When produced externally by filth, the insect is like a small Til-seed with many and is generally found in the hair and clothes. They are called *juka* (lice). They produce small very itchy pimples, and sometimes a large boil.

When *phlegm* produces the worms internally, it is deranged by indigestable food, particularly when taken at improper times, or with much sugar, or sweetmeats, or much liquids, as vinegar or sour food, curdled milk, vegetables, and unleavened flour when taken daily and frequently. A sedentary life, and sleeping during the day predisposes to worms.

When *blood* produces worms many diseases are the consequence. In this case it is caused by improper mixtures, or by the indigestable food, or certain vegetables, etc. The worms are produced in the blood.

मा पिष्टाम्लवणगुड़शाकैः पुरीषजाः।
मांसमत्स्यगुड़क्षीरदधिशुक्तैः कफोद्भवाः॥
विरुद्धाजीर्णशाकादैः शोणितोत्था भवनिहि।
ज्वरो विवर्णता शूलं हृद्रोगः सदनं भ्रमः॥
भक्तद्वेषोऽति सारश्च सञ्जातक्रिमिलक्षणम्।
कफादामाशये जाता वृद्धाः सर्पनिसर्व्वतः॥
पुथुव्रध्ननिभाः केचित् केचिद्गण्डूपदोपमाः।
रुढ़धाशङ्कुराकारा स्तनुदीर्घा स्तथाणवः॥
श्वेतास्ताम्रावभाषाश्चयसतः सप्तधा तु ते।
अन्त्रादा उदरावेष्टा हृदयादा महागुदाः॥

The general symptoms of internal worms are fever, paleness, and discoloration of the surface, severe pain, or *Sul,* especially in the breast, with languor, giddiness, loss of appetite, and diarrhoea. When produced by phlegm they are usually found in the stomach (*Āmāsiya*), and resemble earth-worms, and when very large they pass from one intestine to another. Some of the worms are like rice which have begun to germinate, some are long, others are short, and very small ; some are white, or like nahogany, others are copper-coloured. There are seven varieties of worms found in the stomach. 1st. *Antrada* or the gnawing kind; 2nd. *Udarābesta,* large form ; 3rd. *Rhidayada,* produces a gnawing pain in the breast ; 4th. *Mahāgada,* with a large tail ; 5th. *Chara,* like flattened rice ; 6th. *Durbakusama,* like the flower of a certain grass, and 7th. *Sugandha,* which has a pleasant smell. These seven kinds of worms produce nausea, a copious discharge of saliva, indigestion, and want of appetite ; fainting, dozing, vomiting and fever ; constipation of urine and faces, and weakness, sneezing, and discharge of mucus from the nose.

The worms in the blood have no feet, some have a round figure and red colour (red globules of the blood), and they are so small that they cannot be distinctly seen. Their names are

परवो दर्मकुसुमाः सुगन्धास्त्ये कुर्व्वते।
हृल्लासमास्यश्रवण मविकमरोचकम्।
मूर्च्छाछर्द्दिज्वरानाह कार्श्यक्षवथुपीनसान्।।
त्रक्तवाहिशिराग्यान रक्तजा जन्तवोऽणवः।
अपादा वृत्तताम्राश्च रक्षात् केचिद्दर्शनाः।।
केशादा रोमविध्वंसा रोमद्दीपा उडुम्वराः।
राट् ते कुष्ठैककर्म्माणः सह सौरस मातरः।
पक्काशये पूरीषोत्था अन्तेऽधो विसर्पिणः।
बृद्धास्ते सार्न्मवेयुश्च ते यद्दामाशयोन्मुखाः।
हास्योद्गारनिश्वामविड्गन्धानुविधायिनः।।
पृथुवृत्ततनुस्थूलाः ह्यवपीतसितासिताः।।
ते पञ्च नाम्ना क्रिमयः ककेरुकमकेरुकाः।

1. *Kāysāda:* this form eats the roots of the hair of the head which drop out. 2. *Romabidhansa :* this form eats the roots of the hair over the body. 3. *Romadipa :* this variety produces elevations at the roots of the hair. 4. *Arambara,* are like the seeds of the wild fig ; these worms may produce the (*kustha*), leprosy. 5. *Saurasa,* (father,) and 6. *Mātrī*, (mother.) These two pass quickly from one relation to another, or are hereditary.

Sushruta enumerates other kinds of worms generated in the blood ; as, *Nakāda,* which destroys the nails.

Dantāda, which produces the caries of the teeth.

Kīkīsa, which always accompanies leprosy.

When worms form in the small and large intestines they are called *Parisajya,* which are produced in the faeces, and are discharged by the anus. When these worms grow and ascend in the abdomen frequent eructations occur, which have the smell of the dejection. They are large, round, thick or thin, and are sometimes of a gray colour, or of a yellow white or dark colour. There are five kinds of such worms, 1. *Kakīraka ;* 2. *Makīraka ;* 3. *Sausurāda,* producing much pain ; 4. *Sasulākiya ;* 5. *Sailika,*

सौसुरादाः सशूलाख्या लेलिहा जनयन्त्यि हि॥
विङ्भेदशूलविष्टम्भ-कार्श्यपारुष्यपाण्डुताः॥
रोमहर्षाग्निसदनं गुदकण्डुर्व्विमार्गगाः॥

पाण्डुकामला-कुम्भकामला-हलीमक-निदानम्

पाण्डुरोगाः स्मृताः पञ्च वातपित्तकफैस्त्रयः।
चतुर्थः सन्निपातेन पञ्चमो भक्षणान्मृदः॥
व्यायाममम्लं लवणानि मद्यः, मृदं दिवास्वप्नमतीवतीक्ष्णम्।
निषव्यमाणस्य प्रदूष्य रक्त्वं दोषास्त्वचं पाण्डुरतां नयन्ति॥
त्वक्स्फोटन-ष्ठीवन-गात्रस्वाद-मृद्भक्षण-प्रेक्षण कुटसोथाः।
विन्मूत्रपीतत्वमथाविपाको भविष्यतस्तस्य पुरः-सराणि।
त्वङ्भूत्रनयनादीनां रुक्षकृष्णारुणाभताः।
वातपाण्ड्वामये तोद कम्पानाह भ्रमादयः।

which licks the intestines. These worms produce diarrhoea, pain in the stomach, dryness of the faeces, constipation, weakness, roughness, and dryness of the surface of the body, which is of a dirty yellow colour. There is loss of appetite with an itchiness towards the anus.

The thirteen first kinds of internal worms are curable, but the seven last are very difficult, or are incurable.

JAUNDICE (*Pandu*)

This disease is produced by excesses in venery, eating earth, sour or salt food, or drinking much wine. It is likewise produced by sleeping during the day, and eating very hot things, which derange the air, bile, and phlegm.

There are five kinds of this disease produced by deranged air, bile, or phlegm; when these three are deranged together, and when produced by eating earth, especially chalk. When the air, bile, or phelgm are diseased, they derange the blood; and produce the pale or yellowish white colour of the skin. Before the disease appears the skin feels as if pinched, the

पीतमूत्र शकृन्नेत्रो दाहतृष्णाज्वरान्वितः।
भिन्नविट्कोऽतिपीताभः पिततपाण्ड्वामयी नरः।
कफप्रसेकश्वयथुतन्द्रालस्यातिगौरवैः।
पाण्डुरोगी कफाच्छुक्लैस्त्वङ्मूत्रनयनाननैः।
ज्वरारोचकहृल्लास-छर्दि-तृष्णाकलमान्वितः॥
पाण्डुरोगी त्रिभिर्द्दोषै स्त्याजाः क्षीणो हतेन्द्रियः।
मृत्तिकादनशीलस्य कुप्यत्यन्यतमो मलः।
कषाया मारुतं पित्तं उषरा मधुरा कफम्।
कोपयेन्मन्द्रसादींश्च रौक्षाद्भुक्तञ्च रुक्षयेत्।
पूरयत्य विपक्वैव स्त्रोतांसि निरुणद्ध्यपि।

sputa is red, the person cannot do any work, and has a desire to eat earth his eyelids swell, the dejections and urine are yellow, and whatever is eaten is not digested.

1. When air is deranged producing this disease, the skin, urine, and eyes, or other parts, are rough, dark-coloured, and brownish with shaking, pain over the body, and the dejections and urine are constipated, with giddiness.

2. When the *bile* is deranged, the urine, dejections, and eyes are of a yellow colour, the body is hot, with thirst, and fever, there are frequent dejections, and the surface of the body is very yellow.

3. Phlegm. In this form the phlegm proceeds from the mouth and nose, the person often dozes and complains of lassitude and heaviness of the body; the skin, eyes, and faces are of a whitish colour; the urine is also pale.

4. When the *air, bile,* and phlegm are at the same time deranged, there is fever, no appetite, retching and vomiting, the person complains of thirst, and the body feels painful and tired. When such a person is very weak and insensible the person will die.

5. When produced by eating earth there are three kinds;

इन्द्रियाणां बलं हत्वा तेजोवीर्य्यौजसी तथा।
पाण्डुरोगं करोत्याशु बलवर्णाग्निनाशनम्।
शूनाक्षिकूटगण्डभ्रूः शूनपान्नाभिमेहनः।
क्रिभिकोऽष्ठोतिसार्य्यैत मलं सासृक्कफान्वितम्।।
पाण्डुरोगश्चिरोतपन्नः खरोभूतो न सिध्यति।
कालप्रकर्षाच्छूनानां यो वा पीतानि पश्यति।
वद्धाल्पविट् सहरितं सकफं योऽति सार्य्यते।।
दीनः शेतादिदिग्धाङ्गश्छर्द्दिमूर्च्छातृडर्द्दितः।
स नास्तासृक्क्षयाद् यश्च पाण्डुशेतत्वमाप्नुयात्।।
पाण्डुदन्तनखो यस्तु पाण्डुनेत्रश्च यो भवेत्।
पाण्डुसंधातदर्शी च पाण्डुरोगी विनश्यति।
अन्तेषु शूनं परिहीनमध्यं म्लानन्तथ्यन्तेषु च मध्यशूनम्।

one deranging the air, another the bile, and third the *phlegm.* Astringent earth (*kasāya mritika*) also deranges air; salt-earth (*usara*), deranges *bile*; and sweet-earth (*madhura*), deranges the *phlegm*. When earth deranges the elements of the body, and whatever is eaten remains undigested, the blood which is formed stops the mouths of the vessels of the intestines that carry the chyle, blood, etc., and they derange the senses. The strength of the body is impaired, and the surface becomes pale and yellow, and it produces dyspepsia. In this form of *Jaundice* the person feels drowsiness, languor, cough, has difficulty in breathing, pain in the belly, and feels no appetite: his cheeks and eyelids swell, also the legs, umbilicus, and penis; *diarrhoea* occurs, and the dejections are as if they consisted of a mixture of blood and phlegm, with worms.

Prognosis. When there is much fever with dyspepsia, nausia, vomitting, thirst, and languor occur; when the person is very weak and insensible, or when caused by the derangement of the three humours, or when very chronic, with rough skin and swelling over the body the prognosis will be unfavourable.

गुदे च शेफस्यथ मुष्कयोश्च, शूनं प्रताम्यन्तमसंज्ञककल्पम्।
विवर्ज्जयेत् पाण्डुकिनं यशोर्थी, तथातिसारज्वरपीड़ितञ्च।।
पाण्डुरोगी तु योऽत्यर्थं पित्तलानि निषेवते।
तस पित्तमसृक्मांसं दग्ध्वा रोगाय कल्पते।।
हारिद्रनेत्रः स भृसं हारिद्रत्वङ्नखाननः।
रक्तपीतशकृन्मूत्रो मेकवर्णो हतेन्द्रियः।
दाहाविपाकदौर्व्वबलामदनारुचिकर्षितः।
कामला बहुपित्तैषा कोष्ठ शाखाश्रया मता।
कालान्तरात् खरीभूता कृच्छ्रा स्यात् कूम्भकामला।।
कृष्णपीतशकृन्मूत्रो भृशं शूनश्च मानवः।।
म रक्ताक्षिमखच्छर्द्दविन्मूची यश्च ताम्यति।

Should the patient see every thing yellow he will not soon get well. When constipated, when the dejections are yellow and mixed with bile, when accompanied with diarrhoea and much fever, restless and thirst, and when the eyes, teeth and nails become yellow, the prognosis must be unfavourable. In like manner, when the extremities are swollen, and the trunk is thin, or when the trunk is swollen and the extremities are small; or when there is much swelling about the anus, penis and scrotum, the prognosis must be guarded. When the patient suffers much, when senseless, or when attacked at the same time with dysentery and fever, such patients the physician should not treat.

A variety of Jaundice is named *kāmalā*, which is produced by eating much sour, salt, and other indigestable articles of food after an attack of Jaundice. In this case the bile is much affected, and produces yellowness, particularly of the face, accompanied with drowsiness, loss of strength, and the other symptoms above stated.

If in *kāmalā*, there is swelling and pain in the joints, then it is called *kumbha-kāmalā* (from *kumbha,* a water-pot, and

दाहारुचितृड़ानाह तन्द्रामोहसमन्वितः।
नष्टाग्निसंज्ञः क्षिप्रं हि कामलावान् विपद्यते।
छदर्द्यरोचकहृल्लास-ज्वरक्लमनिपीड़ितः।
नश्यति शासकासार्त्तो विड्भेदी कूम्भकामली॥
यदा तु पाण्डोर्व्वर्णः स्याद्धरितः श्यावपीतकः।
बलोत्साहक्षयस्तन्द्रा मन्दाग्नित्वं मृदुज्वरः।
स्त्रीष्ठहर्षोऽङ्गमर्दश्च दाहतृष्णारुचिभ्रमः।
हलीमकं तदा तस्य विद्यादनिलपित्ततः॥

रक्तपित्तनिदानम्

धर्मव्यायामशोकाध्वव्यवायैरतिसेवितैः।
तीक्ष्णोष्णक्षारलवणैरम्लैः कदुमिरेव च॥

kāmalā, Jaundice). In this case the dejections and urine are of a dark or yellow colour : the body is swelled, and the eyes and mouth are of a red colour. When vomiting takes place the matter vomited is of a red colour, as also the dejections and urine.

In some cases the patient is delirious, his body is hot, he has no appetite, is thirsty, and the dejections and urine become constipated : such cases are unfavourable. In other cases the person dozes, and the internal fire and the understanding, are much affected. Such persons will soon die ; as will be the case when there is vomiting with no appetite, fever, debility, noise in breathing, cough, and frequent dejections.

Another form of Jaundice is called *Halimaka* or *Lācorokaka*. This variety is produced by air and bile, and is characterized by fever, pain over the body, giddiness, languor, drowsiness, emaciation of the body, with the symptoms of the form of Jaundice produced by *air* and *bile*.

HAEMORRHAGIA (*Raktapitta.*)

This order of disease is divided into those which occur from the mouth, nose, ears, eyes; from the anus, urethra or vagina, or from the skin.

पित्तं विदग्धं स्वगुणौर्ब्बिदहत्याशु शोणितम्।
ततः प्रवर्त्तते रक्तभूर्द्ध्ञ्चाधो द्विधापि वा।
ऊर्द्धं नासाक्षिकर्णास्यै मेंदूयोनिगुदैरधः।
कूपितं रोमकूपैश्च समस्तैस्तत् प्रवर्त्तते।
सदनं शीतकामित्वं कण्ठधूमायनं वमिः।।
लोहगन्धिश्च निश्वासो भवत्यस्मिन् भविष्यति।।
सान्द्रं सपाण्डु सस्नेहं पिच्छिलञ्च कफान्वितम्।
श्यावारुगां सफेनञ्च तनुरुक्षञ्च वातिकम्।।
रक्तपित्तं कषायाभं कृष्णं गोमूत्रसन्निभम्।
मेचकागारधूमाभमञ्जनाभञ्च पैत्तिकम्।
संसृष्टलिङ्ग संसर्गात्रिलिङ्गं सान्निपातिकम्।।

Haemorrhage is caused by anger, grief, fear, wrestling, and other severe exercises ; too much intercourse with women; or too free use of hot things, as pepper and salt, or sour articles, when taken in considerable quantities. The improper mixtures of food, or exposure to the heat of the sun, or to fire. By these means the chyle is deranged, which irritates the bile, and this mixing with the blood produces *Rakta-pitta*. It may thus occur from above downwards, or from the surface of the body. This blood usually proceeds from the spleen or liver.

Immediately before the disease occurs the patient is languid, the body is weak, cold, and cool things are desired. His throat is burning hot, as if he had swallowed smoke, with vomiting. The breathing has the smell of quenched iron. When produced by deranged *air, bile,* and *phlegm,* it is known from the blood discharged being very thick, of a yellow colour, shining, and slippery, and mixed with phlegm of a grey colour, of a thick consistence, and with a yellow froth. In other cases it is thin. When bile is deranged in this disease, the blood has an astringent taste, and is of a dark colour, or of the colour of cow's urine, and as if mixed with different colours, as of the colour of smoke, or of a dark colour.

ऊर्द्धगं कफसंसृष्ट मधोगं पवनानुगम्।
द्विमार्गं कफवाताभ्यामुभाभ्यामनुवर्त्तते।
ऊर्द्धव् साध्यमधो याप्यमसाध्यं युगपद्गतम्।
एकमार्गं बलवतो नातिवेगं नवोत्थितम॥
रक्तपित्तं सुखे काले साध्यं स्यान्निरुपद्रवम्।
एकदोषानुगं साध्यं हिदोषं यान्यमुच्यते॥
यत्रिदोषमसाध्यं स्यात् मन्दाग्नेरतिवेगवत्॥
व्याधिभिः क्षीणदेहस्य वृद्धख्यानश्च तश्च यत्॥
दौर्बल्य-शास-कास-ज्वर-वग्रथु-ग्रदापाण्डुता दाह मूर्च्छा,
भुक्ते घोरो विदाहरुत्वधृतिरति सदा हृद्यतुल्य च पीड़ा।
तृष्णा कोष्ठस्य मेदः शिरसि च तपनं पूतिनिष्ठीयनत्वम्॥
भक्तच्छेषाविपाकौ विकृतिरपि भवेत् रक्तपित्तोपसर्गाः॥
मांसप्रक्षालणाभं क्कथितमिव च यत् कर्दमाम्नीनिभं वा,

The symptoms which terminate this order of diseases are weakness, difficult breathing, cough, fever, vomiting, and slight head-ache ; sometimes the patient faints, and his skin is yellow, hot, and after eating, the pit of the stomach burns. He is restless, and has severe pain in the chest, with hoarseness, headache, and the discharge of fecal matter from the mouth ; he has no appetite, is languid, and what is eaten is not digested.

The unfavourable symptoms in this disease are when the hoemorrhage is like the water in which flesh had been washed, or like a vegetable decoction ; is of a liver colour, or like water mixed with mud. When it resembles pus mixed with blood, when it is dark like the fruit of the *Jambu* tree (black-berry), or of a variegated colour, like the rain-bow, such cases are fatal.

When there is a frequent vomiting of blood ; when eructations have the taste of blood, when the eyes are red, and every thing appears the colour of blood, the case is hopeless.

When *phlegm* is deranged the blood is evacuated by the

मेदः पूवयास्त्रकल्पं यकृकदवि यदि वा पक्कजम्बुफलाभम्।
यत् कृष्णं यच्च नीलं भृशमतिकूणप यत्र चोत्का विकारा,
स्तद्दजं रक्तपित्तं सुरपतिधनुषा यच्च तुल्यं विभाति॥
येन चोपहतो रक्तं रक्तपित्तेन मानवः।
पश्येदृश्यं वियच्चैव तच्चासाध्यसमंशयम्।
लोहितं छर्दयेद् यस्तु बहुशो लोहितेक्षणः।
लोहितोद्गारदर्शी च म्रियते रक्तपैत्तिकः॥

राजयक्ष्म-शोष-क्षतक्षीण-निदानम्

वेगरोधात् क्षयाच्चैव साहसाद्विषमाशनात्।
त्रिदोषो जायते यक्ष्मागदो हेतु चतुष्टयात्।
कफप्रधाने र्दोषैस्तु रुद्धेषु रसवर्त्मषु।
अतिव्य्यवायिनो वापि क्षीणे रेतस्यनन्तराः।
क्षीयन्ते धातवः सर्व्वे ततः शुष्यति मानवः॥

mouth; when *air* is deranged it is by the anus ; and when the two are deranged, the blood is evacuated above and below. When the blood passes above, the person may be cured ; but not so when below. When evacuated both ways, it is incurable. When the person is strong, the disease recent, and not severe, and only occurs one way; and when the person in general feels will, with no other bad disease, it will be cured.

CONSUMPTION (*Phthisis Pulmonalis*)

Raj Jakshyā, (the prince of disease;) *Shosha, Kshyā, Khina,* (emaciation;) *Kshata,* (rapture or ulcer of the respiratory organs).

The mythological origin of this disease is that the moon married seven sisters, but attaching himself to one, the others complained to their father, who punished the moon, by declaring that he should be afflicted with consumption. This origin; and the precepts in the treatment, proclaim his frequent,

शासाङ्गमर्द-कफ-संस्रव-तालुशोष-
वम्यग्निसाद-मदपीनस-कास-निद्राः।
शीषे भविष्यति भवन्ति स चापि जन्तुः,
शुक्लेक्षणो भवति मांसपरो रिरंसुः।
स्वप्नेषु काकशुकशल्लकिनीलकण्ठा
गृध्रास्तथैव कपयः कृकलासकाश्च।
तं वाहयन्ति सनदीविजलाश्च पञ्चेच्छ-
ष्कांस्तरुन् पवनधुमदवार्द्दितांश्च॥
अंशपार्श्वाभितापश्च सन्तापः करपादयोः।
ज्वरः सर्व्वाङ्गगश्चेति लक्षणं राजयक्ष्मणः।
स्वरभेदोऽनिलाच्छूलं संधोचश्चांसपार्शयोः।
ज्वरो दाहोऽतिसारश्च पित्ताद्रक्तस्य चागमः॥

and fatal nature. It is characterised by coughing accompanied with bloody expectoration.

It is produced by grief, by the evacuations being retained when nature endeavours to expell them ; by great loss of the humors of the body ; by performing unusual and unnatural actions, as ineffectually endeavouring to raise heavy weights ; and by running, swimming, or other violent exercise. Consumption is produced, by eating bad food, or at unusual times, and in unusual quantities, by fasting, by boils and sores in the chest, and by old age. Is also supposed to be produced by diminishing the mental and bodily strength, by blunting the senses, by producing difficulty in breathing, by altering the voice, by producing vomiting with expectoration, by a discharge from the eyes, nose, and mouth. In such cases the body dries, and the surface appears dirty.

When the air, phlegm, and bile, are deranged in the above disease ; the chyle vessels are stopped by the humours, but particularly phlegm, and the other parts of the body are not nourished. Another form is produced by excessive venery, from

शिरसः परिपूर्णत्वमभक्तच्छन्द एवच।
कासः कण्ठस्य चोध्वंसो विज्ञेयः कफकोपतः॥
एकादशभि रेभिर्व्वा षड्भिर्वापि समन्वितम्।
जह्याच्छोषार्द्दितं जन्तु मिच्छून् सुविमलं यशः॥
कासातिसारपार्शार्त्ति स्वरभेदारुचिज्वरैः।
चिभिर्व्वा पीड़ितं लिङ्गैः कासश्वासासृगामयैः॥
सर्व्वैरर्द्धैस्त्रिभिर्वापि लिङ्गैर्मांसवलक्षये।
युक्तो वर्ज्जश्चिकित्स्यस्तु सर्व्वरूपोऽन्यतोऽन्यथा।
महाशनं क्षीयमानमति सारनिपीड़ितम्॥
शूनमुष्कोदरञ्चैव यक्ष्मिगां परिवर्ज्जयेत्॥

the great discharge of semen, by which all the other elements are deranged. The disease commences by the person becoming emaciated and debilitated ; difficult breathing and pain over the body comes on with cough, and a discharge of mucus, from the mouth and nose. The palate is dry, vomiting and loss of appetite takes place, from the internal heat being diminished. There is also derangement of the mind, jaundice, cough with expectoration, and the loss of taste, and smell. The patient sleeps continually, the eyes become of a pearl white colour. The person is fond of animal food, and is desirous of intercourse with women. The following symptoms indicate the presence of this disease ; when the patient's voice changes, he sees in his dream crows, parrots, porcupines, peacocks, vultures, monkeys, and lizards ; and he supposes he is mounted upon these animals. He sees also dry beds of river dry trees, as if destroyed by storms, and by fire.

The characteristic symptoms are pain in the shoulders, and sides of the chest. A burning feverish feel of the palms of the hands and soles of the feet is felt, which extends over the body.

Consumption is sometimes produced by derangements

उपक्रामेदात्मवन्तं दीप्ताग्निमकृशं नरम्।
शुक्लाक्षमन्नद्वेष्टार मूर्द्धशाग निपीड़ितम्।
कृच्छ्रेण बहु मेहन्तं यक्ष्मा हन्तीह मानवम्॥
व्यवाय-शोकवार्धक्य व्यायामाध्वप्रशोषितान्।
व्रणोरःक्षतसधौ च शोषिणौ लक्षणै शृणु॥
व्यवायशोषी चारय धाय। प्रध्यानशीलः स्त्र.....
शाकशीषापि तादृशः। जराशीषी कृशो मन्दः
वीर्य्यबुद्धि...... कम्पनोऽरुचिमान् भिन्नकांस्यनद्धत स्वरः॥
ष्ठीनां..... हीनंगौरवारतिषीडितः॥

of one of the three humours. The symptoms produced by derangement of the air are hoarseness ; pain, particularly in the shoulders and sides of the chest, and a bent form of the body. The symptoms of bile are fever, the body burning diarrhoea, and hemoptisis. The symptoms of phlegm are a fulness and heaviness of the head, no appetite, cough, and the windpipe is painful as if bruised, with a change in the voice. When all the above symptoms are present at the same time, and in the same person ; or when there is cough, diarrhoea pain of the chest and sides, hoarseness, loss of appetite and fever, or when cough, asthma, and the discharge of blood is present, with emaciation, the person will die. When these bad symptoms are absent the physician may attend the person, but when the person has a strong appetite, the food does not produce strength, flesh, or diarrhoea ; or when the testicles or stomach swell, the person will not recover. When the person is strong, the disease recent, and he has slight fever ; when he can work, has a good appetite, is equal to the treatment, and follows the judicious instructions of the physician, such a person may recover.

When the eye is white, when there is no appetite, with great derangement of breathing; when there is a great secretion of urine, with pain, the person will not recover. The other form

सम्पस्त्रुता स्यानासाक्ष शुष्करूचमलच्छवि॥
अध्वशोषी न स्योदिर मंमद परुषन्हाविः।
.....गाव्यवयताः शुष्कक्लीमगनाननः॥
वाग्यटा म शेषी।
...... लिङ्गणरद्धतकृत बुद्धिक्षतं विना।
रक्तज्ञययाहेदनाभिस्तथैवाहारयन्त्रणात्।
व्रणितसा भवे श्छोषः स चा साध्यतमो मतः॥
धनुषायांस्यातोऽर्थं भारमुद्दहते गुरुम्।
युध्यमानस्य बलिभिः पततो विषमोर्च्चतः॥
वृषं हयं वा धावन्तं दम्यं वान्यं निगृह्नतः।

of consumption is produced by excessive venery, grief, old age, great fatigue, by taking long journies on foot, by the debility produced by old ulcers, and by the rupture of the organs of respiration, by which the body will become thin, and the disease declare itself. By excessive venery the body becomes emaciated, debilitated, with the other symptoms of diminished semen, such as pain in the scrotum and penis, impotency, or a slight discharge of semen, mixed with blood, when the body becomes yellow, and the other humours are diminished.

When consumption is produced by *grief* the person remains complaining, with the other symptoms of the last form; but without the evacuation and the symptoms of deranged semen. When the disease is produced by old age the body beocmes very thin, the person cannot labour, his organs of sense and strength are diminished, his body shakes, he has no appetite, and his voice is like a broken pewter-plate when struck. There is always a flow of saliva from the mouth, weakness, and heaviness ; and his eyes, nose, and mouth discharge mucus. The dejections, and surface of the body are in these patients dry and rough. When the body is thin from great fatigue, or walking ; the person cannot get up, his body changes in colour, is painful and some parts lose their sensibility. The palate, throat,

शिला काष्ठाश्मनिघातान् क्षिपतो निघ्नतः परान्।।
अधीयानस्यवात्युच्चैर्दूरं वा व्रजतो द्रुतम्।
महानदीर्व्वा तरतो हयैर्व्वा सह धावतः।
सहसोत्पततो दूरं तूर्णं प्रनृत्यतः।।
तथान्यैः कर्मम्भिः क्रूरेर्भृशमभ्यहतस्य वा।
विक्षते वक्षसि व्याधि र्बववान् समुदीर्य्यते।
स्त्रीषु चातिप्रसक्तस्य रुक्षाल्पप्रमिताशिनः।।
उरो विरुच्यतेऽत्यर्थ्यं भिद्येतऽथ विभज्ज्यते।
प्रपीड्येते ततः पार्षे शुष्यात्यङ्ग प्रवेपते।।
क्रमाद्वीर्या बलं वर्णो रुचिरग्निश्च हीयते।

and mouth are dry. When produced by other kinds of violent exercise or by a rupture of the lungs, the symptoms are the same as above.

When old ulcers debilitate the body, by the great loss of blood, when there is much pain, and there is little nourishment in the food which is taken, the disease is incurable. When consumption is produced by a rupture of the respiratory organs, as by the frequent use of the bow and arrow, by carrying great weights, when a weak person fights with a strong man, when jumping from a great height, or when a person attempts to run after and seize an ox, a horse, or a docoit, or pull at a bow, or throw pieces of wood or stone, the disease is dangerous. In like manner, loud reading, walking quickly and to a great distance, or swimming much, much horse exercise, or running up a height or to a great distance, dancing quickly, or other bad customs, eating very dry articles, or very little food, or only one kind of food, will produce the disease. When this disease is present there is great pain in the breast as if it was wounded, pain in the sides, and body dries up, and shakes. By degrees the spirit and strength fail, and the colour of the skin is diminished or unnatural, there is no appetite, with fever, pain, dejection of mind, diarrhoea and loss of appetite. The sputa is

ज्वरो व्यथा मनोदैन्यं बिड्भेदाग्निवथावपि॥
दुष्टः श्यावः दुर्गन्धः पीतो विग्रथिती वहुः।
कासमानस्य चाभीक्ष्णं कफ सासृक् प्रवर्तते।
सक्षतः क्षयतेऽप्यर्थ्यं तथा शूक्रो जसो क्षयात्।
अव्यक्तं लक्षणं तस्य पूर्व्वरूपमिति स्मृतम्॥
उरोरुक् शोणितछर्द्दिः कासो वैशेषिकः क्षते।
क्षीणे सरक्त्व मूत्रत्वं पार्थपृष्ठकटीग्रहः॥
अल्पलिङ्गस्य दीप्ताग्नेः साध्यो बलवतो नवः॥
परिसंवत्सरो याप्यः सर्व्वलिङ्गन्तु वर्ज्जयेत्॥

कासनिदानम्

धूमोपधाताद्रसतस्तथैव व्यायामरुक्षान्ननिषेवणाच्च।
विमार्ग गत्वाच्च हि भोजनस्य वेगावरोधात् क्षवथोस्तथैव॥

of a light blue or yellow colour, with a bad smell, and like the knot of a piece of rope, being unequal. At other times the sputa is mixed with blood. These symptoms increase daily, with pain in the chest, more blood is vomited, and cough becomes more severe. When the body is much emaciated from the drying up of the juices, indicated by the parched dry mouth, etc., the urine has the colour of blood, and the sides, back and thighs are painful. Consumption often occurs in the progress of other diseases, and is always accompanied with danger, being cured with much difficulty. When the internal heat is natural, and the symptoms not severe, and remain but a few days, the person will be cured. If it continues one year the cure will not be accomplished, and when the severe symptoms above enumerated are present the person will die.

COUGH (*Kāsa*)

This disease is produced, by smoke or dust entering the mouth and nostrils, by fighting, by great fatigue, by dry food,

प्राणो ह्युदानानुगतः प्रदुष्टः संभिन्नकांस्यस्वन-तुल्यघोषः।
निरेतिवक्तात् सहसो सदोसो मनीषिभिः कास इति प्रदिष्टः॥
पञ्च कासाः ष्मृता वातपित्तश्लेष्मत्ततक्षयैः।
क्षयायोपेक्षिताः सर्व्वे वलिनश्चोत्तरोत्तरम्।
पूर्व्वरूपं भवेत्तेषां शूकपूयर्णगलास्याता॥
कण्ठे कण्डुश्च भोज्यनामवरोधश्च जायते॥
हृच्छ्रूङ्खमूर्द्धोदरपार्थशूलौ क्षामाननः क्षीणबलस्वरौजाः।
प्रसक्तवेगस्तु समीरणेन भिन्नस्वरः कासति शुष्कमेव।
उरोविदाहज्वरवक्तशोषै रभ्यार्द्दि तरितक्त मुखस्तृषार्त्तः।
पित्तेन पीतानि वमेत् कटूनि कासेत् सपाण्डूः परिदह्यमानः॥

by articles of food entering the air passages, by sneezing, or by resisting the calls of nature. These causes derange the vital air (*Prān-bāyu*) in the chest, and the *Udān-bāyu* which is situated in the trachea, by which the air which passes through the air passage to the mouth, produces a peculiar noise, like a broken metallic vessel.

The disease may likewise be produced by air, bile, and phlegm, by ruptures of the respiratory organs, or by the loss of particular humours. All these varieties of cough, pass to consumption if neglected. The disease commences with a feeling in the mouth and throat as if it was covered with some irritating substance. It feels itchy, or there is a stinging which prevents the passage of the food into the stomach.

The symptoms of cough are produced by deranged *air*, the change of voice, the dry and frequent cough, distresses the patient, with pain in the temples, head, stomach, and chest. The face becomcs sallow, and the person becomes weak.

When *bile* is deranged the mouth is dry and bitter, and the breath is hot with fever ; the person complains of thirst, and severe pain over the body ; the expectoration is sour, and of a yellowish colour, and the skin becomes yellow and hot.

प्रलिप्यमानेन मुखेन सीदन् शिरोरुजार्त्तः कफपूर्ण देहः।
अभक्तरुग् गौरवस्वादयुक्तः कासेद्धयशं सान्द्रकफः कफेन॥
अतिव्यवायभाराध्व-युद्धाश्वगजविग्रहैः।
रुक्षस्योरः क्षतं वायर्गृहीत्वा कासमाचरेत्।
स पूर्व्वं कासते शुष्कं ततःष्ठीवेत् सशोणितम्॥
कण्ठेन रुजतात्यर्थं विरुग्नेनेव चोरसा।
सूचीभिरिव तीक्ष्णाभि स्तुद्यमानेन शूलिना॥
दुःखस्पर्शेन शूलेन भेदपीड़ाभितापिना।
पर्व्वभेद-ज्वरशास-तृष्णावैषर्य्यपीड़ितः॥
पारावत इवाकूजन् कासवेगात् क्षतोद्भावात्॥
विषमासात्म्यभोज्याति ब्यवायाद्वेगनिग्रहात्।
घृणिनां शोचतां नृणां व्यापन्नेऽग्नौ त्रयो मलाः॥

When *phlegm* is deranged, the mouth is full of mucus with head-ache, loss of appetite, languor, frequent cough, with thick mucus expectoration. The person cannot labour, has frequent fits of coughing, the body is heavy and weak, he has no appetite, the frequency of coughing increases, and much phlegm is expectorated.

Katazoā Kāsa is caused by excessive venery, fatigue, carrying heavy weights, going great distances when unaccustomed, and violent exercise upon horseback or elephants. By these causes the air passages are injured or ulcerated, when the patient is first affected with dry cough followed by spitting of blood, much pain in the throat and chest, which is increased by pressure. The joints and other parts of the body are painful, as if pins were penetrating it ; pain in the muscles, fever, difficulty of breathing, thirst, hoarseness, and change in the voice, so that it resembles that of wild pigeon.

Khyā Kāsa (Pneumonia) This form of the disease is produced by taking improper food, at improper, or unusual times ; excessive venery, and neglect of the calls of nature. In

कुपिताः क्षयजं कासं कुर्य्युद्दिहक्ष्ययप्रदम्॥
सगात्रशूल-ज्वर-दाहमोहान् प्राणक्षयञ्चोपलभेत कासी।
शूष्यन् विनिष्ठीवति दुर्व्वलस्तु प्रक्षीणमांसो रुधिरं संपूयम्॥
तं सर्व्वलिङ्गं भृशदुश्चिकित्स्यं चिकित्सितज्ञाः क्ष्ययजं वहन्ति॥
इत्येष क्ष्ययजः कासः क्ष्रीणानां देहनाशनं॥
साध्यो बलवतां वा स्याद् याप्य स्तेवं क्षतोत्थितः।
नवौ कदाचित् सिध्येतामपि पादगुणान्वितौ।
ख्यविराणां जरा कासः सर्व्वो यान्यः प्रकीर्त्तितः।
त्रीन् पूर्व्वान् साधयेत् साध्यान् पथ्यैर्यान्यांस्तु यापयेत्॥

हिक्कानिदानम्

विदाहि गुरु विष्टम्भि रुक्ष्याभिष्यन्दि भोजनैः।

other cases the disease is produced by grief, by food which has a bad taste, or produces disgust by which the internal heat is diminished and deranged, with the air, bile, and phlegm. This disease is characterized by the person being affected with severe pain and emaciation of the body, fever, and a burning sensation of the body. His intellect becomes affected and the person loses his strength. The cough is at first dry, is accompanied with vomiting, and is followed by purulent and bloody expectoration. When these symptoms are present they are rarely cured ; and in weak persons the disease is generally fatal, unless when recent. In old age the cough *(Jarā Kāsa)*will remain, and not be removed.

When *Kātazoa* and *Khyā Kāsa* are recent, with the assistance of a good physician, and proper remedies, a cure may be obtained. When air, bilc and phlegm produce these diseases separately, it may be cured.

HICCUP *(Hikka)*

This disease is produced by nearly the same causes as *Swāsa* (asthma), and *Kasa* (cough). Such as heavy and

शीतपानाशनख्यान-रजो-धूमातपानिलैः।
व्यायायामकर्म-भाराध्व-वेगाघातापतर्पगौः॥
हिक्का शासश्च कासश्च नृणां समुपजायते।
मुहुर्मुहु र्वायुरुदेति सश्वनो यकृतप्लिहान्त्राणि मुखादि वा क्षियपन्।
सघोष वानाशु हिनस्त्यसून् यतस्ततस्तु हिक्केत्यभिधीयते बुधैः॥
अन्नजां यमलां क्षुद्रां गम्भीरां महतीं तथा॥
वायुः कफेनानुगतः पञ्चहिक्काः करोति हि।
कण्ठोरसोर्गुरुत्वञ्च वदनस्य कषायता।
हिक्कानां पूर्व्वरूपानि कुक्षेराटोप एव च॥
पानान्नैरतिसंयुक्तैः सहसा पीड़ितो निलः।
हिक्कयत्यूर्द्धगो भूत्वा तां विद्यदन्नजां भिषक्॥

indigestable food, or roasted, hot, and dry food ; or much food, or an improper mixture of food, or articles that increase cough, etc., so as to produce constipation. In other cases very dry things, cold things, or situations, exposure to dust, smoke entering the mouth or nostrils ; or much heat, as exposure to the sun, and hot air. Violent exercise, as shooting arrows, carrying heavy loads, walking great distances, not attending to the calls of nature, or long fasting produce this disease. It is called *hikka*, because the air comes to the mouth frequently, with a peculiar noise, and the spleen, liver, and intestines seem to be coming up to the mouth. This disease quickly debilitates, and destroys the *prāna* (life).

The precursory symptoms are a heaviness of the throat and chest, an astringent taste in the mouth, and a rumbling noise in the belly. There are five kinds of hiccup, in all of which air and phlegm are deranged.

1. ***Unnugā.*** This form is produced by taking too much food and drink, which deranges the air, and produces the disease.

चिरेण यमलैर्वेगंर्था हिक्का सम्प्रवर्त्तते।
कम्पयन्ती शिरो ग्रीवां यमलां तां विनिर्द्दिशेत्।
विकृष्टकालैर्या वेगैर्ग्मन्दैः समभिवर्त्तते।
क्षुद्रिका नाम सा हिक्का जत्रुमूलात् प्रधाविता।।
नाभिप्रवृत्तः या हिक्का घोरा गम्भीरनादिनी।
अनेकोपद्रववती गम्भीरा नाम सा स्मृता।।
मर्मण्युत् पीड़यन्तीव सततं या प्रवर्त्तते।
महाहिक्केति सा ज्ञेया सर्व्वं गात्रविकम्पिनी।।
आयम्यते हिक्कतो यस्य देहो दृष्टिश्चोर्द्धं नाम्यते यसा नित्यम्।
क्षीणोऽन्नद्दिट् क्षौति यश्चातिमात्रं तौ द्वौ चान्त्यौ वर्ज्जयोद्धिक्कमानौ।
अतिसञ्चितदोषस्य भक्तच्छेदकृशस्य च।।
व्याधिभिः क्ष्यीणदेस्य तृद्धस्थातिव्यवायिनः।
आसां या सा समुत्पन्ना हिक्का हन्त्याशु जीवितम्।

*2. **Jumulā.*** In this form the passage of air proceeds, after a considerable time, with eructations of air, and the head and neck shake at the moment; hence the name.

*3. **Khudrā.*** (hiccup) takes place slowly, is not strong, and proceeds from the scrobiculus cordis.

*4. **Gambirā.*** In this form the hiccup, commences from the navel, is strong, and very noisy, and is always accompanied with other severe or fatal symptoms.

*5. **Mahatī.*** There is frequent hiccup, which produces pain in the vital parts, and shakes the whole body. The unfavourable symptoms are when hiccup is accompanied with fixed eyes, as if drawn up by some one ; when there is great weakness, and patient's arms and legs are thrown out, with frequent sneezing. When the person is very weak and old, or becomes weak after excessive venery, with no appetite, and a cough, it will soon prove fatal. When combined with other diseases, as delirium, fainting, great thirst, etc., it will be fatal. When the person is

यमिका च प्रलापार्त्ति मोह तृष्णा समन्विता।
अक्ष्यीणश्चाप्यदीनश्च स्थिरधात्विन्द्रियश्च यः।
तस्य साधयितुं शक्या यमिका हन्त्यतोऽन्यथा।।

श्वासनिदानम्

महोर्ध्वछिन्नतमकक्षुद्रभेदैस्तु प्रञ्चधा।
भिद्यते स महाव्याधिः श्वास एको विशेषतः।
वाताधिको भवेत् क्षुद्र स्तमकस्तु कफोद्भवः।
कफ वाताधिक सैव संसृष्टः छिन्नसंज्ञकः।।
श्वासो मारुतसंसृष्टो महानूर्द्ध स्ततो मतः।
प्रागूरूपं तस्य हृत्पीड़ा शूलमाधानमेव च।।
आनाहो वक्त्रवैरस्यं शङ्कनिस्तोद एव च।।
यदा स्त्रोतांसि संरुध्य मारुतः कफपूर्व्वकः।

strong, has a good constitution, hiccup may be cured. Thus when the patient is not thin, when his memory is good, his tissues and senses are healthy, the person will recover.

ASTHMA *(Swāsa)*

This disease is produced by the same causes as produce hiccough. It is by the *Prān-bāyu* changing its place, and being confined in its passage by phlegm, which produces the difficulty in breathing. There are the following five varieties of asthma :–

*1. **Swāsa*** is a severe disease, and has only slight varieties. It is ushered in with pain in the chest and sides, loss of appetite, restlessness, tightness of the abdomen, a bad taste in the mouth, and a constipation of the bowels and bladder.

*2. **Mahā-swāsa.*** The air is confined in the air passages by the phlegm, and thus produces Asthma. The patient respires with difficulty, and with a noise like that of a wild bullock. He becomes low-spirited, his eyes are always moving about ; his

विश्वग्व्रजति संरुद्धस्तदा श्वामान् करोति सः॥
उद्धयमानवातो यः शब्द वहुःखितो नरः।
उच्चैः श्वसिति संरुद्धो मत्तर्षभ इवानिशम्॥
प्रनष्ट ज्ञानविज्ञानस्तथा विभ्रान्तलोचनः।
विवृताक्षन्यननो वद्धमूत्र वर्च्चा विशीर्णवाक्।
दीनः प्रश्वसितञ्चास्य दूराहिज्ञायते भृशम्।
महाश्वासोपसृष्टस्तु खिप्रमेव विपद्यते।
ऊर्द्धं श्वसिति यो दीर्घं न च प्रत्याहरत्यधः॥
श्लेष्मावृतमुखस्त्रोता क्रुद्धगन्धवहार्द्दितः॥
ऊर्द्धदृष्टिर्विपश्यंस्तु विभ्रान्ताक्ष्य इतस्ततः।
प्रमुह्यन् वेदनार्त्तश्च शुक्लास्येऽरतिपीड़ितः।
ऊर्द्धश्वासे प्रकुपिते ह्यधःश्वासो निरुध्यते॥
मुह्यते स्ताम्यतश्चोर्द्धं श्वास स्तस्यैव हन्त्यसून्।
यस्त श्वसिति विच्छिन्नं सर्व्वप्राणेन् पीड़ितः॥
न वा श्वसिति दुःखार्त्तो मर्म्मच्छेदरुगर्द्दितः॥

mouth open, with constipation of urine and faeces ; he speaks with difficulty, and his distress may be observed from a distance.

3. ***Urdha-swāsa.*** The patient in this disease respires with difficulty and with an effort; the air passages being closed by phlegm, and air trying to escape gives much pain. His eyes are directed upwards, he cannot see, and different objects appear before the eyes; sometimes he faints, his mouth remains dry with restlessness and severe pain over the body. The respiration becomes more difficult, and he dies.

4. ***China-swāsa.*** This form occurs in fits at irregular intervals. In these cases he is sometimes still, and cannot breathe. The vital parts are much affected, and very painful. He is constipated in his bowels, with much perspiration and drowsiness. He complains of much pain in the bladder, which is very hot, his eyes are always rolling about, and red ; great

आनाह स्वेद-मूर्च्छार्त्तो दह्यमानेन वस्तिना।
विप्लताक्षः परीखिणः श्वसन् रक्तैकलोचनः।।
विचेताः परिशुष्कास्यो विवर्णः प्रलपन्नरः।
छिन्नश्वासेन विच्छिन्नः स शीघ्रं विजहात्थ सून्।
प्रतिलोमं यदा वायुः स्त्रोतांसि प्रतिपद्यते।
ग्रीवां शिरश्च संगृह्य श्लेष्माणं समुदीर्य्य च।।
करोति पीनसं तेन रुद्धोघुर्घुरकं तथा।
अतीवतीव्रवेगञ्च श्वासं प्राणप्रपीड़कम्।
प्रताम्यति स वेगेन तृष्यते सन्निरुद्धते।
प्रमोहं कासमानश्च स गच्छति मुहुमूहुः।
श्लेष्मण्यमुच्यमाने तु भृशं भवति दुःखितः।।
तस्यैव च विमोक्षान्ते मुहुर्त्तं लभते सुखम्।
तथास्योध्वंसते कण्ठः कृच्छ्राच्छक्नोति भाषितम्।
न चापि लभते निद्रां शयानः श्वासपीड़ितः।।
पाश्र्वे तस्यावगृह्णाति शयानस्य समीरणः।
आसीनो लभते सौख्यमुष्णञ्चैवाभिनन्दति।।

debility, low spirits, mouth dry, bad colour of the skin, and delirium. Such persons quickly die.

5. ***Tamaka*****-** **sw*āsa.*** In this variety the air passes in, but is not discharged easily. The vessels of the neck and air passages are affected, with a collection of mucus in the air passages. Catarrh is produced, as indicated by yellow sputa from the mouth, and snoring, with great uneasiness and difficulty in breathing. When he coughs he often faints, but on mucus being discharged he feels easier. At times he cannot speak, does not sleep, and when he does he complains of much pain in the sides and chest. He is easiest in the sitting position, and likes hot things. His eyes are turned upwards, he perspires much in the forehead, his mouth is dry, and the body swings about as if he was riding upon an elephant. From time to time his breathing

उच्छ्रिताक्षो ललाटेन स्विद्यता भृषमर्त्तिमान्
विशुष्कास्यो मुहुःश्वासो मुहुश्चैवावधम्यते।
मेधाम्बुशीतप्राग्वातैः श्लोष्मलैश्च विवर्द्धते।
स याप्यस्तमक श्वासः साध्योवास्यन्नवोत्थितः॥
ज्वरमूर्च्छापरीतस्या विद्यात् प्रतमकन्तुतम्।
उदावर्त्तरजोजौर्ण क्लिन्नकायनिरोधजः॥
तमसा वर्द्धतेऽत्यर्थं शीतैश्चाशु प्रशाम्यति॥
मज्जतस्तमसीवास्य विद्यात् सन्तमकन्तु तम्॥
रुक्षायासोद्भवः कोष्ठे क्षुद्रो वात उदीरयन्।
क्षुद्रश्वासो न सोऽत्यर्थं दुःखेनाङ्ग प्रवाधकः॥
हिनस्ति न स गात्राणि नच दुःखो यथेतरे।
नच भोजनपानानां निरुणद्धयुचितां गतिम्॥
नेन्द्रियाणां व्यथां नापि काञ्चिदापादयेद्रुजम्।
स साध्य उक्तो बलिनः सर्व्वे चाव्यक्तलक्षणः।
क्षुद्रः साध्यमतस्तेषां तमकः कृच्छ्र उच्यते।
त्रयः श्वासा न सिद्धन्ति तमको दुर्व्वलस्य च।

is difficult. This disease is increased in cloudy, rainy, and cold weather ; especially during the prevalence of easterly winds. Whatever increases phlegm, is liable to increase the disease. This form of disease may be cured if recent, but in the old, or when it has continued for some time, it is not curable. When this form is combined with fever, and dozing, it forms *Pratamaka*. When produced or increased by *Udabarta,* (constipation,) *Ajirna,* (dyspepsia,) *Rajah*, (or dust) and darkness. In this form cold things give relief, and the person sees imperfectly like one in darkness. This is called *Sangtamaka*.

6. ***Khudra-swāsa.*** It is produced by dry food and exercise. In this form there is less difficulty in breathing, and there is no pain or uneasiness. It does not prevent diglutition, nor the action of the senses, and only produces difficulty in breathing

कामं प्राणहरा रोगा बहवो नतु ते तथा।
यथा श्वासश्च हिक्का च हरतः प्राणमाशु च।

स्वरभेद-निदानम्

अत्युच्चभाषण-विषाध्य यनाभिधात-संदूषणैः
प्रकुपिताः पवनादयस्तु। स्त्रोतःसुप्ते स्वरवहेषु गताः प्रतिष्ठां,
हन्युः स्वयं भवति वापि हि षड्विधः मः।
वातादिभिः पृथक् सर्व्वेर्मेदसा च क्षयेण च।
वातेन कृष्णनयनामन्-भूचवर्च्चा भिन्नं शनै र्वदति गर्द्दभवत् स्वरञ्च।
पित्तेन पोतनयनानन मूत्रवर्च्चा ब्रूयादग्लेन स च दाह समन्वितेन।
ब्रूयात् कफेन सततं कफरुद्धकष्ठः
स्वलपं शनैर्वदति चापि दिवा विशेषात्।
सर्वात्मके भवति सर्वतिकारसम्पत् तच्चाप्यसाध्मृषयः स्वरभेदमाहः।।

on running, etc. No other disease is produced by this one, and it is curable unless when combined with some other disease.

HOARSENESS *(Swarabheda)*

The causes of this disease are loud speaking, poison, long continued reading, external injuries, exposure to cold, etc. When air, bile and phlegm are deranged in the air-passages they produce the six varieties of hoarseness. One is produced by derangements of the air, bile, or phlegm ; by the combination of the three ; by fatness ; and by weakness.

1st. ***Air*** when deranged produces this disease, when the person's eyes, mouth, urine, and dejections become black, and his tone of speaking is slow, and like an ass braying.

2nd. When ***bile*** is deranged, the eyes, mouth, urine, and dejections are of a yellowish colour, and the patient speaking from the throat, with a sense of burning pain in the part.

3rd. ***Phlegm*** when deranged, the throat is filled with

धूप्येत वाक् क्षयकृते क्षयमाप्नुयाच्च वागेष चापि हतवाक् परिवर्ज्जनीयः।
अन्तर्गतं खरमञ्चक्ष्यपदं चिरेण भेदोऽन्वयाहदति दिग्धगलस्तृषार्त्तः।
क्षीणस्या वृद्धस्य कृशस्य वापि चिरोत्यितो यश्च महोपजातः।
मेदस्विनः सर्वासमुद्भवश्च स्वरामयो यो न स सिद्धिमेति।

अरोचक-निदानम्

वातादिभिः शोकभयातिलोभ-क्रोधैर्मनोघ्नाशनरूपगन्धैः
अरोचकाः स्युः परिहृष्टदन्तः कषायवक्तश्च मतोऽनिलेन
कट्वम्लमुष्णं विरसञ्च पूति पित्तेन विद्याल्पवणञ्च वक्त्रम्।
माधुर्य्यपैच्छिूलागुरुत्वशैत्य-विवद्धसंभवद्धयुतं कफेन॥
अरोचके शोक-भयाति लोभ क्रोधाद्यहृद्याशुचिगन्धजे स्यात्।
स्वाभाविकञ्चास्यमथारुचिञ्च चिदोषजे नैकरसं भवेत्तु॥
हृच्छूलपीड़नयुतं पवनेन पित्तात् तृड्दाहचोषबहलं सकफप्रसेकम्।
श्लेष्मात्मकं बद्धरुजं बहुभिश्च विद्यादैगुव्य मोहजड़ताभि रथापरञ्च॥

mucus, and the person speaks little and that slowly and with difficulty, particularly at night.

When air, bile, and phlegm are deranged, the combined symptoms of the three varieties are present ; and the patient speaks so indistinctly that he cannot be understood. This form is incurable.

4th. When weakness or diminution of the essential parts (*dhātu*) produce the disease, the patient cannot speak, and when he tries, smoke appears to proceed from the mouth, with pain. He speaks very little. This form is also incurable.

5th. When it is produced by *fatness* the person's speaking is indistinct, and he thinks his throat and palate are covered with something. Such disease will not be cured when the person is weak, old, thin; when it has been of long continuance, and is congenital. In fat people, and when produced by the combination of the three humours it is also incurable.

छर्द्दिनिदानम्

दुष्टैर्दोषैः पृथक् सर्व्वैर्वीभत्सालोचनादिभिः।
छर्द्दयः पञ्च विज्ञेया स्तासां लक्षणमुच्यते॥
अतिद्रवैरतिश्निग्धैरहृद्यैर्लवणैरति।
अकाले चातिमात्रैश्च तथासात्म्यैश्च भोजनैः॥
श्रमाद्भयात्तथोद्वेगादजोर्णात् क्रिमिदोषतः।
नार्य्याश्चापन्नसत्वायास्तथातिद्रतमश्नतः।
वीभत्सैर्हेतुमिश्चान्नैर्द्रुतमुत्क्लेशितो वलात्॥
छादयत्याननं वेगैरर्द्दन्नङ्गभञ्जनैः।
निरुच्यते छर्द्दिरिति दोषो वक्तं प्रधावितः॥
हृल्लासोद्धारोधौ च प्रसेको लवणस्तनुः।
देवोऽन्नपाने च भृशं वमीनां पूर्व्वलक्षणम्॥
हृत्पार्श्वपीड़ा मुखशोष-शीर्ष-नाभ्यर्त्ति-कास-स्वरभेदतोदैः
उद्गारशब्दं प्रबलं सफेनं विच्छिन्नमुष्णं तनुकं कषायम्॥
कृच्छेण चाल्पं महता च वेगेनार्त्तोऽनिलाच्छर्द्दयतीह दुःखम्।
मूर्च्छा पिपासा मुखशोषमूर्द्ध ताल्वक्षिसन्तापतमो भ्रमार्त्तः॥
पीतं भृशोष्णं हरितं सतिक्तं धूम्रञ्च पित्तेन वमेत् सदाहम्।

VOMITING (Chardi)

Deranged air, bile, and phlegm, produce this disease ; as also when the three humours are deranged, or when the person takes too much fluid, or bad articles of food. When disgusting objects are seen, smelt, or eaten, it may produce this disease. In other persons it is produced by eating food too fast, or at unusual times, and by great fatigue, grief, indigestion, and worms. The state of pregnancy likewise produces vomiting.

Before vomiting occurs, the person complains of nausea, a cessation of belching, a watery and saltish discharge from the mouth, he dislikes food, becomes weak and unsteady in walking, which is followed by vomiting.

When produced by air the vomiting is frothy and scanty,

तन्द्रास्य माधुर्य्य-कफप्रसेक-सन्तोषनिद्रारुचिगौरवार्त्तः॥
स्निग्धं घनं स्वादु कफाद्दिशुद्धं सरोमहोर्षोऽल्परुजं वमेत्तु।
शूलाविपाकारुचिदाहतृष्णा श्वासप्रमेहप्रवला प्रसक्तम्॥
छर्दिस्त्रिदोषाल्पवणाम्ल-नीलसान्द्रोष्णरक्तं वमतां तृष्णां स्यात्॥
विट्स्वेदमूत्राम्वु-वहानि वायुः स्त्रोतांसि संरुद्ध्य यदोर्द्धमेति।
उत्सन्नदोषस्य समाचितं तं दोषं समुद्धूय नरस्य कोष्ठात्॥
विश्भू त्रयो तत्समगन्धवर्णं तृट्-श्वासाहिक्कार्त्तियुतं प्रसक्तम्॥
प्रश्थछद्रद्दैवयैदुष्टमिहातिवेगात्तयर्द्दि तश्चाशु विनाशमेति॥
वीभत्सजा दौर्द्वदजामजा च असात्म्यजा च क्रिमिजा च या हि।
सा पञ्चमी ताञ्च विभाभयेच्च,
दोषोच्छ्रयेणैव यथोक्तमादौ शूलहृल्लासबहुला क्रिमिजा च विशेषतः॥
क्रिमिहृद्रोगतुल्येन लक्षनेन च लक्षिता॥
क्षीणस्य या छर्द्दिरतिप्रसक्ता सोपद्रवा। शोणितपूययुक्ता।
सचन्द्रिकां तां प्रवदेदसाध्यां साध्याश्चिकित्सेन्निरुपद्रवाञ्च॥

तृष्णानिदानम्

भयश्रमाभ्यां बलसंक्षयाहा ऊर्द्धवश्चितं पित्तविवर्द्धनैश्च।
पित्त्वं सवातं कुपितं नराणां तालुप्रपन्नं जनयेत् पिपासाम्।
स्त्रोतः-स्वपां वाहिषु दूषितेषु दोषैश्च तृट् संभवतीह जन्तोः।

much pain is felt in the back, and sides of the abdomen ; great exhaustion, and vomiting occurs, with a loud noise, and an astringent taste in the mouth. When *bile*, produces vomiting, the person feels faint, thirsty, the mouth is dry and the head, palate, and eyes hot. He sees indistinctly as if he was in darkness, his body turns round, and he vomits a bitter matter of yellow, hot, green, or sour nature. When phlegm is the cause the patient is heavy and dozes, his mouth is sweet, phlegm is discharged, thick, white and copiously mixed with mucus, and a horripilation is felt. The person has no appetite, and the fluid vomited is neither salt, sour, nor bitter. When air, bile, and phlegm are deranged, all the above symptoms are present.

तिस्त्रः स्मृतास्ताः क्षतजा चतुर्थी क्षयात्तथह्यामसमुद्भवा च।
भक्तोद्भवा सप्तमिकेति तासां निवोध लिङ्गान्यनुपूर्व्वशस्तु।
क्षामास्यतामारुतसद्भवायां तोदस्तथा शङ्ख शिरःसु चापि।
स्त्रोतोनिरोधो विरसश्च वक्तं शीताभिरद्भिश्च विवृद्धिभेतिं।
मूर्च्छान्नविद्वेष विलापदाहा रक्तेक्षणत्वं प्रततश्च शोषः॥
शीताभिनन्दा मुखतिक्ता च पित्तात्मिकायां परिदूयनञ्च।
वाष्पावरोधात् कफसंतृतेऽग्नौ, तृष्णा बलासेन भवेत्तथा तु॥
निद्रा गुरुत्वं मधुरास्यता च तृष्णार्द्दितः शुष्यति चातिमात्रम्।
क्षतस्य रुक्शोणितनिर्गमाभ्यां तृष्णा चतुर्थी क्षतजा मता तु॥
रसक्षयाद्याक्षसम्भवा सा तयाभिभूतश्च निशादिनेषु।
पेपीयतेऽम्नः ससुखं न याति तां सन्निपातादिति केचिदाहुः॥
रसक्षयोक्तानि च लक्षणानि, तस्यामशेषेण भिषग्व्यवस्येत्।
त्रिदोषलिङ्गामसमुद्भवा च हृच्छलनिष्ठीवन सादकर्त्री।
स्निग्धं तथाम्लं लवणञ्च भुक्तं मुर्व्वन्नमेवाशु तृषां करोति॥
दीनस्वरः प्रताम्यन् दीनः संशुष्ककण्ठगलतालुः॥
भवति खलु योपसर्गात् तृष्णा सा शोषिणी कष्टा॥
ज्वर मोहक्षयकासप्रवासाद्युपसृष्टःदेहानां
सर्व्वस्त्वतिप्रसक्ता रोगकृशानां वमिप्रयुक्तानाम्॥
घोरोपद्रवसंयुक्ता तृष्णा मरणाय विज्ञेया।

When produced by the sight of disagreeable objects, pregnancy or worms, the humours will be deranged, and the variety of the disease will be distinguished by their peculiar symptoms. When produced by worms, there is frequent eructations, and much pain, accompanied with the symptoms of those diseases of the chest which are produced by worms.

The unfavourable symptoms are great debility, and the matter vomited being mixed with blood and pus, or resembles the variegated colour of the pecock's tail. There is also frequent vomiting in other dangerous disease. All the varieties of vomiting are produced by disorders of the stomach.

मूर्च्छाभ्रमनिद्रासंन्यासनिदानम्

क्षीणस्य बहुदोषस्य विरुद्घाहारसेविनः।
वेगाघातादभीघाताद्धीनसत्वस्य वा पुनः॥
करणयतनेषूग्रा वाह्येष्वभ्यन्तरेषु च।
निविषन्ते यदा दोषास्तदा मूर्च्छन्ति मानवाः॥
संज्ञावहासु नाड़ीषु पिहिताव्यनिलादिभिः।
तमोऽभ्युपैति सहसा सुखदुःखव्यपोहकृत्।
सुखदुःखव्यपोहाच्च नरः पतति काष्ठवत्॥
मोहोमूर्च्छेति तामाहुः षड़िवधा सा प्रकीर्त्तिता।
वातादिभिः शोणितेन मद्येन च विषेण च॥
षट्स्वप्येताषु प्रित्तन्तु प्रभुत्वेनावतिष्ठते॥
हृत्पीड़ा जृम्भणं ग्लानिः संज्ञा दौर्व्वल्यमेव च।
सर्व्वासां पूर्व्वरूपाणि यथास्वञ्च विभावयेत्।
नीलं वा यदि वा कृष्णमाकाश्चमथवारुणम्।
पश्यंस्तमः प्रविशति शीघ्रञ्च प्रतिबुध्यते॥
वेपथुश्चाङ्गमर्द्दश्च प्रपीड़ा हृदयस्य च।
कार्श्य श्यावारुणा च्छाया मूर्च्छायां वातसम्भवे॥
रक्तं हरितवर्णं वा वियत् पीत्मथापि वा।
पश्यंस्तमः प्रविशति सखेदश्च प्रबुध्यति॥

SWOONING *(Murchhā)*

When the person is weak, or when the *air, bile* and *phlegm* are very much deranged, by eating improper mixtures of food, such as milk and fish, or flesh, etc., by constipation, etc., this disease is produced ; in which the organs of sense, both external and internal are deranged, with faintness.

When the derangements of *air, bile* and *phlegm* close the passages of the vessels, the person cannot see, and falls down as a piece of wood : this disease is called *Mūrchhā* or *moha*.

सपिपासः ससन्तापः रक्तपीतारुणेक्षणः।
संभिन्नवर्च्चाः पीताभो मूर्च्छायां पित्तसम्भवे।
मेघसङ्काशमाकांशमावृतं वा तमोघनैः।
पश्यंस्तमः प्रविशति चिराक्ष प्रतिबुध्यते॥
गुरुभिः प्रावृतैरङ्गैर्यथैवार्द्रेण चर्म्मणा।
सप्रसेकः सहुल्लासो मूर्च्छायां कफसम्भवे॥
सर्व्वाकृतिः सन्निपातादपस्मार दूवागतः।
स जन्तुं पाययत्याशुविना वीभत्सचेष्टितैः॥
पृथिव्यापस्तमोरूपं रक्तगन्धस्तदन्वयः।
तस्माद्रक्तस्य गन्धेन मूर्च्छन्ति भुवि मानवाः॥
द्रव्यस्वभाव दूत्येके दृष्ट्वा यदभिमुह्यति
गुणस्तीव्रतरत्वेन स्तितास्तु विषमद्ययोः।
तएव तस्मात्ताभ्यन्तु मोहौ स्यातां यथेरितौ।
स्तब्धाङ्गदृष्टिस्त्वसृजा गूढ़ोच्छासश्च मूर्च्छितः॥
मद्येन विलपन् शेते नष्टविभ्रान्तमानवः।
गात्राणि विक्षिपन् भूमौ जरां यावन्न याति तत्।
वेपथुस्वप्रतृष्णाः सुस्तमश्च विषमूर्च्छिते।
वेदितव्यं तीव्रतरं यथास्वं विषलक्षणम्॥
मूर्च्छा पित्ततमः प्राया रजःपित्तानिलाद्भ्रमः।
चक्रवद् भ्रमतो गात्रं भूमौ पतति सर्व्वदा॥

There are six varieties of this disease, but in all the bile is deranged. The six are produced by derangements of *air, bile* or *phlegm,* by blood, by drinking spirits, and by poison.

The approach of this disease is known by pain in the breast, gaping, languor, loss of sense, and strength. These symptoms are the same in all the varieties.

When produced by derangements of *air,* every thing appears of a dark-blue or red colour, or like the sky. The person

भ्रमरोग इति ज्ञेयो रजपित्तानिलात्मकः।
तमोवातकफात्तन्द्रय निद्रा श्लेष्तभोभवा॥
इन्द्रियार्थेष्वसंवित्ति गौरवं जृम्भणं क्लमः।
निद्रार्त्तस्येव यस्येहा तस्य तन्द्रां विनिर्द्दिशेत्॥
देषेषु मदमूर्च्छाया हृतवेगेषु देहिनाम्।
स्वयमेवोपशम्ययन्ति संन्यासो नौषधैर्व्विना।
वाग्देहसनसां चेष्टामाक्षिप्यातिबला मलाः।
सन्यस्थन्ताबलं जन्तुं प्राणयतनमाश्रिताः॥
स ना सन्याससन्यस्तः काष्ठीभूतो मृतोपमः।
प्राणै र्व्विमुच्यते शीघ्रं मुक्त्वा सद्यःफलां क्रियाम्॥

पानात्यपरमदपानाजीर्णपानविभ्रमनिदानम्

ये विषस्य गुणाः प्रीक्लास्तेऽपि मद्ये प्रतिष्ठिताः।
तेन मिथ्योपचारेन भवत्युग्रो मदात्ययः॥
किन्तु मद्यं स्त्रभावेन यथैवान्नं तथा स्मृतम्।
अयुक्तियुक्त रोगाय युक्तियुक्त यथास्मृतम्॥
प्राणाः प्राणभृतामन्नं तद्रयुक्त्या निहत्यासून्।
विषं प्राणहरं तच्चयुक्तियुक्तं रसायनम्॥
विधिना मात्रया काले हितैरन्नैर्यथाबलम्।
प्रहृष्टो यः पिवेमन्द्यं तस्त्य स्यादमृतोपमम्॥
स्निग्धैस्तदन्नैर्म्मांसैश्च भक्षैश्च सह सेवितम्।

cannot see, and faints, but the senses soon return. There is shivering, pain of the body and breast, weakness, and the skin becomes dirty, and of a reddish or green colour.

Bile. The person sees every thing of a yellow, or green colour ; he cannot see, and faints. He is soon restored to his senses, with perspiration. When he recovers, the skin becomes yellow, the body becomes hot, eyes red, and dejections yellow.

भवेदायुःप्रकर्षाय बलायोपचयाय च॥
काम्यता सनसस्तुष्टि स्तेजो विक्रम एव च।
विधिवत् सेव्यमाने तु मद्ये सन्निहिता गुणाः।
बुद्धि-स्मृति-प्रीतिकरः सुखश्च पान्नान्न-निद्रा-रति-वर्द्धनश्च।
संपाठ गीतस्वरवर्द्धनश्च प्रोक्तोऽतिरम्यः प्रथमो मदो हि।
अव्यक्त बुद्धिप्सृतिवाग्विचेष्टः सोन्मत्तलीलाकृतिरप्रशान्तः।
आलस्यनिद्राभिहतो मुहुश्च मध्येन मत्तः पुरुषो मदेन॥
गच्छ्रेदगम्यां न गुरुंश्च मन्येत् खादेदभक्षाणि च नष्टसंज्ञः॥
ब्रूयाच्च गुह्यानि हृदि ख्यितानि मदे तृतीये पुरुषोऽस्वतन्त्रः॥
चतुर्थे तु मदे मूढ़ो भग्नदार्व्विव निष्क्रियः।
कार्य्यकार्य्यविभागज्ञो मृतादप्यवयो मतः।
को मदं तादृशं गच्छेदुन्मादमिव चापरम्।
बुहुदोषमिवामूढः कान्तारं स्ववशः कृती।
निर्भक्तमेकान्तत एव मद्यं निषेब्यमानं मनुजेन नित्यम्।
आपादयेत् कष्टतमान् विकारानापादयेच्चापि शरीरभेदम्॥
क्रुद्धेन भीतेन पिपासितेन शोकाभितप्तेन कुभुक्षितेन।
व्यायामभाराध्वप्ररिक्षतेन वेगावरोभिहतेन चापि॥
अत्यम्वुभक्षावततोदरेण साजीर्णभुक्तेन तथावलेन।
उष्णाभितप्तेन च सेव्यमानं करोति मद्यं विविधान् विकारान्॥
पानात्ययं परमदं पानाजीर्णमथापि वा।
पानविभ्रममुग्रञ्च तेषां वक्ष्यामि लक्षणम्॥

Phlegm. He sees every thing of the colour of clouds ; the sky appears misty and dark, followed by fainting, in which sensation remains long absent. The body feels like as if a piece of soaked leather had been put upon it : phlegm is discharged from the mouth and nose, followed by nausea and vomiting.

When these three humours are deranged at the same time, they produce all the symptoms of the three separate diseases ;

हिक्का श्वासशिरःकम्प पार्श्वशूलप्रजागरैः।
विद्याद्वहुप्रलापस्य वातप्रायं मदात्ययम्।
तृष्णादाहज्वरस्वेद-मोहातिसारविभ्रमैः॥
विद्याद्धरितवर्णस्य पित्तप्रायं मदात्ययम्।
छर्द्यरीचकहृल्लासः-तन्द्रा-स्तैमित्यगैरवैः।
विद्याच्छीतपरीतस्य कफप्रायं मदात्ययम्॥
ज्ञेय स्त्रिदोषजश्चापि सर्व्वलिङ्गै र्मदात्ययः।
श्लेष्मोच्छ्रयोऽङ्गगुरुता विरसास्यता च
विन्मूत्रसक्तिरथ तन्द्रिररोचकश्च॥
लिङ्गं परस्य च मदस्य वदन्ति तज्ज्ञा
स्तृष्णा रुजा शिरसि सन्धिषु चापि भेदः।
आध्मानमुग्रमथ चोद्गिरणं विदाहः
पाने जरां समुपगच्छति लक्षणानि।
हृद्गात्रतोद कफसंस्त्रवकण्ठधूमा,
मूर्च्छावमि ज्वर शिरोरुजनप्रदाहाः।

but without the symptoms of Epilepsy. When these diseases occur, and the person does not feel when needles are thrust into his flesh, red hot irons put upon the surface, or hot substances put into his mouth, the person will soon die.

Seeing *blood* often produces swooning from its containing earth and water, which possess the properties of *tamoguna,* the cause of darkness. In this manner the occurrence of fainting, on seeing blood, by the quality of darkness which it possesses.

When swooning is produced by *poison* there is shivering drowsiness, thirst, followed by weakness and insensibility. There are various kinds of this variety, but all produce these symptoms. Fainting is generally produced by deranged bile, when mixed with *tamoguna,* or darkness. When bile and air are mixed with *rajoguna,* it produces swooning, and drowsiness ; coma is produced when air and phlegm are mixed with *tamoguna ;* and phlegm and *tamoguna* when mixed together produce sleep.

द्वेषः सुरान्नविकृतेष्वपि तेषु तेषु तं
पान विभ्रम मृशस्त्यखिलेन धीराः।
हीनत्तरौष्ठमतिशशीतममन्ददाहं
तैलप्रभास्यमपि पानहतं त्यजेत्तु।
जिह्वौष्ठदन्तमसितस्वथ वापि नीलं
पीतञ्च यस्य नयने रुधिरप्रमे वा।
हिक्काज्वरौ वमथु-वेपथु पार्श्वशूलाः
कासभ्रमावपि च पानहतं भजन्ते॥

दाहनिदानम्

त्वचं प्राप्तः स पानीस्मा पित्तरक्ताभिमूर्च्छितः।
दाहं प्रकुरुते घोरं पित्तवत्तत्र भेषजम्॥
कृत्स्नदेहानुगं रक्त्वमुद्रिक्त्वं दहति ध्रुवम्।
स उष्यते तृष्यते वा ताम्राभ

Drinking spirits derange the *air, bile* and *phlegm,* and produce swooning, which continues until the effects of the spirit ceases.

Another form of this disease is called *sangnyāsa* (apoplexy). It is produced by the deranged air, bile and phlegm, which pass to the place in which life is retained, and overpowers all the functions of both mind and body, and the person suddenly falls down, and remains as if dead, or like a piece of wood. If not immediately, and properly treated, such a person will die.

BURNING OF THE BODY (*Dāha.*)

This is generally a symptomatic disease attended with fever. The blood of the whole body is affected in this disease, the body becomes hot, and the patient complains of a burning sensation over the body, as if hot charcoal was applied to the surface which becomes of a red colour like copper. The eyes of such a person are red, and his breath is like hot iron.

There are seven forms of this disease, one being produced by bile, another by blood, the third by external injury of the trunk, the fourth by not quenching thirst, the fifth by the injury

स्ताम्रलोचनः लोहगन्धाङ्गवदनो वह्निनेवावकीर्य्यते।
पित्तज्वरसमः पित्तात् च चाप्यस्य विधिः स्मृतः।
तृष्णानिरोधदव्धातौ क्षीणी तेजः समुद्गतम्।
अवाह्याभ्यन्तरं देहं प्रदहेन्मन्दचेतसः॥
संशुष्कगलतालोष्ठो जिह्वां निष्कृष्य वेपते।
असृजः पूर्णकोष्ठस्य दाहोऽन्यः स्यात् सुदुस्तरः।
धातुक्षयक्त्वो यो दाहस्तेन मूर्च्छातृड़र्दितः॥

of vital parts, the sixth by excess in drinking, and the seventh by the loss of the essential parts of the body, as chyle, blood, etc.

1st and 2nd. When produced by *bile,* it is accompanied with fever. When *blood* is affected the body, eyes, etc., become red, and he complains of a burning sensation over the body.

3rd. when any viscus is injured, and is filled up with blood, and affects a *dāha* which is difficult to cure.

4th. When produced by excessive drinking the internal heat comes out externally, and is increased by the derangement of bile and blood. It then produces great burning of the body.

5th. If a foolish person does not drink water, when he is very thirsty, the watery part of the body is diminished ; and the internal heat is increased, producing a burning of the external and internal parts of the body ; his throat, palate, tongue and lips, become dry, and the tongue protrudes, with shaking of the body,.

6th. When the essential fluids of the body are diminished by any cause, as an excess in venery, too much exercise, copious evacuation of any of the fluids, the body feels very hot, and the patient faints, has much thirst, his voice becomes low and altered, he cannot move his body, and soon dies.

7th. When any vital part is injured, as the bladder, heart, or brain, it produces a burning sensation over the body which is incurable.

क्षामण्वरः क्रियाहीनः स सीदेद्धशपीड़ितः।
मर्म्माभिघातजोऽप्यस्ति सोऽसाध्यः सप्तमो मतः।
सर्व्व एव च वर्ष्यः स्युः शीत गात्रेषु देहिनः॥

उन्माद-भूतोन्मादनिदानम्

मदयन्तुद्गता दोषा यस्मादुन्मार्गमागताः।
मानसोऽयमतो व्याधिरुन्माद इति कीर्त्तितः॥
एकैकशः सर्व्वशश्च दोषैरत्र्थमूर्च्छितैः॥
मानसेन च दुःखेन स च पञ्चविधो मतः।
विषाद्भवति षष्ठश्च यथास्वं तत्र भेषजम्॥
च चाप्रवृद्ध स्तरुणो मदसंज्ञां विभर्त्ति च॥
विरुद्धदुष्टाशुचिभोजनानि प्रधर्षणं देवगुरुद्विजानाम्।
उन्मादहेतु र्भयहर्षपूर्व्वो मनोऽभिघातो विषमाश्च चेष्टाः।
तैरल्पसत्वस्य मलाः प्रदुष्टा बुद्धेर्निवासं हृदयं प्रदुष्य।

When the body feels cold to another while the patient is suffering from an internal burning, it is always a very unfavourable symptom in this kind of disease.

Burning of the feet (Pāda-dāha) is a variety of this order; and is a peculiar, severe and very untractable disease.

MADNESS (*Unmāda.*)

The causes producing this disease are improper food, endeavouring to perform impossibilities, strong passions of the mind, cursing the gods, brāhmans, and spiritual guides ; eating poison, etc.

The *air, bile and phlegm* are affected by the above causes, which deranged knowledge (*satwagun*), affects the seat of understanding and the heart, and pass through the vessels conveying sense(*mana*) when the person becomes mad, speaks foolishly, is restless, and his eyes are continually moving about.

There are six kinds of madness. Three being produced

स्त्रोतांस्यधिष्ठाय मनोवहानि प्रमोहयन्त्याशु नरस्य चेतः॥
धीविभ्रमः सत्वपरिप्लवश्च पर्य्याकुला दृष्टिरधीरता च।
अवद्धवाक्त्वं हृदयञ्च शून्यं सामान्यमुन्मादगदसा लिङ्गम्॥
रुक्षाल्प शीतान्नविरेक-धातुक्षयोपवासैरनिलोतिवृद्धः॥
चिन्तादिदुष्टं हृदयं प्रदुष्य बुद्धिं स्मृतिञ्चापुप्यहन्ति शीघ्रम्।
अस्थानहास्यस्मित नृत्यगीत-वागङ्गविक्षेपण-रोदनानि॥
पारुष्यकार्श्यरुणवर्णता च, जीर्णे बलञ्चानिलजस्य रुपम्।
अजीर्णाकट्वम्लविदाहशीतैं भोज्यैश्चितं पित्तमुदीर्णवेगम्॥

by derangements of air, bile and phlegm ; one by the combination of these ; another by the violent actions of the passions ; and the last by poison.

Air is deranged and the mind is thus affected by the use of dry, cooling, articles of food ; by food in small quantities ; by strong purgatives ; by the causes diminishing the humours (*dhātu*), or by fasting. By these causes the air is deranged, producing madness ; in which the man laughs, dances, and sings unreasonably, and moves his limbs about. At other times he cries without cause ; the skin of his body becomes dry, rough, and of a dark-red colour. These symptoms are more violent after the digestion of food ; and the patient becomes greatly emaciated.

When *bile* is generally deranged by the use of indigestible food, and the use of pungent and heating substances, the symptoms it produces are impatience of control, and anger ; the person wishes to use violence to others ; he remains naked, prefers cooling food, and wishes to live under the shade, or in water. The body is yellow and hot.

When *phlegm* is deranged by the usual causes, as a too sedentary life, and taking too much nourishing food ; by which the phlegm is deranged, affecting the functions of the heart, and producing the following symptoms : A love of solitude, taciturnity, and loss of appetite ; the person has a desire for

उन्मादत्युग्रमनात्मकस्य हृदि स्थितं पूर्व्ववदाशु कुर्य्यात्।
अमर्षसंरम्भाविमग्नभावा: सन्तर्ज्जनातिद्रवणौष्णरोषा:॥
प्रच्छाय शीतान्नजलाभिलाषा: पीतता च भा पित्तकृतस्य लिङ्गम्।
सम्पूणौ र्मन्दविचेष्टितस्य, सोष्मा कफोमर्म्मनि सम्प्रदुष्ट:।
बुद्धिं स्मृतिञ्चापुप्यहत्य चित्तं प्रमोहयन् संजनयेद्विकारान्॥
वाक्चेष्टितं मन्दकरोचकश्च नारी विविक्तप्रियता च निद्रा।
छर्द्दिश्च लाला च बलञ्च भुङ्क्ते नखादिशौक्लञ्च कफात्मके स्यात्॥

women, enjoys deep sleep, and has vomiting, or expectoration. After eating any thing the symptoms are very violent, and the body as well as the nails and countenance are whitish.

When *air, bile, and phlegm* are deranged together, all the separate symptoms are produced, and the disease becomes of very difficult cure.

When the disease is produced by the passions ; as when frightened by a robber, a tyrannical official, etc.; by the loss of wealth, and friends, or by the love of particular women, the symptoms are characterized by talking, laughing, singing, and sometimes crying. This variety terminates in idiocy.

When madness is produced by poison, the person becomes faint, from the sudden loss of strength ; his eyes become red, and the countenance and the body become yellow or blue. The unfavourable symptoms are when the person is weak and emaciated, remains in one position, and is always looking downwards, or upwards. When the patient has no sleep, and is so courageous that he will throw himself from a height, the disease will be fatal.

POSSESSED PERSONS, OR DEVIL-MADNESS, (*Bhutonmāda*).

There are two kinds of spiritual being, a good and a bad spirit, which are supposed to enter the body, and to produce disease. These are called *Bhutonmāda, (Devil-Madness)*; and *Debonmāda,* (madness produced by good spirits).

यः सन्निपातप्रभतोऽतिघोरः सर्व्वैः समस्त्यैः स च हेतुभिः स्यात्॥
सर्व्वाणि रूपाणि विभर्त्ति तादृग्विरुद्धभैषजा विधि र्विवर्ज्यः॥
चोरैर्नरेन्द्रपुरुषैररिभिस्तथान्यै र्वित्रासितस्य धनवान्धवसंक्षयाद्वा।
गाढ़ क्षते मनसि च प्रियया रिरंसो र्जायेत चोत्कटतरो मनसो विकारः॥
चित्रं व्रवीति च मनोऽनुगतं विसंज्ञो गायत्यथो हसति रोदिति चापि मूढः।
रक्तेक्षणी हतबलेन्द्रियभाः सुदीनः श्वावाननो विषकृतेऽथ भवेद्विसंज्ञः।

When produced by attack of devils, the person shows his aversion to every thing divine, is very strong, and has much knowledge ; and when from the entrance of good spirit or (*Debtā*) the person has a pleasure in flowers and good smells , becomes pure and holy, and is inclined to speak Sanskrit. He obeys *brāhmans* with strictness, and looks courageous. There are no intermissions in these forms of madness.

Devils know the present, the future, and what is hid or unknown. They are never at rest ; and they are employed in different kinds of business. An unclean or wounded person, or those who do not perform their ceremonies, may be injured by devils. They are very numerous and powerful, and are usually considered as the attendants, or servants of *Shiva*. This explains how the energy, and work of the affected person, is much beyond that of man ; his mind is now powerful, his knowledge extensive, and he understands the *shāstras*. Sometimes the person appears sane, and at another time is mad. Such madness is produced by a devil, which is known by the unnatural motion of the person's eyelids.

There are eight principal devils that torment the human species.

1. When *Debagraha*, of good spirit, enters a body, the person is always happy and contented, remains clean in his person, and wears garlands of the sacred flowers, etc.; his person has a pleasant smell, and he has no sleep. He speaks Sanskrit correctly. The person is strong, his eyes remain fixed,

अवाञ्ची वाप्युदञ्ची वा क्षीणमांसबलो नरः।
जागरूकी ह्यसन्द हेमुन्नदिन विनश्यति॥
अमर्त्यवाग्विक्रमवीर्य्यचेष्टो ज्ञानादि-विज्ञान-बलादिभिर्यः।
उन्मादकालोऽनियतश्च यस्य भूतोत्थसुन्मादमुदाहरेत्तम्।
सन्तुष्टः शुचिरतिदिव्यमाल्यगन्धो निस्तन्द्री रवितथ-संस्कृत प्रभाषी।
तेतस्वी स्वियरनयनो वरप्रदाता ब्रह्मण्यो भवति नरः स देवजुष्टः॥
संस्वेदी द्विज गुरुदेवदोषवक्ता जिह्माक्षो विगतभयो विमार्गदृष्टिः।
सन्तुष्टो न भवति चान्नपानजातैर्दुष्टात्मा भवति स देवशत्रजुष्टः॥

and he blesses those who approach him. He has a great love for *brāhmans*, and performs the prescribed ceremonies and attends to old customs of his ancestry.

2. *Asuragraha*. They are the enemies of the *Debtās*. When the person is possessed with them, he perspires much, speaks of the bad conduct of *brāhmans*, and the *Debtās*. His eyes are turned and fixed, he has no fear, and is always performing bad actions. He is a glutton, is not pleased with his food and drink, and is always mischievous.

3. *Gandarbagraha*. The person possessed with this devil is slways happy, prefers living in an island, near the bank of a river, or in the jungle ; and his conduct is good. He is fond of singing, of sweet smells, and of looking at flowers. He is fond of dancing, and laughing. Those are the choristers of heaven (demigods) who wear sacred flowers, put marks on their person, and have a great love for adorning their persons. They speak little but properly, and agreeably.

4. *Jakshyagraha*. This class of demigods are fabled to superintend the treasures, and gardens of heaven. When he enters the body, the person's eyes become yellowish red like copper. They wear thin red clothes, talk little, but are profoundly intelligent, and have much patience ; such a person walks fast, is never revengeful, though very strong, and is always wanting to bestow his means upon others.

हृष्टात्मा पुलिनवनान्तरोपसेवी स्वाचारः प्रियपरिगीतगन्धमाल्यः।
नृत्यन् वै प्रहसति चारु चाल्पशब्दं गन्धर्व ग्रहपरिपीड़ितो मनुष्यः।
ताम्राक्षः प्रियतनु-रक्तवस्त्रधारी गम्भोरो द्रुतगतिरल्पवाक् सहिष्णुः।
तेजस्वी वदति च किं ददामि कस्मै यो यक्षग्रहपरिपीड़ितो मनुष्यः॥
प्रेतानां स दिशति संस्तरेषु पिण्डान् शान्तात्मा जलमपि चापसव्यवस्त्रः।
मांसेप्सुस्तिलगुड़पायसाभिकामः स्तद्भक्तो भवति पितृग्रहाभिजुष्टः॥
यस्तुर्व्यां प्रसरति सर्पवत् कदाचित्
सृक्कण्यौ र्विलिहति लिह्वया तथैव॥
क्रोधालु र्गुड़मधुदुग्धपायसेप्सु र्ज्ञातव्यो भवति भुजङ्गमेन जुष्टः।
मांसासृग्विविधसुराविकारलिप्सु र्निर्लज्जो भृशमतिनिष्ठुरोऽतिशूरः॥

5. *Pitrigraha*. These are spirits which are separated after death from the bodies of mankind. When an ancestor thus enters the body, the person is always preparing prayers for them, and performing the different ceremonies *(shrāddha)* for ancestors. Such a patient is quiet and peaceable, and is fond of animal food, and sweetmeats.

6. *Sarpagraha*. When the serpent-devil enters the body, the person walks irregularly, or from one side to another, like a serpent ; his tongue is thrust from one side of the mouth to the other ; and he is passionate, and fond of treacle, honey, and sweetmeats.

7. *Rākshyasagraha*, or cannibal-devil. When one of these devils enters the body of a person, he is fond of eating flesh, blood, and wine. He has no shame, his appearance is disagreeable, and he is very strong, and passionate. Such a person walks about at night, is unclean, and is always performing bad actions.

8. *Pishācha*, or fiend, is known to have entered the body, by the person always stretching out his hands. His body is thin, and is disagreeable to look upon, and he speaks fast, and without meaning. His body has a disagreeable smell, and he is

क्रोधालु र्विपुलबलो निशाविहारी
शौचद्विड़ भवति स राक्षसै र्गृहीतः।
उद्धस्तः कृशपरुषोऽचिरप्रलापी दुर्गन्धो भृशमशुचि स्तथातिलोलः॥
बह्वाशी विजनवनान्तरोपसेवी ब्याचष्टन् भ्रमति रुदन्, पिशाचजुष्टः॥
ख्यूलाक्षो द्रुतमटनः स फेनलेही निद्रालुः पतति कम्पते च यो हि।
थश्चाद्रि द्विरदनगादिविच्युतः स्यात्।
सोऽसाध्यो भवति तथा त्रयोदशाब्देः॥

unclean, restless, and covetous. Such a person eats much, prefers living in jungles, and retired places; he walks with an unnatural motion of the limbs and is sorrowful, and frequently cries.

The unfavourable symptoms of such persons possessed with devils are ; his eyes are swollen, he walks fast, and his tongue is passed rapidly, and continually, from one side of the mouth to the other ; he is always sleep and sometimes falls down; and at other times he is affected with severe shivering. When the madness is produced by falls from high places, such as from elephants, or trees, they are more difficult to cure. It is also dangerous in old age, and when hereditary. When the disease has continued 13 years it will not be cured.

The devils invade the body of persons on different days according to the species. *Debtā* invade at full moon, and devils *(Asur)*, enter in the morning and evening. The *Gandarba* enters on the eighth, and *Jakshya* on the first day of the moon. *Sarpagraha,* or serpent-devils, enter on the fifth day after new and full moon. *Rākshyasa* enter at night. *Pishācha* enter on the 15th day after new and full moon. We cannot see when a spirit enters the body, in the same manner as the soul enters, and leaves the body without being seen ; as light enters the water in a glass, or as heat or cold enters a body, without our being aware how it takes place. *Unmāda, and Bhūtonmada,* are said to be cured when the functions of the sense, judgment,

देवग्रहाः पौर्णमास्यामसुराः सन्ध्यायोरपि।
गन्धर्व्वाः प्रायशोऽष्टम्यं यक्षाश्च प्रतिपद्यत॥
पित्र्यः कृष्णक्षये हिंस्यः पञ्चम्यमपि चोरगाः।
रक्षांसि रात्रौ पिशाचाश्चतुर्दश्यां विशन्ति हि।
दर्पणादीन् यथा च्छाया शीतोष्ण प्राणिनो यथा।
स्वमणिं भास्कराच्चिर्चश्च यथा देहञ्च देहधृक्।
विशन्ति च न दृश्यन्ते ग्रहास्त्वहच्छूरीरिणः॥

अपष्मारनिदानम्

तमःप्रवेशः संरम्भो दोषोद्रेकहतस्मृतेः।
अपस्मार इति ज्ञेय गदो घोरश्चतुर्व्विधः।
हृतकम्पः शून्यता स्वेदो ध्यानं मूर्च्छा प्रमूढ़ता।

and heart, are restored to a perfect state, and the tissues are natural.

Persons not liable to be afflicted by devils are, prophets, charitable persons, those who speak the truth, and those who attend to the orders of the *shāstras*, and perform particular duties, and employ proper terms in addressing holy men. Those who have the eight qualities of the body, are always pure, humble, and wise, visit holy places, always govern their passions, and speak the truth ; and those who pray, and attend to the prescribed ceremonies and are charitable, over such persons devils have no power. Devils only go about at night, and they live, under their eight chiefs, on blood, fat, flesh, and disgusting animals.

EPILEPSY (*Apasmara or Mrigi*)

Generic character. Sudden loss of sense, loss of sight, and the person falls down with convulsions. These eymptoms are preceded by palpitation of the heart, lightness and hollowness of the chest and body, perspiration, inaccurate thinking, dullness of sense, and loss of sleep.

निद्रानाशश्च तस्मिंश्च भविष्यति भवत्यथ।
कम्पते प्रदशेद्दन्तान् फेनोहामी श्वसित्यपि।
परुषारुणकृष्णानि पश्येद्रूपाणि चानिलात्।।
पीतफेनाङ्गवक्त्राक्षः पीतासृग्रूपदर्शकः।।
सतृष्णोष्णानलव्याप्तलोकदर्शी च पैत्तिकः।
शुक्लफेनाङ्गवक्त्राक्षः शीतहृष्टाङ्गजो गुरुः।।
पश्यन् शुक्लानि रूपाणि श्लैष्मिको मुच्यति चिरात्।
सर्व्वैरेतैः समस्तैश्च लिङ्गैर्ज्ञेयस्त्रिदोषजः।।
अपस्मारः स चासाध्यो यः क्षीणस्यानवश्च यः।
प्रस्फुरन्तं सुबहुशः क्षीणं प्रचलितभ्रुवम्।
नैत्राभ्याञ्च विकुर्व्वाणमपस्मारो विनाशयेत्।।

When air, bile, and phlegm are deranged by grief, sorrow, or the like, they pass into the vessels immediately communicating with the heart, and produce this disease, with the loss of sense and memory.

Exciting causes. This disease is produced by the improper use and indulgence of the senses ; as too much, or too little listening, seeing, tasting, smelling, etc.; the improper mixtures of food, or putrified articles of food ; the neglect of the calls of nature, connection with women during the flow of the menses, and by such passions, as sorrow, grief, and anger. By these causes the mind is so effected as to produce epilepsy.

There are four kinds of disease, one being produced by the derangement of each of the three humours, and the fourth by the combination of the three.

When *air* is deranged, the symptoms of epilepsy are followed by shivering, grinding of the teeth, foaming at the mouth, hurried respiration, and to the patient every object appears obscured, red, and confused.

When *bile* is deranged the symptoms are accompanied

पक्षाद्वा द्वादशाहाद्वा मासाद्वा कुपिता मलाः।
अपस्माराय कुर्व्वन्ति वेगं किञ्चिदथान्तरम्॥
देवे वर्षत्यपि यथा भूमौ वीजानि कानिचित्।
शरदि प्रतिरोहन्ति तथा व्याधिसमुच्छ्रयाः॥

वातव्याधिनिदानम्

रुक्षशीताल्पलध्वन्न-व्यवायातिप्रजागरैः।
विषमादुपचाराञ्च दोषासृक् स्त्रवणादपि॥

with a yellowness of the body and countenance. To the patient every thing appears of a yellowish colour, the sputa is of the same colour, and the eyes appear red. The patient has great thirst, and every thing feels hot, and as if enveloped in flames.

When *phlegm* is deranged the symptoms are whiteness of the countenance and body, the saliva and foam are of the same colour, the body is cold, and the patient shivers. The person sees every thing white, and as it appears to approach near him he faints. These fits cease very slowly.

Whe *air, bile,* and *phlegm* are deranged together, all the symptoms of the spearate forms are present. This disease is incurable if not recent, as the person becomes weak and emaciated, and the fits are frequent, and accompanied with severe convulsive movements of the body. The eye-brows contract frequently with the eyelids, and the eyes move rapidly. In such cases the patient will die. The fits come after ten days, a fortnight, or monthly. In other cases they occur very often. As some seeds thrown in the ground during the rains do not germinate for a long time after, so in this disease the deranged air, bile, and phlegm produce the disease after long intervals.

NERVOUS DISEASES (*Bāta Byādhi*)

These diseases are produced by the continued use of dry, cold, or light articles of food, taken in unusually small quantities; excessive venery, and watching ; improper and violent exercise;

लङ् घनप्लवनात्यध्व-व्यायामादिविचेष्टितैः।
धातुनां संक्षयाच्चिन्ताशोकरोगातिकर्षणात्॥
वेगसन्धारणादामादभिघातादभोजनात्।
मर्म्मावाधाद्गजोष्टाश्व-शीघ्रयानापतंसनात्।
देहे स्त्रोतांसि रिक्तानि पूरयित्वानिलो बली॥
करोति विविधान् व्याधीन् सव्वांङ्गैकाङ्गसंश्रयान्॥
अव्यक्तलक्षणं तेषां पूर्व्वरूपमिति स्मृतम्।
आत्मरूपन्तु यद्व्यक्तमपायो लघुता पुनः॥
सङ्कोचः पर्व्वणां स्तम्भो भङ्गोऽस्थ्नां पर्व्वणामपि।
रोमहर्षः प्रलापश्च पाणिपृष्ठशिरोग्रहः॥
खाञ्जयपाङ्गुकुञ्जत्वं शोषोऽङ्गानामनिद्रता।
गभशुक्ररजोनाशः स्पन्दनं गात्रसुप्तता॥
शिरोनासाक्षिजत्र्णां ग्रीवायाश्चापि हुण्डनम्।

fasting ; and copious discharges of blood, or other evacuations. They are also produced by much jumping, swimming, or fighting, wearing wet clothes, or wanting to do impossibilities, as raising weights, etc. Any cause producing the absorption of parts by which the individual is weakened, and swoons ; too much thinking, sorrow, grief, fear, and other diseases producing emaciations ; sleeping uncomfortably during the day, or in an unusual position ; anger, or not attending to the calls of nature ; the accumulation of indigestable food, or certain injuries of vital parts, produce these diseases. They are also caused by the person falling from a height, by riding very fast on an elephant, horse, or camel, or whatever goes very fast. These causes derange air, filling the empty vessels in one part, or over all the body, and thus produce the symptoms of the disease.

When air is so deranged it produces the following symptoms : the muscles of the small joints are contracted with rigidity, and cannot be moved. These symptoms are accom-

भेदस्तोदोऽर्त्तिराक्षेपो मुहुश्चायास एव च॥
एवं विधानि रूपाणि करोति कुपितोऽनिलः।
हेतुस्थानविशेषाच्च भवेद्रोगविशेषकृत्॥
तत्र कोष्ठाश्रिते दुष्टे निग्रहो मूत्रवर्च्चसोः।
व्रध्नहृद्रोग-गुल्मार्शपार्शशूलञ्च मारुते॥
सर्व्वाङ्गकुपिते वाते गात्रस्फु रणभञ्जनम्॥
वेदनाभिः परीतश्च स्फुटन्ति वास्य संधयः।
ग्रहो विन्मूत्रवातानां शूलाध्मानाश्मशर्करा:॥
जङ्घोरु-त्रिक-पात् पृष्ठरोगशोषौ गुदे ख्यिते।
रुक् पार्श्वोदर हृन्नमेस्तृष्णोद्गार विसूचिकाः।
कासः कण्ठास्यशोषश्च श्वासश्चामाशयख्यिते॥
पक्वाशयस्ख्योऽम्त्रकुजं शूलाटोपौ करोति च।
कृच्छ्रमूत्र-पुरीषत्व मानाहं त्रिकवेदनाम्।

panied with so much pain, that they seem as if broken by force. The skin becomes rough, the person speaks nonsense, and complains of pain in the joints of the hand, back, and head; he cannot sleep, nor walk with vigour, and is deformed, and the members become thin. When women are so affected, they have miscarriages, and it diminishes the semen, and stops menstruation. The parts affected shake, there is no feeling in the part, the person has severe pain in the head, and no smell ; the eyes become dry and dull, and a painful weight is felt in the pit of the stomach, and stiffness of the nape of the neck. These symptoms are accompanied with spasm of different parts, with loss of sense and great fatigue.

These different causes, and the different parts of the body affected, produce various forms of the disease. When the air is deranged in the abdomen, the dejections and urine are constipated, pain is felt in the abdomen and its sides, and diseases of the heart, hysteria (*gulma*), and piles (*arsha*), are produced. When air is deranged generally there is much pain over the body, which shakes with pain in the joints. They feel

श्रोत्रादिस्विन्द्रियवधं कुर्य्याद्दुष्टसमीरणः॥
त्वग्रुक्षा स्फुटिता सुप्ता कृशा कृष्णा च तुद्यते।
आतन्यते सरागा च पर्व्वरुक् त्वग्गतेऽनिले॥
रुजास्तीव्राः ससन्तापा वैवर्ण्यं कृशतारुचिः॥
गात्रे चारूंसि भुक्तस्य स्तम्भश्चासृग्गतेऽनिले॥
गुर्व्वङ्ग तुद्यतेऽत्यर्थं दण्डमुष्टिहतं यथा॥
समक् श्रमितमत्यर्थे मांसमेदोगतेऽनिले।
भेदोऽस्थिपर्व्वणां सन्धि शूलं मांसबलक्षयः।
अस्वप्नः सन्तता रुक् च मज्जाख्यिकुपितेऽनिले॥
क्षिप्रं मुञ्चति बध्नाति शुक्रं गर्भमथापि वा॥
विकृतिं जनयेच्चापि शुक्रख्यः कुपितोऽनिलः।
कुर्य्याच्छिरागतः शूलं शिराकुञ्चनपूरणम्॥

as if broken. When situated in the pelvis it stops the usual evacuations, with great pain and flatulency, and produces gravel, and the stone. In women it produces deformities in the foetus, and the plurality of children. When air is deranged in the anus, the legs, thighs, *os coccygus*, hands, and breast are painful, and the body is thin. When deranged air is situated in the *stomach,* the sides, back, scrobiculus cordis, and navel are painful, with thirst, belching, and cholera ; the person complains of cough, and the throat and mouth are dry, with asthma. When air is deranged in the small intestines (*paukāshay*), they make a noise, with scanty dejections, and little urine. Such a person has uneasy choliky pains in the abdomen, with pain in the lower part of the back.

When air is deranged in the *organs of sense* it destroys their functions. When deranged in the skin it becomes dry, rough, and has no feeling ; has a black colour, and is painful. In some cases it is stretched over the body without wrinkles, and is of a red colour, accompanied with pains in the joints, and slight chops in the skin over the body.

स वाह्वाभ्यन्तरायामं खलीं कौब्ज्यमथापि वा।
सर्व्वाङ्गैकाङ्गरोगांश्च कुर्य्यात् स्नायुगतोऽनिलः।
हन्तिय सन्धिगतः सन्धीन् शूलटोपौ करोति च॥
प्राणी पित्तावृते च्छर्द्दिर्द्दाहश्चैवोपजायते।
दौर्व्वल्यं सदनं तन्द्रा वैरस्यञ्च कफावृते।
उदाने पित्तयुक्ते तु दाहो मूर्च्छा भ्रमः क्लमः॥
अस्वेदहसौ मन्दोग्निः शीतता च कफावृते॥
स्वेददाहौष्ण्यमूर्च्छाः स्यः समाने पित्तसंवृते॥
कफेन सङ्गे विन्मूत्रे गात्रहर्षश्च जायते।
अपाने पित्तयुक्ते तु दाहौष्ण्यं रक्तमूत्रता॥
अधःकाये गुरुत्वञ्च शीतता च कफावृते।
व्याने पित्तावृते दाहो गात्रविक्षेपणं क्लमः।

When air is deranged in the *blood,* great pain is felt in the body which is hot, and the colour of the skin is unnatural. The body is thin, the person has no appetite, and the skin has red eruptions over it, and after eating the body is unwieldy, and the person cannot work. When air is deranged in the *flesh or fat* the body is heavy, with pain, as if beaten with a stick, and the person is much fatigued.

When air is deranged in the *bones* and *marrow* the long bones and joints are very painful ; his strength and flesh become diminished ; the person has no sleep, and pain is very severe and continued.

When air is deranged in the *semen* it is quickly discharged, or is constipated, and in women it retains the foetus long in the uterus, or abortions are produced. The semen in such cases has an unusual colour, and produces twins.

When air is deranged in the *vessels* it produces painful contraction, or fulness of the vessel.

When air is deranged in the *nerves* (tendons ?) the whole

स्तम्भनो दण्डकश्चापि शूलशोथौ कफावृते।
यदा तु धमनी सर्व्वाः कुपितोऽभ्येति मारुतः।
तदाक्षिपत्याशु मुहुर्मुहुर्देहं मुहुश्चरः॥
मुहुर्मुहुश्चाक्षेपणादाक्षेपक इति स्मृतः।
क्रुद्धः स्वैः कोपनै र्वायुः ख्यानादर्द्ध्वं प्रपद्यते।
पीड़यन् हृदयं गत्वा शिरःशङ्खौ च पीड़यन्॥
धनुर्वन्नमयेद्गात्रन्याक्षिपेन्मोहयेत्तदा।
स कृच्छ्रादुच्छ्रसेच्चापि स्तब्धाक्षोऽथ निमीलकः॥
कपोत इव कूजेच्च निःसज्ञः सोऽपतन्त्रकः।
दृष्टिं संस्तभ्य संज्ञाञ्च हत्वा कण्ठेन कूजति॥
हृदि मुक्ते नरः स्वाख्यं वाति मोहं वृते पुनः।
वायुना दारुणं प्राहुरेके तदपतानकम्॥

body may be diseased, or it may be confined to one situation. It produces episthotonos, with lameness, spasm, and cramps of the leg, with hemiplegia.

When in the *joints* it produces swellings, and pain in the joints.

When the vital air (*prān bāyu*), which is situated in the thorax, is deranged with bile, it produces vomiting with a burning sensation of the parts. When this air is mixed with phlegm it produces weakness, debility, languor, and drowsiness; and the taste for food is deranged.

Vital air in the throat (*udān bāyu*), when mixed with *bile* produces great heat in the body, swooning, fainting, and languor. When mixed with *phlegm* there is no perspiration, horripilation is felt over the body ; the person become melancholy, has little internal heat in the stomach, and the body feels cold.

Vital air in the umbilical region (*samāna bāyu*), when mixed with bile, produces much perspiration, a burning sensation of the body, fainting, and swooning. When mixed

कफान्वितो भृशं वायु स्तास्वेव यदि तिष्ठति॥
दण्डवत् स्तम्भ्येद्देहं स तु दण्डापतानकः।
धनुस्तुलां नमेद् यस्तु स धनुस्तम्भसंज्ञकः।
अङ्गुलीगुल्फजठरहृद्वक्षोगलसंश्रितः।
स्नायुः प्रतानमनिलो यदाक्षिपति वेगवान्।
विष्टव्धाक्षः स्तब्धहनुर्भग्नपार्श्वः कफं वमन्।
अभ्यन्तरं धनुरिव यदा नमति मानवम्॥
तदास्याभ्यन्तरायामं कुरुते मारुतो बली।
बाह्यस्नायु प्रतानख्यो वाह्ययामं करोति च।

with phlegm constipation of the dejections and urine, and a state of goose-skin over the surface may be remarked.

Vital air in the anus (*apāna bāyu*). When mixed with bile the body is very hot, or is only slightly warm, and the urine is bloody. When mixed with phlegm the person has a sense of heaviness in the lower part of the trunk, and the body feels cold.

Vital air over the body (*byān bāyu*), when mixed with bile the body is very hot, and there are convulsions of the extremities, with great fatigue. When mixed with phlegm the person remains stupid, and rigid, and he feels pain, and swelling of the body.

Different varieties of nervous diseases are thus supposed to be produced by the derangements of the air (*bāyu*). In *Bhābaprakāsha* eighty varieties are described. The following may be considered the most important :–

1. When air is much deranged, and passes into the different vessels of the body it produces contractions of the body. This form is called *akhyepaka*, or spasmodic convulsions.
2. When air is deranged, and rises from its situation, it produces pain in the chest, head, and temples. The

तमसाध्यं बुधाः प्राहु व्वक्षःकट्यूरुभञ्जनम्।
कफपित्तान्विते वायु र्वायुरेव च केवलः॥
कुर्य्यदाक्षेपकं त्वन्यं चतुर्थ मभिघातजम्।
गर्भपातनिमित्तश्च शोणिततिश्चवाञ्च यः।
अभिघातनिमित्तश्च न सिद्धत्यपतानकः।
गृहीतार्द्धं तनो र्वायुः शिरास्नायु विशोष्य च।
पक्षमन्यतरं हन्ति सन्धिवन्धान् विमोक्षयन्॥
कृत्स्नार्द्धकाय स्तस्य स्यादकर्म्मण्यो विचेतनः॥
एकांघरोगं तं केचि दन्ये पक्षबधं विदुः।

body and members are bent like a bow ; and it produces convulsions. The person has difficulty in breathing, the eyes are fixed and shut. The person moans, and has little sense. This form is called *apatāntraka* or rigid spasms. In this disease the body is drawn up either backwards or forwards, or to either side.

3. When the eye remains fixed, with loss of sense, the person makes a peculiar noise, the air is dislodged from the chest with relief, and is followed by weakness of the senses ; it is called *dāruna or apantānaka*.
4. When air is mixed with phlegm, and is situated in the vessels, the person is rigid like a stick, hence its name is *dandāpatānaka*.
5. When the body is bent like a bow it is called *dhanus-tambha*.
6. When the air is deranged in the fingers, ankles, belly, chest, or neck, the air contracts the nerves of these parts, and forces the body forward, accompanied with Tetanus, and vomiting of phlegm ; the eyes are fixed, and severe pain is felt in the sides ; this form is called *āmbotreama*.

सर्व्वाङ्गरोग स्तद्वच्च सर्व्वकायाश्रितऽनिले।।
दाहसन्तापमूर्च्छा। स्युर्वायौपित्तसमन्विते।
शैत्यशोथगुरुत्वानि तस्मिन्नेव कफान्विते।
शुद्धवातहतं पक्षं कृच्छ्रसाध्यतमं विदुः।
साधऽमनेऽन संयुक्त मसाध्यं क्षयहेतुकम्।।
उच्चैर्व्याहरतोऽत्यर्थं खादतः कठिनानि वा।
हसतो जृम्भतो वापि भाराद्विषमशायिनः।।
अर्द्दरत्यनिलो वक्त्र मर्द्दितं जनयत्यतः।।

7. When the air affects the veins of the back it produces *apostrotonas (bājhyā-āma) ;* this form is incurable, as the breast and back joints are broken by the violence of the symptoms. This variety of the disease is produced by external injuries, in miscarriages, and great hemorrhages.

8. *Pakshyāghāta* (paralysis, *hemiplegia*). There are two varieties of this disease, one affecting one side of the body, and another affecting one half of the body taken transversely. When air affects the vessels and nerves of one side, it produces this disease ; when the person loses the power of that part, which is without feeling, and with looseness of the joints. When deranged air alone produces *hemiplegia*, the disease will be cured with difficulty. When air and bile, or air and phlegm produce this disease it may be cured ; but when there is great weakness of the essential parts of the body, as after hemorrhagia in parturition or injuries, the disease is incurable.

9. When all the body is palsied it is called *sarbānga-rog*. When air and bile are both deranged, it produces great heat of the body, and fainting. When air is deranged with phlegm, the body is cold, is swelled, and heavy.

वक्रीभवति वक्त्रार्द्धं ग्रीवा चाप्यपवर्त्तते॥
शिरश्चलति वाक् सङ्गो नेत्रादीनाञ्च वैकृतम्॥
ग्रीवाचिवुकदन्तानां यस्मिन् पार्श्वे च वेदना॥
तमर्द्दितमिति प्राहु र्व्याधिं व्याधिविचक्षणाः।
क्षीणस्यनिमिषाक्षस्य प्रसक्ताव्यक्तभाषिणः।
न सिद्धत्यर्द्दितं नाढ त्रिवर्षं वेपनस्य च॥
गति वेगे भवेत् स्वास्थ्यं सव्विेष्वाक्षेपकादिषु॥
जिह्वानिर्लेखुनाच्छष्कभक्षणपादभिघाततः।
कुपितो हनुमूलस्थः, श्रंसयित्वानिलो हनुः॥

10. Arddata, or hanustambha, (Tetanus and Trismus ?) When the air is deranged by a person speaking very loud, or by eating large mouthfuls of meat, or hard things, or laughing much, or gaping or sleeping uncomfortably, or bearing heavy weights, it affects the lower jaw of half the face and neck, which it draws laterally, and the head shakes. The person cannot speak, there is a deformity of the eye, nose, mouth, and neck, with pain in these parts, as also in the chin and teeth, and senses are in an unhealthy state. The dangerous symptoms of this disease are when the person is weak, the pain severe, and he cannot move his eyelids, nor speak distinctly ; when the mouth is turned to one side, and with the shaking of the part of the body, as the head, has continued for three or more years. In all these spasmodic diseases the symptoms for a time disappear, and again recur.

11. Sometimes while cleaning the tongue with the tongue scraper, when eating dry and hard food, or by external injury, the air is deranged in the joints of the jaw, and are sometimes dislocated, when the mouth remains open. In other cases the jaw is locked, when the patient is unable to speak or eat.

करोति विवृतास्यत्वमथवा संवृतास्यताम्।
हनुग्रहः स तेन स्यात् कृच्छ्रच्चर्व्वणभाषणम्॥
दिवा स्वप्नासमख्यान विब्रृतोर्द्धंनिरीक्षणैः।
मन्यास्तम्भं प्रकुरुते स एव श्लेष्मणावृतः॥
वाग्वाहिनीशिरासंख्यो जिह्वां स्तम्भयतेऽनिलः।
जिह्वास्तम्भः स तेनान्त्रप्रानवाक्येप्वनीशता।
रक्तमाश्रित्य पवनः कुर्व्यन्मूर्द्धधराः शिराः।
रुक्षाः सवेदनाः कृष्णाः सोऽसाध्यः स्यात् शिरोग्रहः।

12. When sleeping in the day time, especially in an unnatural attitude, or when regarding intensely an object above the person, *air* may be so deranged, and mixed with phlegm as to produce the stiffness of the neck, which remains straight and rigid. This is called *manyāstambha*.

13. When the air affects the nerve of the tongue, it becomes rigid and immoveable, and person cannot speak, eat, or drink. This disease is named *jihwāstambha*.

14. When air enters the blood-vessels of the head, the vessels becomes dry, black, and painful, producing head-ache or the disease called *shirograha*.

15. When air attacks the buttocks, back, loins, hip, thigh, knees, legs, and feet, it produces pain in these parts ; passes from one to the other, often without the pain being properly defined. In other cases the affected parts shake ; sometimes when air is mixed with phlegm it produces heaviness of the part, dyspepsia and drowsiness. This variety is called *gridhrasi*.

16. Bishwāchī. When air affects the tendons of the back of the hand and arm, it produces this disease, in which there is no motion in the hand or arm.

स्फिक्पूर्व्वा कटिपृष्टोरु जानुजं घापदं क्रमात्।
गृध्रसी स्तम्भरूक तोदैगृह्णाति स्मन्दते मुहुः।
वाताद्वातकफात्तन्द्रा गौरवारोचकान्विता।
तलं प्रत्यङ्गुलीनां या कण्डरा बाहुपृष्ठतः।
वाह्वो कर्मभक्षयकरी विश्वची चेति सोच्यते॥
वातशोणितजः शोथी जानुमध्ये महारुजः।
ज्ञेयः क्रोष्टुकशीर्षस्तु स्थूलः क्रोष्टुक शीर्षवत्।
वायुः कट्याश्रितः रुक्थ्रः कण्डरामाक्षिपेद् यदा।
खञ्जस्तदा भवेज्जन्तुः पङ्गु सक्थ्रोद्वयीर्वधात्।
प्रक्रामन् वेपते यस्तु खञ्जन्निव च गच्छति॥

17. When air and blood are changed in a part, it swells with severe pain. In this manner the knee-joint may be affected, and become large, like a jackal's head. This disease is called *kustakashirsha*.

18. When air is deranged in the sides of the thighs, it draws the tendons of these parts, which contract, and person walks feebly. This disease is called *khanja*.

19. If both sides are affected the person cannot walk, this disease is called *pangu*.

20. When in walking the person limps, his body shakes, or as if the person was walking over *kālai,* a kind of pea, and is feeble, it is called *kalāskhanja* (chorea sanctir viti).[1] in this disease the parts seem as if loosened from their natural binding. The disease is characterized by the person feeling in the commencement a trembling or shivering sensation through his body, accompanied with a dimness of sight, and a pain in the neck, jaw, or teeth, or of the part affected. These symptoms are followed by involuntary twitching of the head, neck, and jaw often of one side, especially of one leg. The patient speaks indistinctly, and then

कलायखञ्जं तं विद्यात् मुक्तसन्धिप्रबन्धनम्॥
रुक् पादे विषमन्यस्ते श्रमाद्वा जायते यदा।
वातेन गुल्फमाश्रित्य तामहुर्वातकण्ठकम्।
पादयोः कुरुते दाहं पित्तसृक्सहितोऽनिलः॥
विशेषश्चंक्रमतः पाददाहं तमादिशेत्॥
हृष्येते चरणौ यस्य भवेताञ्चापि सुप्तकौ।
पादहर्षः स विज्ञेय कफवातप्रकोपतः॥

the involuntary motions extend to the whole voluntary muscles of progression, producing a dancing motion. When the disease extends over the body, and has continued long, it is considered incurable. Its existing cause is considered to be irregularity in the bowels from eating indigestable food, too much walking or laughing, carrying great loads etc.

21. When the ankle joint is strained in walking it produces pain in the ankle with stiffness, it is called *bāta-kantaka*. The pain resembling that of a thorn piercing the flesh.

22. Air, bile, and blood accumulated in the feet produce a burning sensation of the part, particularly when the person is walking, it is called *pādadāha*. This is one of the most distressing and intractable diseases peculiar to this country. It is called "Fever in the feet."

23. When *phlegm* and *air* are deranged in the two feet they become cold, with insensibility, as when sitting very long in a particular position, when the leg feels dead with a disagreeable numb feeling. It is called *pādaharsha* (foot numbness) ; and is a frequent complaint among us, from our sitting on the ground, in often constrained positions.

24. When air is deranged in the shoulder-joint, it dries the ligaments and tendons of the part. They are

अंशदेश-ख्यितो वायुः शेषयेदंसवन्धनम्।
शिराश्चाङ्क्य तत्रस्थो जनयेदववाहुकम्॥
आवृत्य वायुः सकफो धमनीः शब्दवाहिनीः॥
नरान् करोत्यक्रियकान् मूकमिन्मिणगद्गदान्।
अधो या वेदना याति वर्च्चोमूंत्राशयोत्थिता।
भिन्दन्तीव गुदोपस्थं सा तूनी नाम नामतः॥
गुदोपस्थोत्थिता या तु प्रतिलोमं प्रधाविता॥
वेगैः पक्काशयंयाति प्रतीतूनीति सोच्यते।
साटोपभत्युग्ररुज माध्मातमुदरं भृशम्।
आध्मानमिति तं विद्याद्धोरं वातनिरोधजम्।

contracted, and the arm becomes fixed. It is called *apabāhuka,* or stiff arm.

25. When the air is mixed with phlegm, and enters into the air-vessels (*dhamani*) the person cannot speak, or speaks slowly, and indistinctly. This disease is called *mūka* (dumbness), and *minmina and gadgada* (indistinct speech).

26. When pain commences from the bowels and bladder, and passes to the anus and urinary passages, producing great pain in these parts, which feel as if torn asunder, the disease is called *tunie*..

27. When it commences from the anus and urinary passages, and passes up to the intestines with great violence, it is called *pratunie*

28. Swelling and pain, with a rumbling noise of the abdomen, produced by the air being confined in the abdomen, is called *ādhyāna,* or drumb-belly.

29. When the swelling is confined to the stomach with pain and noise, it is called *pratyādhyāna* ; and is produced by the air being mixed with phlegm.

विमुक्तपार्श्वहृदयं तदेवामाशयोत्थितम्।
प्रत्याध्मानं विजानीयात् कफव्याकुलितानिलम्।।
नाभेरधप्तात् संजातः सञ्चारी यदि वा चलः।।
अष्ठोलावद्वनग्रन्थिरुर्द्धमायतः उन्नतः।
वाताष्ठीलां विजानीयाद् वहिर्मार्गावरोधिनीं
एतामेव रुजोयेतां वातविन्मूत्ररोधिनीम्।।
प्रत्यष्ठीलामिति वदेज्जठरे तिर्य्यगुत्थिताम्।
मारुतेऽविगुणे वस्तौ मूत्रं सम्यक् प्रवर्त्तते।
विकारा विविधा श्चात्र प्रतिलोमे भवन्ति च।।
सार्व्वङ्गकम्पः शिरसो वायुर्वेपथुसंज्ञकः।

30. When a hard oblong swelling is felt under the navel, which passes from one part to another, or rests stationary, and becomes prominent, and air, urine, and dejections are constipated, it is called *ashthilā* or *bātashthilā*.

31. When the hard swelling is longitudinal, and is accompanied with much pain, and the urine and dejections are constipated, it is called *pratashthilā*. These derangements of air produce diseases in variour situations ; when deranged in the bladder, it causes the stoppage of urine, etc.

32. When air is deranged in the head, it is always shaking. The disease is called *bapati*.

33. When air is affected in the feet, legs, thighs, and wrist, it produces spasm and is called *kuli*. The other diseases of air are named according to the part particularly affected. In all these nervous diseases it is of importance that the Physician observe whether the symptoms of bile and phlegm, etc. are present, as they will affect his prognosis, and treatment. In *hanu-graha* (lock-jaw), *ardito* (or paralysis of the face),

खल्वो तु पादजंघोरुकरमूलावमोटनी।
ख्याननामानुरूपैश्च लिङ्गैः शेषान् विनिर्दिशेत्।
सर्व्वेष्वेतुषे संसर्गं पित्ताद्यैरुपलक्षयेत्।
हनुस्तश्नार्द्दिताक्षेपपक्षाघातापतानका।
कालेन महताठ्याना यत्नात् सिध्यन्ति वा न वा।
नवान् बलवतस्त्वेतान् साधयेन्निरूपद्रवान्।
विसर्पदाहरुक्सङ्घमूर्च्छारुच्याग्निमार्द्दबैः।
क्षीणमांसबलं वाता घ्नन्ति पक्षबधादयः॥
शूनं सुप्त त्वच्चं भग्नं कम्पाध्मानपीड़ितम्॥
रुजार्त्तिमन्तञ्च नरं वातव्याधि र्विनाशयेत्॥
अव्याहतगतिर्यस्य ख्यानस्थः प्रकृर्तिख्यितः।
वायुः स्यात् सोऽधिकं जीवेद्वीतवरोगः समाशतम्॥

> *akhepokā* (spasmodic diseases), *pakhyāghāta* (hemiplegia), *apatānaka (*epilepsy), our prognosis may be rather favourable, when the person is strong, the disease is recent, and is not accompanied with any bad symptoms. This is particularly the case when the patient is rich, as the treatment will generally be tedious.

The unfavourable symptoms are when the disease is accompanied with erysipelas (*bisarpa*), or with severe burning sensations, with great heat and pain, as if the body was torn, and with constipation, fainting, and loss of appetite, or when the digestion is very weak. In such cases the patient will die. This disease is also dangerous when the person is swollen, when the parts are without feeling, and are accompanied with flatulency and shaking of the body, with great pain and weakness.

Should the air not be deranged, and be confined to its usual situation, the person will live for a hundred years free from disease.

वातरक्तनिदानम्

लवणाम्लकटुक्षारस्निग्धोष्णजीर्णभोजनैः।
क्लिन्नशुष्काम्बूजानूपमांसपिण्याकमूलकैः॥
कुलत्थमाषनिष्पावशाकादिपललेक्षुभिः॥
दध्यारनालसौ वीर शुक्ततक्रसुरासवैः।
विरुद्धाध्यशनक्रोध दिवास्वप्नप्रजागरैः।
प्रायशः सुकुमाराणां मिथ्याहारविहारिणम्।
स्त्यूलानां सखिनाञ्चापि कुप्यते वातशोणितम्।
हस्त्यश्वोष्ट्रै गच्छतश्चाश्नतश्च विदाह्यन्नं सविदाहोऽशनस्य।
कृतस्नं रक्तं विदहत्त्वाशु तच्च दुष्टं स्त्रुतं पादयोश्चीयते तु।

A KIND OF LEPROSY[2] (*Bāta-rakta)*

This disease is produced by the blood being diseased with air (*bayu*). Its exciting causes are using sour food, and alkaline salts. In like manner spices, or other hot articles, indigestable articles of food, putrified, or drymeats, as the flesh or crocodiles, of the buffalo, of the rhinoceros, or the like. Til oil-cake, and other indigestable articles of food, curdled or butter-milk, bad wines, and excess in eating and drinking, the passions, unhealthy and improper mixtures of food, eating too often, or sleeping during the day produce this disease. Delicate constitutions, and fat people, who lead a sedentary life are predisposed to this disease. Long continued riding on horses, elephants, or camels, and whatever produces great heat of the body; by these causes the blood is diseased, and is conveyed by the air to the feet, where it accumulates, and produces this disease, first in the feet, and then in other parts of the body. *Bāta-rakta* is ushered in sometimes by free, at other times by a cessation of perspirations; the body becomes of a dark hue, and parts have no feeling. If there are sores they are very painful; the joints are loose, the person feels languid, and cannot work; and small pimples appear over the body, with pain of a gnawing or

तत्संपृक्तं वायुना दूषितेन तत्प्रावल्यदुच्यते वातरक्तम्॥
स्वेदोत्यर्थं वा कार्ष्णं स्पर्शज्ञत्वं क्षतेऽतिरुक्।
सन्धिशैंशिल्यमालस्यं सदनं पिड़कोद्गमः॥
जानुजङ्घोरुकट्यंस हस्तपादाङ्ग–सन्धिषु।
निस्तोदः स्फुरणं भेदो गुरुत्वं सुप्तिरेव च।
कण्डूः सन्धिषु रुग् भूत्वा भूत्वा नश्यति चासकृत्।
वैवर्णं मण्डलोत्पत्ति र्वातासृक् पूर्व्वलक्षणम्॥
वातेऽधिकेऽधिकं तत्र शूलस्फुरणभञ्जनम्।
शोथस्य रौक्षं कृष्णत्वं श्यावता।
बृद्धिहानयः धामन्यङ्गुलिसन्धीनां सङ्लोचोऽङ्गग्रहोऽतिरुक्॥
शीतद्देषानुपशयौ स्तम्भवेपथुसुप्तयः॥
रक्ते शोथोऽतिरुक् तोद स्ताभ्रश्चिमिचिमायते॥

lancinating kind, as if ants were eating the flesh, or needles thrust into the skin. The knees, legs, thighs, loins, shoulders, hands, and arms, are so affected. The pain intermits, and these parts become heavy, without feeling, and the skin has patches of an unusual colour.

When *air* is much deranged there is severe pain of the body, as if ants were eating the flesh, and the vessles, nails, fingers, and joints are contracted. The patient has no appetite, and if not treated the symptoms increase. The person cannot work, and the body shakes, with rigidity of the joints.

When *blood* is much deranged swelling appears over the body, with much pain. The skin is of copperish colour with slight stinging pain (*chin chin*).

When *bile* is deranged the body feels hot, with a burning, sensation, and dullness of intellect. He perspires much, has fainting fits, with an appearance of drunkenness and thirst; pressure of the part produces great pain, with redness, heat, swelling, and sometimes abscesses are formed.

When *phlegm* is deranged the body is very cold, as if a cold wet cloth was applied over the body, which feels heavy,

स्निग्धरुक्षैः शमं नैति कण्डूक्लेदसमन्वितः॥
पित्ते विदाहः सम्मोहः स्वेदो मूर्च्छा मदस्तृषा।
स्पर्शासहत्वं रुग्रागः शोथः पाको भृशोष्मता।
कफे स्त्यैस्त्यैमित्यगुरुता सुप्तिस्निग्धत्वं शीततां।
कण्डू मंन्दा च रुग्द्वन्दं सर्व्वलिङ्गञ्च सङ्करात्।
पादयोर्मलमाख्याय कदाचिद्धस्तयोरपि॥
आखोर्विषमिव क्रुद्धं तद्देमहुपसर्पति॥
आजानु स्फुटितं यच्च प्रभिन्नं प्रस्रु तञ्च यत्।
उपद्रवैश्च यज्जुष्टं प्राणमांसक्षयादिभिः॥
वातरक्तमसाध्यं स्यात्याप्यं संवत्सरोत्थितम्।
अस्वप्नरोचकश्वास मांसकोथशिरोग्रहाः।

and without feeling. The skin is smooth, shining and itchy, and feels cold, with slight pain.

When two or three of the above humours are affected the symptoms resemble the two or three forms, as above enumerated.

In some cases the ankles and wrists are first affected, and then it extends over the body like the poison of certain animals.

The disease is incurable, when accompanied with a sore from the ankle to the knee, or when it is opened and pus escapes in large quantities. When the person is very weak and reduced the disease will be fatal ; but if the person lives for a year, or it is chronic, he will live. When the disease is severe the person cannot obtain sleep, has no appetite, has a difficulty in breathing, parts of the body slough, he complains of headache, fainting, delirium, pain in the body, thirst, fever, has no sense, with shaking, hiccough, contraction of the fingers and toes, so that he cannot walk nor work, and erysipelas appears with vascular eruptions. Severe pain is felt in the vital parts, tumours appear over the body, want of memory, fatigue, and delirium follow, and precede death. When all the symptoms of

मूर्च्छातिमदरूक्तृष्णा ज्वरमोह प्रवेपकाः॥
हिक्कापांगुल्य वीसर्पपाकतोदभ्रमक्लमाः॥
अङ्गलीवक्रतास्फोटदाहमर्म्माग्रहार्बुदाः।
एतै रूपद्रवैवर्ज्जं मोहेनैकेन वापि यत्।
अकृस्नोपद्रवं याप्यं साध्यं स्यन्निरुपद्रवम्।
एकदोषनुगं साध्यं नवं याप्यं द्विदोषजम्।
त्रिदोषजमसाध्यं स्यात् यस्य च स्युरुपद्रवाः॥

ओरुस्तम्भनिदानम्

शीतोष्णद्रवसंशुष्कगुरुश्निग्धैर्निषेवितैः।
जीर्णाजीर्णे तथायास संक्षोभस्वप्रजागकैः॥
स श्लेष्ममेंदःपवनः साममत्यर्थसञ्चितम्॥
अभिभूयेतरं दोषमूत्र चेत् प्रतिपद्यते।

this severe form of the disease are not present, the disease may not be fatal. If none of the severe symptoms are present, the disease may be cured. When only one of the humours is deranged ; as air, bile, etc., and the disease is recent, it may be cured ; but, if two of the humours are deranged, the disease will remain, when three are affected the disease is incurable, and when all the severe symptoms are present the disease will be fatal.

DISEASES OF THE EXTREMITIES

The diseases of the upper extremities are few, and of little importance, compared to those of the lower extremities ; to which the following remarks are principally confined. These diseases are *Urustambha* and *Slipada*, or swellings of the extremities, diseases of the nails, of the soles of the feet, and ulcers of the axilla, and groin. The other diseases of the extremities have been already considered under those *Bāta-byadhi*.

सक्थ्यस्थिनी प्रपूर्य्यान्तः श्लेष्मणा स्तिमितेन च।
तदा स्तंभाति तेनोरू स्त्रब्धौ शीतावचेतनौ।
परकीयाविव गुरु स्यातामतिभृशव्यघौ।
ध्यानाङ्गमर्द्द स्तैमित्य तन्द्रा छर्दऽरुचि ज्वरैः।
संयुक्तौ पादसदनकृच्छ्रोद्धरणसुप्तिभिः।
तमुरुस्तम्भमित्याहुराढ्यवातमथापरे॥
प्राग् रूपं तस्य निद्रातिध्यानं स्तिमितता ज्वरः।
रोमहर्षोऽरुचिच्छर्द्दिर्जङ्घोरूः सदनं तथा॥
वातशङ्किभिज्ञानात्तस्य स्यात् स्नेहनात् पुनः।
पादयोः सदनं सूप्तिः कृच्छ्रादुद्धरणां तथा॥
जङ्घोरुग्लानिरत्यर्थं शश्यच्चादाह्ववेदने।
पादञ्च व्यथते न्यस्तं शीतष्मर्से न वेत्ति च।
संस्थाने पीड़ने गत्यां चालने चाप्यनीश्वरः।
अन्यनेयौ हि संभग्नाबरू पादौ च मन्यते॥

Urustambha (large abscess). These are produced under the fascia of the thigh by cold, hot, or very liquid or dry food, heavy oleaginous or indigestable food, or other articles of the like kind, fatigue, grief, agitation, sleeping during the day, and watching at night. By these means the air, phlegm, and fat are deranged and mixed with bile, which accumalates in the thighs, and in the external parts of the thigh-bone. The thigh then becomes senseless like a dead part, and is very painful.

This disease produces lowness of spirits, pain over the body, drowsiness, and chilliness, cold, vomiting, loss of appetite and fever. The thigh cannot be moved, and it is raised with difficulty, and as if asleep. Other parctitioners call the disease *Adabāta*.

Before the accumulation of humours in the thigh, the person feels sleepy, is in low spirits, the body cold, with fever, loss of appetite and vomiting. Both legs and thighs are heavy and weak. When the pain is supposed to be rheumatic, and the part is rubbed with oleaginous medicines, the disease increases, affects the feet and prevents the person walking ; and is accompanied with much pain, swelling, and inflammation, followed by

यदा दाहार्त्तितोदर्त्तो वेपनः फुरुषो भवेत्।
उरूस्तन्ध स्तदा हन्यात् साधयेदन्यथा नवम्॥

अमवातनिदानम्

विरुद्धाहारचेष्टस्य मन्दाग्नेर्निश्चलस्य च।
स्निग्धं भुक्तवतोऽह्यन्न व्यायामं कुर्व्वतस्तथा।
वायुना प्ररितो ह्यामः श्लेष्मस्थानं प्रधावति।
तेनत्यर्थे विदग्धोऽसौ धमनीः प्रतिपद्यते॥
वातपित्तकफैर्भूयो दूषितः सोऽन्नजो रसः।
स्त्रोतांस्यभिष्यन्दयति नानावर्णोऽतिपिच्छलः॥
जनयत्याशु दौर्व्वलं गौरवं हृदयस्य च।
व्याधीनामाश्रयो क्ष्येष आमसंज्ञेति दारुणः॥
युगपत् कुपितावन्तस्त्रिकसन्धिप्रवेशकौ।

insensibility, and the leg feels as if it was broken. When there is much lancinating pain, inflammation, and shivering, the patient will die. When these symptoms are absent, or the disease is recent, the patient may be cured by the practitioner, as the disease under this circumstance is not always fatal.

ACUTE RHEUMATISM (*Ambāt)*

This disease is produced in dyspeptic patients who lead a sedentary life, taking improper food, or are intemperate. All indigestable food has this effect ; such as oleaginous articles, particularly when the person, at the same time, takes much exercise. By such causes the chyle is not properly prepared, and indigested food (*Am*) is formed in the stomach. This *Am* is carried into the great abdominal vessels. The deranged chyle produced in this manner, by the morbid condition of air, bile, or phlegm is like mucilage, and deranges all the abdomen. This (*Amras*) morbid chyle is the cause of all the varieties of this disease. The deranged phlegm and air are accumulated in the loins producing pain and rigidity of the body, and hence it

स्तब्धं वा कुरुते गात्र मामवातः स उच्यते।
अङ्गमर्द्दोऽरुचिस्तृष्णा चालस्यं गौरवं ज्वरः।
अपाकशूनताङ्गना मामवातस्य लक्षणम्।
स कष्टः सर्व्वरोगाणां यदा प्रकुपितो भवेत्॥
हस्तपादशिरोगुलफ-त्रिकजानुरुसन्धिषु।
करोति सरुजं शोथं यत्र दोषः प्रपद्यते॥
स देशो रुजाज्यतेत्यर्थं व्याविद्ध इव वृश्चिकैः।
जनयेत् सोऽग्निदौर्व्वल्यं प्रसेकारुचिगौरवम्।
उत्साहहानिं वैरस्यं दाहञ्च बहुमूत्रताम्।
कुक्षौ कठिनतां शूलं तथा विद्राविपर्ज्जयम्॥
तृट्छर्द्दिभ्रममूर्च्छांश्च हृद्ग्रहं विद्विवन्धताम्।
जाड्यान्तकुजमानां कष्टांश्चान्यानुपद्रवान्॥
पित्तात् सदाहरागञ्च सशूलं पवनानुगम्।

is called *Ambāt,* (air, mixed with morbid chyle.) From the loins it extends over all the body.

The general symptoms are pain over the body, loss of appetite, thirst, want of appetite, languor, heaviness, fever, and there is a deadened sensation of the parts. When this disease is in such an aggravated form, it is most difficult to cure.

When the deranged phlegm and air with the morbid chyle passes to the wrist, ankle, neck, hip, knee, loins, it produces a burning sensation, much pain, like the bite of the centipede, with swelling. The person feels great lassitude with a copious flow of urine ; he cannot sleep, and complains of pain in the abdomen, and is distressed with thirst, vomiting, giddiness, fainting, pain in the chest, costiveness, etc.

When bile is much deranged in this disease there is a burning sensation and redness of the parts ; and when air is principally deranged, the pain is very severe. When phlegm is much deranged, the itching and rigidity of the part is consider-

स्तिमितं गुरुकण्डञ्च कफदुष्टं तमादिशेत्॥
एकदोषानुगः साध्यो द्विदोषो याप्य उच्यते।
सर्व्वदेहचरः शोथः सकृच्छ्रः सान्निपातिकः॥

शूलपरिनामशूलान्नद्रवशूलनिदानम्

दोषैः पृथक् समस्तामद्वन्दैः शूलोऽष्टधा भवेत्।
सर्व्वेष्वेतेषु शूलेषु प्रायेण पवनः प्रभुः॥
व्यायामयानादतिमैथुनाच्च प्रजागरात् शीतजलातिपानात्।
कलाय मुद्गाढ़किकोरदूषादत्यर्थ रुक्षाध्यशनाभिघातात्॥
कषाय-तिक्तातिविरूढ़जान्न विरुङ्वल्लुरकशुष्कशाकात्।
विट्शुक्रमूत्रानिलवेगरोधात् शोकोपवासादतिहास्यभाष्यात्॥
वायुः प्रवृद्धो जनयेद्धि शूलं हृतपार्श्वपृष्ठ त्रिकवस्तिदेशे।
जीर्णे प्रदोषे च घनागमे च शीते च कोपं समुपैति गाढ़म्॥

able, and it feels as if it was covered with a wet cloth. When one humour is alone affected, it is curable, when two it is difficult to cure, and when three, and the whole body is affected the cure if very difficult, tedious, and the disease is even fatal in some cases.

GASTROPERIODYNIA *(Sul, Colic)*

This disease is called *Sul*, from the pain resembling that produced by piercing the abdomen with the deadly *Trisula* or three-pointed instrument in the hands of *Shiva,* the destroying power of the Triad, and it is said to be sometimes so incurable that even *Shiva* himself cannot remove it. It frequently happens that the individual, in despair of being cured, commits suicide, as the only means left of relieving himself, and of propitiating the anger of the deity. Such fancies have a pernicious effect upon the progress of medical knowledge, for instead of endeavouring to discover the cause and nature of the disease, and the means of alleviating the sufferings of the afflicted, the practitioner finds a ready excuse for his indifference and ignorance in what he declares to be the will of God.

मुहुर्मुहुश्चोपशम-प्रकोपौ विड्वातसंस्तम्भन तोदभेदैः।
संस्तेदनाभ्यञ्जनमर्द्दनाद्यैः स्निग्धोष्णभोज्यैश्च समंप्रयाति।।
क्षीराततितीक्ष्णोष्णाविदाहि-तैल-निष्पावपिण्याककुलत्थयुषैः।
कट्वम्लसौवीर-सुराविकारैः क्रोधानलायासरविप्रतापैः।।
ग्राम्यातियोगादर्शनैर्विदग्धैः पित्तं प्रकुप्याशु करोति शूलम्।
तृण्मोहदाहार्त्तिकरं हि नाभ्यां संस्वेदमूर्च्छाभ्रम-चोषयुक्तम्।।
मध्यन्दिने कुप्यति चार्द्धरात्रे विदाहकाले जलदात्यये च।
शीते च शीतैः समुपैति शान्तिं सुस्वादुशीतैरपि भोजनैश्च।।

There are eight varieties of *Sul*, produced by derangement of air, bile, and phlegm ; by two being deranged together ; by the three being deranged together, and the last form is by indigestion. In all these forms, however, air is more or less deranged.

1. The causes of Air Colic (*Bāyu-Sul*) are violent exercise, as fighting, riding, frequent intercourse with women, watching at night, drinking too much cold water, eating peas (especially *Kalāi, Mudga, Araki*), dry food, as dry flesh, vegetables, and fish, overeating, or eating too often; injuries, and bitter or astringent food. When rice is eaten, and other grain that have vegetated, or an improper mixture of food is taken, as milk and flesh, etc., or when the calls of nature are not attended to, and the semen, urine, air, faeces are constipated ; or by grief, fasting, much and loud laughing or speaking, they produce *Sul* by deranging the air. When air is so deranged the accession of pain occurs at intervals when the person drinks cold water on an empty stomach, when the food has been digested, towards the evening in the rainy reason, when the sky is overcast, and during the winter months.

   The pain is in the chest, sides of the abdomen, back, in the joining of the lumbar vertebrae with the *os coccygis*, and in the pelvic region. It is accompanied

आनुपवारिजकिलाट-पयोविकारै
मांसेक्षुन्यिकृशरातिलशङ्कुलीभिः।
अन्यैर्वलासजनकैरपि हेतुभिश्च
श्लेष्मा प्रकोपमुपगम्य करोति शूलम्॥
हल्लासकास-सदनारुचि-सम्प्रसेकै
रामाशये स्तिमितकोष्ठ-शिरोगुरुत्वैः।
भुक्ते सदैव हि रुजं कुरुतेऽतिमात्रं
सूर्य्योदयेऽथ शिशिरे कुसुमागमे च॥

with difficulty in breathing, rigidity of the body, and scanty evacuations.

2. When deranged bile produces this disease, it is caused by eating nitre or heating salts of the same kind, hot food like white mustard-seed, pepper, or the like ; different kinds of wines, roasted articles or oils, or shoots of the young bamboo, or oil cake, sour or bitter articles ; great anger, remaining near the fire, exposure to the sun, great fatigue, excess in venery, or any thing that is very heating is to be carefully avoided. These different causes derange bile, and produce that form of *Sul* when it felt in the umbiliacus. In this case it produces thirst, his senses are dull, body hot, with great grief, and severe pain in the umbiliacus. He perspires much, and he is giddy and sometimes faints, with dryness of the mouth, is eager to remain in a cold situation, and to take cold articles of food. Accessions of pain occur at noon and midnight, during great heat of the weather, and at the beginning of the rains. The pain is diminished during the cold hours of the day, when the body is cool ; and when cold or bitter things are taken, especially when they feel grateful they mitigate the symptoms.

3. When deranged phlegm produces *Sul*, it is caused by eating the flesh of the rhinoceros or buffalo, fish or

सर्व्वेषु दोषेषु च सर्व्वलिङ्गं विद्याद्भिषक् सर्व्वभवं हि शूलम्।
सुकष्टमेनं विशवज्रकल्पं विवर्ज्जनीयं प्रवदन्ति तज्ज्ञाः॥
आटोपहृल्लास-वमीगुरुत्व-स्तैमित्य-मानाह-कफप्रसेकैः।
कफस्य लिङ्गेन समानलिङ्ग माभोद्भवं शूलमुदाहरन्ति॥
वस्तौ हृत्पार्श्वपृष्ठेषु सशूलः कफवातिकः
कुक्षौहृन्नाभिमध्येषु सशूलः कफपैत्तिकः।
दाहज्वरकरो घोरो विज्ञेयो वातपैत्तिकः॥
एकदोषोत्थितः साध्यः कृच्छ्रसाध्यो द्विदोषजः।

any kind of food obtained from water, whey, milk, or butter-milk ; or sugarcandy, rice cakes, or sesamum-seed, oil, rice, and other articles of food which are of a cooling or heavy nature, as *Māskalāi*. All these articles increase phlegm, and thus may produce *Sul*. In these cases the patient complains of nausea, cough, languor, and want of appetite, phlegm proceeds from his nose and mouth, the pit of the stomach is cold, and his body is very heavy with head-ache. In such cases after eating great pain occurs, especially at sun-rise, and during the spring or dew months. (*Sishira.*)

4. When air, bile and phlegm are deranged together the symptoms of the three above forms are combined in one person. When so deranged in one spot a physician will know it by examining the part. This form gives much distress, like poison or thunder, and such a person should be avoided by the physician as incurable.
5. When *Sul* is produced by indigestion the symptoms are the same as produced by deranged phlegm. There is a rumbling noise heard in the abdomen, nausea and vomiting, the body feels heavy and cold, as if covered with a wet cloth, and the breathing is difficult. The person can get neither appetite not sleep, he is costive with severe pain in the abdomen, and there is a discharge of phlegm, from the nose, mouth, etc.

सर्व्वदोषोत्थितो घोरस्त्वसाध्यो भूर्युपद्रवः॥
स्वैर्निदानैः प्रकुपितो वायुः सन्निहितस्तदा।
कफपित्ते समावृत्य शूलकारी भवेद्बली॥
भुक्ते जीर्य्याति यच्छलं तदेव परिणामजम्।
तस्य लक्षणमप्येतत् समासेना भिधीयते॥
आध्मानाटोपविष्मूत्र-विवन्धारतिवेपनैः।
स्निग्धष्णोपशमप्रायं वातिकं तद्वदेडिषक्॥
तृष्णादाहारतिस्वेदं कट्वम्ललवणेद्भवम्।
शूलं शीतशमप्रायं पैत्तिकं लक्षयेद्बुधः॥
छर्द्दिहृल्लससन्मोहं स्वल्परुग्दीर्धसन्तति॥

In order to distinguish the different forms of *Sul* the practitioner should know that air is chiefly affected when the pain is principally confined to the pelvic region. When bile is much deranged, the pain is principally felt in the umbiliacal region ; and when phlegm is deranged it produces pain in the breast, sides of the abdomen, and in the scrobiculus cordis. When air, bile, and phlegm and deranged the pain is felt in all the above situations. When phlegm and air are deranged there is severe pain in the pelvic region, sides of the abdomen, and back. When bile and phlegm are deranged the pain is in the scrobiculus cordis, and between the chest and the umbiliacus. When air and bile are deranged there is great heat of the body, and inflammatory fever. *Sul* may be cured when it is produced by either air, bile, or phlegm, being deranged singly. When two are diseased, with difficulty ; but when all the three are deranged at the same time it is incurable. In *Sul* some other forms of disease may accompany and complicate it ; such as severe pain, thirst fainting fits, spasm of the intestines with costiveness, the body is heavy and there is no appetite, with cough, asthma, and hiccough. Other *shāstras* enumerate the following symptoms, severe pain in the abdomen, vomiting, fever, thirst, and the body seems to swim round. When the person becomes thin, and has no strength, he will not recover.

कटुतिक्तोपशान्तौ चं तच्च ज्ञेयं कफात्मकम्॥
संसृष्टलक्षणं बुद्धवा द्विदोषं परिकल्पयेत्।
त्रिदोषज मसाध्यन्तु क्षीणमांसबलानलम्॥
जीर्णे जीर्य्यत्यजीर्णे वा यच्छूल मुपजायते।
पथ्यापथ्यप्रथोगेण भोजनाभोजनेन च॥
न शमं याति नियमात् सोऽन्नद्रव उदाहृतः।
अन्नद्रवावख्यशूलेषु न तावत् स्वास्थ्यमश्नुते॥
वान्तमात्रे जरत् पित्तं शूलमाशु व्यपोहति॥

अदावर्त्तनाहनिदानम्

वातविन्मूत्रजृम्भाश्रुक्षवोद्गरवमीन्द्रियः।

6. *Parinām Sul*[3] is the variety produced during the digestion of food. When air is deranged by the usual causes it affects also bile and phlegm., and *Sul* is the consequence. After eating, when degestion has taken place, severe fever occurs. The symptoms of this variety are, when air is deranged, the abdomen swells, a gurgling noise is heard in the abdomen, the dejections and urine are constipated, with lassitude and shivering. Bile, when much deranged in this form of *Sul*, produces thirst, heat, restlessness, and copious perspirations ; and when sour, pungent, or salt things are eaten the pain is increased, and when cold food is eaten they give relief. When phlegm is much deranged there is vomiting, nausea and dulness of the intellect, with pain, not severe, but remains many hours. When two of these are deranged the respective symptoms are combined, and when three are deranged the person will die. When such a person's flesh, strength and internal fire are much diminished the disease will be fatal.

RETENTION OF DISCHARGES (*Adābarta*)

If a man wish long life he should attend to the calls of nature, while he avoids indulgence of the passions, particularly anger, pride, lust, revenge, and covetousness.

क्षुत्तृष्णीच्छासन्द्रिणां धृत्योदावर्त्तसम्भवः॥
वातमूत्रपुरीषाणां सङ्गाध्मानं क्लमो रुजा।
जटरे वातजायाश्चान्ये रोगाः स्युर्व्वानिग्रहात्॥
आटोपशूलोपरिकर्त्तिकां च सङ्गः पूरीषस्य तथोर्द्धवातः।
पुरीषमास्यादथवा निरेति पुरीषवेगेऽभिहते नरस्य॥
वस्तिमेहनयोः शूलं मूत्रकृच्छ्र शिरोरुजा।
विनामो वङ्लणानाह स्यालिङ्ग मूत्रनिग्रहे॥
मन्या गलस्तम्भशिरोविकारा जृम्भोपधातात् पवनात्मकाः स्युः।
तथाक्षिणासावदनामयाश्च भवन्ति तीव्राः सह कर्णरोगैः॥
आनन्दजं वाप्यथ शोकजं वा नेत्रोदकं प्राप्तसमुञ्चतो हि।

There are thirteen kinds of diseases produced by checking the efforts of nature to relieve herself. As by stopping the evacuation of air, faeces, urine, by yawning, tears, sneezing, belching, vomiting, semen, appetite, thirst and abstaining from liquids, the stopping of breath, watching, and another variety of indisposition is produced by taking bad food. When these are not indulged in, it produces the constipation which forms this class of diseases.

1. When air (*Apanna bāyu*) is stopped in its passage through the anus it produces a swelling in the abdomen, severe pain, difficulty of breathing, head-ache, hiccough, cough, discharge of mucus, difficulty of diglutition and vomiting of bile, phlegm, or faeces with constipation, and severe pain in the anus followed by a discharge of air.

2. *Dejections*. When the faeces are confined a gurgling noise is heard in the abdomen, with pain in the anus, as if the part was cut ; the dejections are confined, as air ascends, and sometimes stercoraceous vomiting occurs.

3. *Urine*. When confined, there is severe pain in the pelvis, urethra, anus, scrotum, groins, navel, and sometimes in the

शिरो गुरुत्वं व्यनामयाश्च भवन्ति तीव्राः सह पीनसेन॥
मन्यास्तम्भः शिरःशूलमर्दिताद्धविभेदकौ।
इन्द्रियाणाञ्च दौर्व्वल्यं क्षवथोः स्याद्विनिग्रहात्॥
कण्ठास्यपूर्णत्वमतीव तोदः कुजश्च वायोरथवा प्रवृत्तिः।
उद्गारवेगेऽभिहते भवन्ति घोरा विकाराः पवनप्रसूताः॥
कण्डुकोठारुचिव्यङ्गशोथपाण्ड्वामयज्वराः।
कुष्ठ वीसर्पहृल्लासा श्छर्दिनिग्रहजा गदाः॥
मूत्राशये वै गुदमुष्कयोश्च शोथो रुजामूत्रविनिग्रहश्च।
शुक्लाश्मरी तत् श्रवणं भवेञ्च ते ते विकारा विहते च शुक्ले॥
तन्द्राङ्गमर्द्दावरुचिः श्रमश्च क्षुधाभिघातात् कृशता च दृष्टैः।

head, when the urine is discharged in small quantities with pain. The bladder swells, and the body remains bent forward.

4. When *gaping* is checked the diseases of the neck, throat, and of the head are produced ; with other diseases of air, such as diseases of the eyes, nose, ears, and mouth.

5. When *tears* are confined they flow when the person is very happy, or very sorrowful; and when confined the head becomes heavy, and various severe eye diseases are produced. In such patients the phlegm discharged from the nose and mouth is without smell or taste.

6. When *sneezing* is confined, diseases of the head, eyes, nose, and ears are produced.

7. When *belching* is confined, the throat and mouth feel as if distended, and very painful ; the person's speech is not intelligible, are is confined by the mouth, anus, etc., and the disease produces the diseases of air.

8. Should *vomiting* be impeded it produces leprosy, loss of appetite, jaundice, fever, great sensibility of the skin and nausea.

9. When *semen* is confined, the bladder, rectum, and testicles swell, and become painful. The urine is confined and

कण्ठास्यशोषः श्रवणावरोध-तृष्णाविघातात् हृदयव्यथा च।
श्रान्तस्य निश्वासविनिग्रहेण हृद्रोगमोहावथवापि गुल्मः।
जृम्भाङ्गमर्द्दोऽक्षिशिरोतिजाड्यं निद्राभिघातादथवापि तन्द्रा।
वायुः कोष्ठानुगो रुक्षैः कषायकटुतिक्तकैः।
भोजनैः कुपितः सद्य उदावर्त्तं करोति च॥
वातमूत्रपुरीषासृक् कफमेदो वहानि वै।
स्त्रोतास्युदावर्त्तयति पुरिषं चातिवर्त्तयेत्॥
ततो हृद्बस्तिशूलार्त्तो हृल्लासारतिपीड़ितः।
वातमूत्रपुरीशाणिकृच्छ्रेन लभते नरः॥

is discharged in small quantities with pain, or the urine has a white deposit, and the semen is discharged involuntary. The other diseases may occur that deranged semen produces.

10. When the *appetite* is not gratified, it is followed by drowsiness, pain as if the part was crushed, loss of appetite, fatigue, and the eye is dim.

11. When the *thirst* is not gratified, the mouth and throat are dry, the hearing becomes dull, and pain is felt in the breast.

12. When the *breathing* is difficult from being confined from the fatigue produced by severe exercise, the food appears to stick in the throat, the understanding is impaired which produces (*Gulma*), and there is a feeling of hard lumps in the abdomen.

13. When *sleep* is not gratified, it is followed by yawning, and pain of the body, as if it was crushed. The eyes and head feel heavy, and coma supervenes.

The air of the stomach when dry, astringent, sour, or bitter food is eaten, produces quickly *Udābarta,* and deranges the canals of air, urine, faeces, blood, phlegm, fat, and the vessels which feed them. Air closes these canals and produces pain in the breast and pelvis, with heaviness of the body, and no appetite, with scanty evacuations.

श्वासकास-प्रतिश्याय-दाहमोहतृषा ज्वरान्।
वमि-हिक्काशिरोरोग मनः श्रवणविभ्रमान्॥
बहुनन्यांश्च लभते विकारान् वातकोपजान्॥
आमं शकृद्वा निचितं क्रमेण भूयो विवद्धं विगुणानिलेन।
प्रवर्त्तमानं न यथास्वमेनं विकारमानाहमुदाहरन्ति॥
तन्मिन् भवन्त्यामसमुद्भवे तु तृष्णा प्रतिश्वायशिरोविदाहाः।
आमाशये शूलमथो गुरुत्वं हृतस्तम्भ-उद्‌गारविघातनञ्च॥
स्तम्नःकटी पृष्ठपुरीषमूत्रे शूलोऽथ मूर्च्छा शकृतश्च छर्द्दिः।
शोथश्च पक्काशयजे भवन्ति तथालसोक्तानि च लक्षणानि॥

गुल्मनिदानम्

दुष्टा वातादयोऽत्यर्थं मिथ्याहारविहारतः।
कुर्व्वन्ति पञ्चधा गुल्मं कोष्ठान्तर्ग्रन्थिरूपिणम्॥

The retention of the above discharges produces pain of the chest and abdomen, nausea, laziness, and the air, urine, and dejections are evacuated with pain. If produced by phlegm there is difficult and noisy breathing, and the phlegm is discharged from the mouth and nose. (*Coryza*). In this case there is neither taste nor smell ; and the body feels hot, with dejection of mind. The person is insensible, and complains of thirst, fever, vomiting, hiccough, and head-ache. The person is deaf, the body swims round, followed by the other symptoms produced by deranged air. The life of such a person should be considered hopeless, when there is much thirst, great weakness, and languor, severe pain in the abdomen, and stercoraceous vomiting.

SWELLINGS IN THE ABDOMEN *(Gulma)*

When air, bile, and phlegm are deranged by eating bad food, at irregular times, or by unsuitable exercise, this disease is produced, which resembles a ball in the abdomen. There

तस्य पञ्चविधं स्थानं पार्श्व हृन्नाभिवस्तयः।
हृन्नाभ्योरन्तरे ग्रन्थिः सञ्चारी यदि वाचलः॥
वृत्तश्चयापचयवान स गुल्म इति कीर्त्तितः।
स व्यस्तैर्जायते दोषैः समस्तैरपिचा चोच्छितैः॥
पुरुषाणां तथा स्त्रीणां ज्ञेयो रक्तेन चापरः।
उद्गारबाहुल्यपुरीषवन्ध स्तप्त्यक्षमत्वान्त्र-विकुजनानि॥
आटोपमाध्नानमपक्तिशक्ति रासन्नगुल्मस्य वदन्ति चिह्नम्।
अरुचिः कृच्छ्रविण्मूत्र-वाततान्त्रविकुजनम्॥
आनाहश्चोर्द्धवातत्वं सर्व्वगुल्मेषु लक्षयेत्॥
रुक्षान्नपानं विषमातिमात्रं विचेष्टनं वेगविनिग्रहश्च।
शोकोऽभिघातोऽतिमलक्षयश्च निरान्नता चानिलगुल्महेतुः॥

are five kinds and situations of this disease. One in either side of the abdomen, one in the umbiliacus, another in the pelvis, and one between the chest and the abdomen, (scrobiculus cordis,) sometimes the swelling is fixed, and at other times it is moveable[4] there are four kinds of this disease in the male, three by the derangement of air, bile, and phlegm, another by the morbid mixture of the three, and the fifth kind is peculiar to females from the retention of the menses.

Gulma is ushered in by much belching, costiveness, loss of appetite, difficulty of making water, fulness of the body, with flatulence, and indigestion. These symptoms are followed by others produced by the use of food and drink of a dry nature, by a kind of wine which produces roughness of the surface of the body, by improper food, or by eating it at irregular times, or eating too much, by taking unsuitable exercise, and by neglecting the calls of nature, such as sneezing, and dejections, grief, accidents, bruises, or by too great evacuations or fasting. The symptoms of *Gulma*, produced by air, are its being situated in the abdomen, in the umbiliacus, or sides, and its moving about. It is sometimes small, and at other times large ; some-

यः स्थानसंख्यानरुजा विकल्पं विड्वाततङ्ग गलवक्त्रशोषम्॥
श्यावारुणत्वंशिशिरंज्वरञ्च हृत्कुक्षि-पार्श्वांस-शिरीरुजञ्च॥
करोति जीर्णे त्वधिकं प्रकोपं भुक्ते मृदुत्वं समुपैति यश्च।
वातात् स गुल्मो न च तत्र रुक्षं कषायक्तिं कटु चोपशेते॥
कट्वम्लतीक्ष्णोष्ण विदाहिरुक्ष क्रोधारिमद्यार्क-हुताशसेवा॥
आमाभिघातो रुधिरञ्च दुष्टं पैतस्य गुल्मस्य निमित्तमुक्तम्॥
ज्वरः पिपासा वदनाङ्ग रागः शूलं महज्जीर्य्यति भोजने च।
स्वेदो विदाहो व्रणवच्च गुल्यः स्पर्शासहः पैत्तिकगुल्मरूपम्।
शीतं गुरु स्निग्ध मचेष्ठनञ्च संपूरणं प्रस्वपनं दिवा च॥
गुल्मस्य हेतुः कसम्भवस्य सर्व्वस्तु दुष्टो निचयात्मकस्य।
स्तैमित्य-शीतज्वरगात्रसाद-हृल्लासकासारुचिगौरवाणि।
शैत्यं रुगल्पा कठिनोन्नतत्वं गुल्मस्य रूपाणि कफात्मकस्य॥
निमित्तरूपाण्युपलभ्य गुल्मे द्विदोषजे दोषबलावलञ्च॥
व्यामिश्रलिङ्गानपरांश्च गुल्मांस्त्रीनादिशेदौषधकल्पनार्थम्।

times round, at other times long ; sometimes the pain is slight, at other times severe, with constipation, dryness of the throat and mouth ; the skin of the body having a dark yellow colour and fever commencing with chilliness. The pain in the breast and sides of the abdomen, shoulders, or head are considerable, particularly after the food is digested, but the person feels better immediately after eating. Astringent, dry, bitter, or pungent things increase the complaint.

Bile. When the disease is produced by eating sour, bitter, hot, or other things of the same kind; by living on dry food ; by anger ; by drinking much wine, remaining much in the sun, or near the fire ; by collections of indigested food, or diseased blood in the abdomen, the bile is deranged producing the *Pitta Gulma*, with the following symptoms. The disease commences with fever, thirst, and a red colour of the mouth and skin. When digestion is going on, there is much pain, and perspiration,

महारुजं दाहपरीतमश्ववद्द्धनोन्नतं शीघ्रविदाहि दारुणम्॥
मनः शरीराग्निवलापहारिणं त्रिदोषजम् गुल्मम साध्यमादिशेत्॥
नवप्रसूताहितभोजना या या चामगर्भं विसृजेदृतौ च॥
वायुर्हितस्य्ः परिगृह्य रक्तं करोति गुल्मं सरुजं सदाहम्॥
पैत्तस्थ लिङ्गेन समानलिङ्गं विशेषणञ्चात्यपरं निवोध।
यः स्पन्दते पिण्डित एव नाङ्गैश्चिरात् सशूलः समगर्भलिङ्गः।
स रौधिरस्त्वीभव एव गुल्मो व्यतीते दशभे चिकित्साः॥
सञ्चितं क्रमशो गुल्मो महावास्तुपरिग्रहः।
कृतमूलः शिरानद्धो यदा कूर्म्म इवोत्थितः।
दौर्व्वल्यारुचिहृल्लासकासछर्द्यरति ज्वरैः।

with a severe burning sensation in the pit of the stomach, which is tender on being touched, or it is followed by a swelling in the stomach, which is painful like a boil.

Phlegm is deranged by cold, or by eating indigestable or oleaginous articles of food; particularly when the person does not take exercise, eats too much, and sleeps too long during the day. When *phlegm* is thus deranged it produces coldness and languor of the body, with low fever, nausea, cough, no appetite, and heaviness of the body, without much pain. The ball gradually becomes harder, and larger.

When air, bile, and phlegm are deranged, and are produced by the causes given above, there will be severe pain, great heat of body, and the *Gulma* or swelling feels hard like a stone, and is large, and quickly produces the heat of the body; so severe is this form of the complaint that the person is in great distress. His body becomes thin, with a bad colour, and he has not appetite, nor strength. Such a disease is incurable.

There is a king of *Gulma*, so like pregnancy that it may deceive physicians, unless they observe the precaution of not giving medicine until after the tenth month, (the supposed time of utero-gestation.)[5]

तृष्णा तन्द्रा प्रतिश्यायैर्युज्यते स न सिद्ध्यति॥
गृहीत्वा सजरं श्वास छर्द्यतीसारपीड़ितम्॥
हृन्नाभि हस्तपादेषु शोथः कर्षति गुल्मिनम्॥
श्वासः शूलं पिपासान्नविद्वेषो ग्रन्थिमूढ़ता।
जायते दुर्व्वलत्वञ्च गुल्मिनो मरणाय वै॥

. हृद्रोगनिदानम्

अत्युष्णगुर्व्वन्नकषायतिक्त-श्रमाभिघाताध्यशनप्रसङ्गैः।
संचिन्तनैर्वेगविधारगौश्च हृदामयः पञ्चविधः प्रदिष्टः॥
दूषयित्वा रशं दोषा विगुणा हृदयं गताः।

The unfavourable symptoms of *Gulma* are its enlarging so as to fill the abdomen ; and the increase being rapid, and the swelling being surrounded by vessels, with much pain in the breast, as well as in the part. When the swelling is of the figure of a turtle, when there is much debility, loss of appetite, nausea, cough, vomiting, restlessness, fever, thirst, coma, and the discharge of mucus from the mouth and nose, without either taste or smell, such a person will not recover.

When a person with *Gulma* has fever, asthma, vomiting, diarrhoea, and swelling of the breast, umbiliacus, with swelling of the hand or feet, the disease will be fatal.

When after asthma, cough, thirst, with no appetite, much pain, and the swelling has suddenly disappeared with much weakness, the person will soon die.

DISEASES OF THE HEART

Painful affections of the heart *Ridraga* (Angina pectoris ?) are produced by want of attention to the calls of nature, the use of hot and dry food ; the improper mixture of food ; an intemperance in eating, or unusual food ; which causes indigestion, and deranges the humours. The impure chyle is

हृदि वाधां प्रकुर्व्वन्ति हृद्रोगं तं प्रचक्षते॥
आयम्यते मारुतजे हृदयं तुद्यते यथा।
निर्म्मथ्यते दीर्यते च स्फोट्यते पाट्यतेऽपि च॥
तृष्णोषादाह चोषाः स्युः पैत्तिके हृदयक्लमः॥
धुमायनञ्च मूर्च्छा च स्वेदः शोषो मुखस्य च।
गौरवं कफसंस्त्रावोऽरुचिस्तम्भोऽग्निमार्द्दवम्॥
माधुर्य्य मपि चास्यस्य बला सावतते हृदि।
विद्यार्तिदोषन्त्वपि सर्व्वलिङ्ग
तीव्रार्तितोदं क्रिमिजं सकण्डुम्।
उत्क्लेदः ष्ठीवनं तोदः शूलं हृल्लासकस्तमः।
अरुचिः श्यावनेत्रत्वं शोथश्च क्रिमिजे भवेत्।
क्लमः सादो भ्रमः शोषो ज्ञैयास्तेषामुपद्रवाः।
क्रिमिजे क्रिमिजातीनां श्लेष्मिकानाञ्च ये मताः॥

received into the heart, and produces this painful disease ; of which there are five varieties. When produced by deranged air the patient feels various acute kinds of pains, sometimes it is lancinating, at other times as if the heart was cut or torn. When produced by deranged *bile* there is much pain in the heart, with thirst, heart-burning and dryness. This is succeeded by fainting, much sweating, dryness of the mouth, and smoke appears to come out of the mouth. When produced by *phlegm* the patient feels a heaviness of the heart, a discharge of mucus from the mouth and nose, loss of appetite, and a sweet taste in the mouth.

When produced by *worms* there is a lancinating, or piercing pain in the region of the heart ; nausea, vomiting, belching and loss of appetite. The eyes become dark greenish, with emaciation of the body. All these diseases of the heart terminate in emaciation, languor, loss of appetite and strength, with giddiness.

मूत्रकृच्छ्रनिदानम्

व्यायाम-तीक्ष्णौषध-रुक्षमद्य प्रसङ्गनित्य-द्रुतपृष्ठयानात्।
आपूपमांसाध्यशनादजीर्णात् स्युर्मूत्रकुच्छ्राणि तृष्णां तथाष्टौ।
पृथक् मलाः स्वैः कुपिता निदानैः सर्व्वेऽथवा कोपमुपेत्य वस्तौ।
मूत्रस्य मार्ग परिपीडयन्ति यदा तदा मूत्रयतीह कृच्छ्रात्॥
तीव्रार्त्तिरुग्वङ्‌वणवस्तिमेढ्रेस्वल्पं मुहुर्मूत्रयतीह वातात्

STRANGURY (*Mutrakrichchhra*)[6]

This disease is produced by wrestling, or other violent kinds of exercise, hot spices, dry food, wines, excessive venery, riding on horseback very quickly ; eating the flesh of the buffaloes, or the rhinoceros, etc., or other indigestable food ; another cause is eating too frequently, or it may be produced by bad digestion.

There are eight forms of this disease. The derangements of air, bile and phlegm separately or combined, when they occur in the bladder, produce this and diseases in the urinary passages, when the urine is discharged with pain. This disease is also produced by injuries of the parts, by constipation of the bowels, and by calculi.

1. When the deranged air produces the disease it causes severe pain in the pelvis, in the testicles, and in the penis. The patient has a frequent desire for making water, and the urine passes in drops accompanied with pain.
2. When the bile of the part is deranged the urine is of a yellow or red colour. There is much scalding or burning pain in the passages, the urine is discharged in small quantities frequently, accompanied with heat and uneasiness.
3. When the phlegm is deranged the pelvis, bladder, urinary passages, and testicles feel heavy ; they are

पीतं सरक्तं सरुजं मदाहं कृच्छ्रं मुहुर्मूत्रयतीह पित्तात्।
वस्ते सलिङ्गस्य गुरुत्वशोथौ मूत्रं सपिच्छं कफमूत्रकृच्छ्रे॥
सर्व्वाणि रूपाणि तु सन्निपातात् भवन्ति तत् कृच्छतमं हि कृच्छम्।
मूत्र वाहिषु शल्येन क्षतेष्वभिहतेषु वा॥
मूत्रकृच्छं तदाघाताज्जायते भृशदारुणम्।
वातकृच्छ्रेण तुल्यानि तस्य लिङ्गानि निर्द्दिशेत्॥
शकृतन्तु प्रतीघाताद्वायुर्विगुणतां गतः।
आध्मानं वातशूलञ्च मूत्रसङ्गं करोति च॥
अश्मरीहेतु तत्पूर्व्वं मूत्रकृच्छ्र मुदाहरेत्।
शुक्रे दोषैरुपहते मूत्रमार्गे विधाविते॥

swelled, and the urine is cold, shining like oil, and soon dries up.

4. When the air, bile, and phlegm are deranged the separate symptoms of each variety appear in the same person, and is cured with difficulty.
5. ***Salajah.*** When the parts are injured by external violence, the disease is accompanied with much pain, followed by other symptoms of deranged air.
6. ***Sakripratikatajah,*** when the bowels are very costive, from air being deranged, it is accompanied with much swelling and pain in the abdomen, with difficulty in mictirition.
7. ***Asarijah*** is produced by calculi, with a difficulty and pain in mictirition.

When a person runs quickly or jumps, is much fatigued, is fasting, or the part is injured, the bladder rises out of the pelvis of a round form, and large like the gravel uterus. It is accompanied with much pain and moves from side to side, and the urine is very hot, and passes in drops. If the swelling is

सशुक्रं मूत्रयेत् कृच्छात् वस्तिमेहन शूलवान्।
अश्मरी शर्करा चैव तुल्य सम्भवलक्षणे॥
विशेषं शर्करायाश्च शृणु कीर्त्तयती मम।
पच्य मानाश्मरी पित्तात् शीष्यमाना च वायुना।
विमुक्तकफसन्धाना क्षरन्ती शर्करा मत।
हृत्पीड़ा वेपथुः शूलं कुक्षावग्निश्च दुर्व्वलः।
तया भवति मूर्च्छा च मूत्रकृच्छ्रश्च दारुणम्।
मूत्र वेगनिरस्ताभिः प्रशमं याति वेदना।
यावदस्थाः पुनर्नेति गुड़िका स्त्रोतसो मुखम्॥

pressed, above the pubis, the urine passes easily, and in a continued stream. When the person cannot move, it is called *Bastikundala*, and is a severe and dangerous disease.

When bile produces the disease it is incurable ; when phlegm it may be cured, especially if it continues to be discharged, except in the case of "*Kundalī bāta.*" When the bladder is round above pelvis, with thirst and insensibility and noisy breathing, it is incurable.

8. ***Sarajah,*** when the semen is affected by deranged humours, and carried into the passage of the the urine, it is discharged with much difficulty and pain.
9. ***Asari*** and ***Sakarā*** produced by stone or gravel. They are produced by the same causes, and the symptoms of both are the same. When the stone is broken and dried up with bile and air, it is discharged through the urethra. When stone is retained in the bladder, it forms the peculiarity of the two diseases.

In ***Sakarā*** therc is shivering with severe pain in the chest and sides, loss of appetite, and fainting. This is followed by a fit of strangury, which is a severe disease, the pain being only mitigated when the urine is not discharged, and the suffering is very acute, as the gravel is passing through the urethra.

मूत्राघातनिदानम्

जायन्ते कुपितै दोषै मूत्राघातास्त्रयोदश।
प्रायो मूत्रविधातद्यैर्व्वातकुण्डलिकादयः।
रौक्षाद्वेगविधातादद्वा वायुर्व्वस्तौ सवेदनः।
मूत्रमाविश्य चरति विगुणः कुण्डलीकृतः॥
मूत्रमल्पाल्प मथवा सरुजं संप्रवर्त्तते।
वातकुण्डलिकां तान्तु व्याधिं विद्यात् सुदारुणम्॥
आध्मापयन् वस्ति गुदं रुद्धा वायुश्चलोन्नताम्॥
कुर्य्यातीव्रात्तिष्ठीलां मूत्रविणमार्गरोधिनीम्॥
वेगं विधारयेत् यस्य मूत्रस्याकुशलोः नरः।
निरुणद्धि मुखं तस्य वस्तेर्वस्ति गतोऽनिलः।
मूत्रसङ्गो भवेत्तेन वस्तिकुक्षिनिपीड़ितः।
वातवस्ति स विज्ञेयो व्याधिः कृच्छप्रसाधनः॥
चिरं धारयतो मूत्रं त्वरया न प्रवर्त्तते।

SUPPRESSION OF URINE (*Mutraghata.*)

The derangements of air, bile, and phlegm in the bladder produce the thirteen forms of this disease.

Bātakundalikā. This disease is produced by eating dry articles of food, by retention of the natural discharges ; by which air is deranged in the bladder, which mixes with the urine producing pain, and they turn round in a circle, and the urine is retained, or it is discharged in drops. The person is very fearful in this disease.

Astila. When the air is deranged between the rectum and bladder it forms a large ball like a stone (prostate gland?) and produces suppression of the urine, faeces, and air ; and is accompanied with swelling in the bladder and much pain. This disease is also called *Bātastila*.

Bātabasti. When an ignorant person stops the evacuation of the urine or dejections, which deranges the air stops up the

मेहमानस्य मन्दं वा मूत्रातीतः स उच्यते।
मूत्रस्य वेगेऽभिहते तदुदावर्त्तहेतुकः।
अपानः कुपितो वायुरुदरं पूरयेद्भृशम्॥
नाभेरधस्तादाध्मानं जानयेत्तीव्रवेदनम्।
तन्मूत्रजठरं विद्यादधोवस्तिनिरोधनम्॥
वस्तौ वाप्यथवा नाले मणौ वा यस्य देहिनः॥
मूत्रं प्रवृत्तं सज्ज्येत सरक्तं वा प्रवाहतः।
स्रवेच्छनै रल्पमल्पं सरुजं वाथ नीरुजम्।
विगुणानिलजो व्याधिः स मूत्रीत्सङ्गसञ्ज्ञितः॥
रुक्षस्य क्लान्तदेहस्य वस्तिस्थौ पित्तमारुतौ।
मूत्रक्षयं सरुग्दाहं जनयेत्तां तदाह्वयम्॥
अन्तर्वस्ति मुखे वृत्तः स्थिरोऽल्पः सहसा भवेत्।
अश्मरी तुल्यरुग्ग्रन्थिर्मूत्रग्रन्थिः स उच्यते॥
मूत्रितस्य स्त्रियं यातो वायुना शुक्र मुद्धतम्।
ख्यानाच्युतं मूत्रयतः प्राक् पश्चाद्वा प्रवर्त्तते॥
भस्मोदकप्रतीकाशं मूत्रशक्रं तदुच्यते।

neck of the bladder, and produces retention. This disease produces pain in the pelvis, and in the sides ; which form is cured with much difficulty.

When a person allows the urine to flow for some time, and then stops, it produces the disease called *Mutrātita,* or retention, when the urine is only discharged in small quantities.

When urine is retained by such causes as produced the same effect as the retention of air, which is situated near the rectum, it produces swelling of the abdomen, with much pain under the umbiliacus. This disease is called *Mutrajathara*.

When the urine stops by impediments in the urethra, near the glans penis or elsewhere; or when expelled with great force mixed with blood, sometimes with much pain, in other cases with no pain. This variety is calley *Mutrasanga*.

व्धायामाध्वातपैः पित्त वस्ति प्रान्यनिलान्वितम्।
वस्तिं मेढ्रं गुदञ्चैव प्रदहेत् स्त्रावयेदधः॥
मूत्रं हारिद्रा मथवा सरक्तं रक्तमेव वा।
कृच्छ्रात् पुनः पुनर्जन्तोरुष्णवातं ब्रुवन्ति तम्॥
पित्तं कफो द्वावपि वा संहन्येतेऽनिलेन चेत्॥
कृच्छ्रान्मूत्र तदा पीतं श्वेत रक्तं धनं सृजेत्॥
सदाहं रोचना शङ्खं चूर्णवर्णं भवेत्तु तत्।
सुष्कं समस्तवर्णं वा मूत्रसादं वा वदन्ति तम्॥
रुक्षदुर्व्वलयो वातेनोदावर्त्त शकृद् यदा॥
मूत्रस्त्रोतोऽनुपद्येत विट्संसृष्टं तदानरः।
विड्गन्धं मूत्रयेत् कृच्छ्रात् विड्विघातं विनिर्द्दिशेत्॥
द्रुताधलङ्घनायासै रभिघातात् प्रपीड़नात्।
स्वस्थानाहस्तरुद्वत्तः स्थूलस्तिष्ठति गर्भवत्॥
शूलस्प्रन्दनदाहार्त्तो विन्दुं विन्दुं स्त्रवत्यपि।

When the body is dried up by the free use of stimulants, and dry food, and great fatigue, the air and bile are deranged in the bladder, and the urine, which becomes scanty is of a black colour, and produces severe pain and heat. This disease is called *Mutrakia*.

When there is a small hard round ball at the neck of the bladder, accompanied with much pain, it may prevent the passage of the urine, and produce the symptoms of stone. It is called *Mutragrinti*.

When at the proper time urine is not discharged, and the patient has connection with woman, the semen is discharged with the urine, sometimes before, and in other cases after the urine. This urine is of a white colour, as if mixed with chalk, and the disease is called *Mutrasukra*.

When violent exercise is taken, as in fighting, travelling, or great heat, the bile is deranged in the bladder with air, which

पीड़ितस्तु सृजेद्धारां संस्तमोद्वेष्टनार्त्तिमान्।।
वस्तिकुण्डलमाहुस्तं घोरं शस्त्रविषोपमम्।।
पवनप्रवलं प्रायो दुर्निवार मबुद्धिभिः।
तस्मिन् पित्रान्वितेदाहः शूलं मूत्रविवर्णता।।
श्लेष्मणा गौरवं शोथः स्निग्धं मूत्रं घनं सितम्।
श्लेष्मरुद्धविलो वस्तिः पित्रोदीर्ण न सिध्यति।
अविभ्रान्तविलः साध्यो नतु यः कुण्डलीकृतः।
स्याद्वस्तौ कुण्डनीमूते तृन्मोहः श्वास एव च।

अश्मरीनिदानम्

वातपित्तकफैस्तिस्त्रश्चतुर्थी शुक्रजापरा।
प्रायः श्लेष्माश्रयाः सर्व्वा अष्मर्य्य सुर्यमोपमा।

passes mixed with urine, and produces a burning pain in the bladder, penis, and anus. The urine becomes yellow as if mixed with tamarinds, or blood ; it is discharged with difficulty, and is called *Usnabāta*.

When deranged air produces this disease it is accompanied with great pain and heat, on its being discharged.

When the urine is yellow from bile, it causes in its passage a burning pain in the part, and there is much sediment.

When phlegm produces the disease the urine is white, like the powder of shells, and is of different consistence. This variety is called *Mutrakasāda*.

When the body is very dry and weak, and the faeces is collected for some time, it may be evacuated with the urine, have the smell of faeces, and pass with difficulty and much pain. This is most probably the recto-vaginal fistula, which is only described in modern books; and is called *Bierbigāta*.

URINARY CALCULI (Ashmari)

When air, bile, and phlegm are deranged it produces different forms of calculi ; and another kind is produced from

विशोषयेद् वस्तिगतं सशुक्रं मूत्रं सपित्तं पवनं कफं वा।
यदा तदाश्मर्युपजायते तु क्रमेण पित्तेष्विव रोचना गोः॥
नैकदोषाश्रयाः सर्व्वाः अथासां पूर्व्वलक्षणम्।
वस्त्याध्यानं तदासन्नदेशेषु परितोऽतिरुकः॥
मूत्रे वस्त्वं सगन्धित्वं मूत्रकृच्छ्रं ज्वरोऽरुचिः।
सामान्यलिङ्ग रुङ्नाभिसेवनी वस्तिमुर्द्धसु॥
विशीर्ण धारमूत्रः स्यात् तया मार्गनिरोधने।
तद्व्यपायात् सुखं भेहेदच्छं गोमेदकोपमम्॥
तत्संक्षोभात् क्षते सास्त्रमायासाश्चातिरुग् भवेत्।
तत्रवाताद्भृशं चार्त्तो दन्तान् खादति वेपते।
गृह्णाति मेहनं नाभिं पीड़यत्यनिशं क्कणन्।
सानिलं मुञ्चति शकृत् मुहु र्मेहति विन्दुशः।
श्यावारुगाश्मरी चास्य स्थाच्चिताकण्ठकैरपि॥
पित्तेन दह्यतेः वस्तिः पच्यमान इवोष्मवान्।
भल्लातकास्थिसंस्थान रक्तपीतासिताश्मरी।
वस्ति र्निस्तुद्यत इव श्लेष्मणा शीतलो गुरुः॥
अश्मरी महती श्लक्ष्णा मधुवर्णा खरा सिता॥
एता भवन्ति बालानां तेषामपि च भुयसा।

semen. Phlegm is the chief cause of the disease in all its different forms.

This disease is produced in those who live on hard indigestable food, and do no use evacuating remedies, by which the phlegm is deranged, and mixing with urine passes into the bladder and forms the stone.

Others suppose that the calculi are produced by collections of the impurities of the urine which sink down and form, by being dried with the internal fire, calculi in the bladder. Others suppose they are formed as hailstones are formed in the sky.

आश्रयोपचयाल्पत्वात् ग्रहण हरणे सुखा॥
शुक्राश्मरी तु महतां जायते शुक्रधारणात्।
ख्यानाच्च्युत ममुक्तं हि मुष्कयोरन्तरेऽनिलः॥
शोषयत्युपसंगृह्य शुक्रं तच्छुक्रमश्मरी।
वस्तिरुङ्मवकृच्छ्रत्वं मुष्कस्वयथुकारिणी।
तस्यामुतपन्नमात्रायां शुक्रमेति विलीयते॥
पीड़िते त्ववकाशेऽस्मिन्नश्मर्य्येव च शर्करा।
अणुशी वायुना भिन्ना सा तष्मिन्ननुलोमगे।
निरेति सह मूत्रेण प्रतिलोमे निरुध्यते।
मूत्रस्त्रोतः प्रवृत्ता सा शिक्ता कुर्यायिदुपद्रवान्॥
दौर्व्वल्यं सदनं कार्शं कुक्षिशूल मथ्यरुचिम्।
पाण्डुत्वमुष्णवातञ्च तृष्णां हृत्पीड़नं वमिम्॥
प्रसूननाभिवृषणं वद्धमूत्रं रुजातुरम्॥
अश्मरीक्षपयत्याशु सिकता शर्करान्विता॥

प्रमेह–मधुमेह–पीड़का–निदानम्

आस्वासुखं स्वप्लसुखं दधीनि ग्राम्यदकानुपरसाः पयांसि।
नवान्नपानं गुड़वैकृतञ्च प्रमेहहेतुः कफकुच्च सर्व्वम्॥
भेदञ्च मांसञ्च शरीरजल क्लेदं कफो वस्तिगतं प्रदुष्य।

This disease is ushered in by pain in the bladder, especially in its neck, scrotum, and penis. In some cases languor and fever are present, and the urine has to smell of goat's urine. When formed the pain is in the umbiliacus, bladder, perineum, penis, particularly during micturition. The urine does not pass in a stream, but in drops : it also stops suddenly. It is sometimes mixed with blood, in other cases it is clear or mixed with gravel. The pain is increased by walking, jumping, and riding.

Four different forms of this disease are observed. The following are the peculiarities of each form.

करोति मेहान समुदीर्ण मुष्णैस्तानेव पित्तं परिदुष्य चापि।
क्षीणेषु दोषिष्वक्कृष्य धातुन् संदुष्य मेहान् कुरुतेऽनिलश्च॥
साध्याः कफोत्था दश पित्तजाः षट् याप्या न साध्यः पवनाच्चतुष्कः।
समक्रियत्वाद्विषमक्रियत्वा न्महात्थयत्वाच्च यथाक्रमं ते॥
कफः सपित्तः पवनश्च दोषा मेदोऽस्त्र शुक्राम्बु-वसालसीकाः।
मज्जारसौजः पिशितञ्च दूष्याः प्रमेहिणं विंशतिरेव मेहाः॥
दन्तादीनां मलाठ्यत्वं प्राग्रूपं पाणिपादयोः।
दाहश्चिक्कणतां देहे तृट् स्वाहास्यञ्च जायते॥
सामान्यं लक्षणं तेषां प्रभूताविलमूत्रता।
दोषदुष्या विशेषेऽपि तत् संयोगविशेषतः।
मूत्रवर्णादिभेदेन भेदो मेहेषु कल्प्यते॥
अच्छ्रं बहुसितं शीतं निर्गन्धमुदकोपमम्।
मेहत्युदक मेहेन किञ्चिदाविल-पिच्छिलम्॥
इक्षोरस मिवात्यर्थं मधुरेञ्चेक्षु मेहतः॥
सान्द्री भवेत् पर्युषितं सान्द्रमेहेन मेहति॥
सुराभेहि सुरातुला मुपर्य्यच्छ्रमधोघनम्।
संहृष्टरोमा पिष्ठेन पिष्टवत् बहुलं सितम्॥
शुक्राभं शुक्रंमिश्रं वा शुक्रमेही प्रमेहति।
मुर्त्तानुन् सिकतामेही सिकतारूपिणी मलान्॥
शीतमेही सवहुशो मधुरं भृशशीतलम्।

When produced by *air* it is always accompanied with deranged phlegm, and this forms the stone. This stops near the neck of the bladder, and suddenly impedes the flow of urine; and is accompanied with much pain. To assist the evacuation of the urine the patient presses the parts particularly the umbiliacus, penis, and anus. The colour of the calculi are black, rough, and unequal; and are surrounded with elevations like the *kadam*.

शनैः शनैः शैन मेही मन्दं मन्दं प्रमेहति।
लालातन्तुयुतं मूत्रं लालामेहेन पिच्छिलम्।।
गन्धवर्णरसष्पशैः क्षारेण क्षारतोयवत्।
नीलमेहने नीलाभं कालमेही मसीनिभम्।।
हारिद्रमेही कटुकं हरिद्रासन्निभं दहत्।
विस्त्रं माञ्जिष्ठमेहेन मञ्जिष्ठासलिलोपमम्।।
विस्त्रमुष्णं सलवणं रक्ताभं रक्तमेहतः।।
वसामेहौ वसामिश्रं वसाभं मूत्रयेन्मुहुः।
मज्जाभं मज्जमिश्रं वा मज्जमेष्ही मुहुर्मुहुः।।
कषायं मधुर रुक्षं क्षौद्रमेहं वदेद्बुधः।
हस्ती मत्त इवाजस्त्रः मूत्रं वेगविवर्जित्तम्।।
सलसीकं विवद्धञ्च हस्तीमेही प्रमेहति।।
अविपाकोऽरुचिश्छर्द्दि र्निद्रा कासः सपीनसः।
उपद्रवाः प्रजायन्ते मेहानां कफजन्मनाम्।।
वस्तिमेहे नयो स्तोदो मुष्कावदरणं ज्वरः।
दाहतृष्णाम्लिका मूर्च्छा विड्भेदः पित्तजन्मनाम्।।
वातजानामुदावर्त्तः कम्पहृद्ग्रहलोलताः।।
शूलमुन्निद्रता शोषः कासः श्वासश्च जायते।।

Bile. In this case the bile being mixed with deranged phlegm, become a thick mass, increases in size, passes to the neck of the bladder, and prevents the passage of the urine. In the bladder there is a burning pain, as if produced by the application of heat. The air from the anus is hot, and the stone is yellow and sometimes red, black, or greyish, and resembles the stone of the "marking-nut."

Phlegm. A person who eats much of those articles of diet which produce diseases of phlegm is liable to have this form of stone. In such cases the phlegm becomes thick, and a stone is formed in the bladder. It produces a sudden stop of the flow of

यथोक्तोपद्रवारिष्टमतिप्रस्रुतमेव च।
पिड़कापीड़ितं गाढ़ं प्रमेहो हन्ति मानवम्॥
जातः प्रमेही मधुमेहिना वा न साध्य उक्तः स हि वीजदोषात्।
ये चापि केचित् कुलजा विकारा भवन्ति तांश्च प्रपदन्त्यसाध्यान्॥
सर्व्वे एव प्रमेहास्तु कालेनाप्रतिकारिणः॥
मधुमेहत्वमायान्ति तदासाध्या भवन्ति हि॥
मधुमेहे मधुसमं जायते स किल द्विधा।
क्रुद्धे धातुक्षयाद्वायौ दोषावृतपथेऽथवा॥
आवृतो दोषलिङ्गानि सोऽनिमित्तं प्रदर्शयन्।
क्षणात् क्षीणः क्षणात् पूर्णो भजते कृच्छसाध्यताम्।
मधुरं यच्च मेहेषु प्रायो मध्विव मेहति।
सर्व्वेऽपि मधुमेहाख्य माधुर्य्याच्च तनोरतः॥
शराविका कच्छपिका ज्वालिनी विनतालजी।
मसूरिका सर्षपिका पुत्रिणी सविदारिका॥

the urine, with severe pain in the bladder, and the person feels as if beaten. The bladder feels heavy and cool; and the stone is white, shining, large, like the appearance of a hen's egg.

The fourth kind of stone is produced by excesses in venery, or by the stoppage of semen which collects between the scrotum and penis. There it dries, and stops the passage of urine. This produces pain in bladder and scrotum, and a difficulty in micturition. In such cases the scrotum sometimes swells.

The three first forms frequently attack children, and old people ; by sleeping during the day, and using improper food and sweetmeats. The stone is easily extracted in the young, as the parts are small. In old people the disease is produced by derangements of air, bile and phlegm.

Stone is a dangerous disease, being like poison, or thunder. When recent it may be cured by medicines ; but when of long standing an operation is required.

विद्रधिश्चेति पिड़का: प्रमेहोपेक्षया दश।
सन्धिमर्म्मसु जायन्ते मांसलेषु च धामसु॥
अन्तोन्नता तु तद्रूपा निम्नमध्या शराविका।
गौरसर्षसंख्याना तत् प्रमाना च सर्षपी।
सहादा कूर्म्मसंस्थाना ज्ञेया कच्छपिका बुधै:।
ज्वालिनी तीव्रदाहा तु मांसजालसमावृता।
अवगाढ़रुजा, क्लेदा पृष्ठे वाप्युदरेऽपि वा।
महती सरुजा नीला विनता नाम सा स्मृता।
महत्यल्पचिता ज्ञेया पिड़का चापि पुत्रिणी॥
मसूराकृतिसंख्याना विज्ञेया तु मसूरिका॥

प्रमेहनिदानम्

रक्तासिता स्फोटचिता विज्ञेया त्वलजी भवेत्।
विदारीकन्द्रवद्वृत्ता कठिना च विदारिका॥

DISEASES OF THE URINARY ORGANS

Under this head will be considered the diseases of the Urine, Bladder and Urethra.

MORBID SECRETION OF URINE (*Prameha*)

This disease is produced by a sedentary life, as sitting, lying down, sleeping in the day time, using too much curdled milk, various kinds of fish, amphibious animals, or the flesh of buffaloes, new rice, or new water, such as rain or fresh rivern water, or food with different preparations of jagry, or whatever produces phlegm. It is also produced by the deranged phlegm of the bladder which affects the fat, flesh, or serum of the body; but particularly the region of the bladder. The bile is deranged by its peculiar causes, and in like manner the air may produce the disease, when the other humours are deranged, and convey them to the bladder.

There are twenty varieties of diseased urine ; of which

विद्रधे र्लक्षणैर्युक्ता ज्ञेया विद्रधिका तु सा।
ये यन्मयाः स्मृता मेहा तेषामेतास्तु तन्मयाः॥
विना प्रमेहमपेत्या जायन्ते दुष्टमेदसः।
तावच्चैता न लक्ष्यन्ते यावद्वास्तुपरिग्रहाः॥
गुदे हृदि शिरस्यंसे पृष्ठे मर्म्मसु चोत्थिताः।
सोपद्रव दुर्व्वलाग्नेः पिड़काः परिवर्ज्जयेत्॥

phlegm forms ten varieties which are curable, bile forms six varieties which are cured with great difficulty, but do not destroy life ; and air forms four varieties, which are incurable. The causes of the different degrees of facility of removing these different varieties are that all the forms are accompanied with deranged phlegm, and when combined with deranged bile the cure of the disease is difficult, as those remedies which diminish bile will increase the phlegm. In like manner those remedies which decrease the air increase the phlegm therefore the cure is difficult; and on this account the disease produced by air is dangerous even from the beginning. These twenty kinds of disease are produced by derangements of air, bile and phlegm, fat, blood, semen, serum (*Amba*), lymph (*Basā*), the essential parts of all the humours (*Ozzo*), the flesh and the chyle.

This order of diseases is ushered in by the appearance of morbid secretions about the teeth, ears, nose, and eyes. The hands and feet are very hot and burning, and the surface of the skin is shining as if oil had been applied to it. This is accompanied with thirst, and a sweet taste in the mouth. The different varieties of this disease are distinguished from each other by the symptoms of deranged humours, and by the colour of the urine.

In the disease produced by phlegm, insects approach the urine ; the person is languid, his body becomes fat, and there is a discharge of mucus from the nose and mouth, with dispeptic symptoms, and looseness of the skin. He is always sleepy, with cough and difficult breathing.

When the disease is produced by bile, there is a cutting pain in the scrotum, bladder, and penis, with fever, dispepsia, vomiting, heat of the body, thirst, want of sleep, and yellowness of the exceretions. In some cases it is accompanied with jaundice.

When produced by diseased air there is pain in the chest, the patient has a desire to eat everything, there is watching, shivering pain and costiveness. The following are the names and characteristic symptoms of the twenty varieties of diseased urine :–

1. ***Udakameha.*** In this disease the urine is nearly of the natural colour, without any sediment. It is white, cold, has no smell, and is like water.

2. ***Ekhyumeha.*** The urine is like the juice of sugar-cane in colour and taste.

3. In ***Sāndrameha*** the urine becomes thick after standing sometime.

4. When the urine is of a white colour, is thin and pure above, and thick belows, it is named ***Surāmeha.***

5. ***Pishtameha.*** At the time of micturition the hair over the body is erect, and the urine has a copious white powder; as if flower had been mixed with it.

6. ***Sukrameha.*** In this variety the urine is the colour of semen, which sometimes appears mixed with it.

7. When the urine lets fall a hard and small deposit like sand it is called ***Sikatameha.***

8. In ***Swetameha*** there is a copious secretion of urine which is sweet and cold.

9. When there are frequent calls to make urine, which is discharged in small quantities, the disease is called ***Shanairmeha.***

10. ***Lālameha.*** When the urine is like mucilage, and has long adhesive fibrous matter mixed with it, the disease is named ***Lālameha.***

11. In ***Khārmeha*** the urine has the colour, taste, and smell of potassa, and is like it to the touch.

12. In ***Nilameha*** the urine is of a blue colour.

13. In ***Kālameha*** the urine is of a black colour, like ink.

14. In ***Haridrameha*** the urine is bitter and of a yellow colour like tamarind water, and there is great heat in passing the urine.

15. In ***Manjistameha*** the urine has the smell of indigested food, and is of the colour of the water of madder.

16. ***Raktameha.*** The smell is like that of indigested food, is hot, is saltish to the taste, and is of a red colour.

17. ***Basāmeha.*** The urine in this variety is of a light colour like fat, and seems as if mixed with it. It is discharged frequently.

18. ***Majjāmeha.*** the urine in this form is like the colour of marrow, and appears as if mixed with it. It is discharged frequently.

19. ***Kandrameha.*** The urine is astringent and sweet to the taste. It has a troubled appearance.

20. ***Hastimeha.*** In this disease there is an incontinence of urine, which is discharged involuntary. It appears mixed with fat.

The unfavourable symptoms of the above varieties of disease are when they are congenital; when the seven forms of diseased air, bile, and phlegm are present; when accompanied with a great discharge of the humours; when accompanied with large deep-seated abscesses; and when accompanied with *Madhumeha*, or sweet urine. These forms destroy the patient. All hereditary diseases being incurable, the congenital forms are such. All these different forms of *Prameha* if not properly treated, terminate in *Madhumeha;* or sweet urine, and they are then incurable.

The following forms of *Prameha* may be cured; when the urine is of the natural colour, is neither shining on the surface, nor white, and is of the usual taste, or is bitter and pungent.

The following eruptions and abscesses may occur in the course of this disease in joints, and in vital or sensible parts; as the temples, or where there is much muscle.

1. ***Sarābika***; with a central hollow, with high edges
2. ***Kachchhapika*** are hot, and are in the form of a turtle, in appearance.
3. ***Jwalini*** is hot, and part appears irregular in its surface.
4. ***Binatā*** eruption is of a blue colour, and is accompanied with severe pain. It appears in the back or abdomen, and is accompanied with a copious secretion of urine.
5. ***Alagi*** is of red and dark colour, in spots.
6. ***Masurikā*** is of small figure with a central depression of a yellow colour.
7. ***Sarsapika*** is of a light yellow colour, and has the figure of mustard seed.
8. ***Patirni*** is elevated, and is surrounded with small eruptions.
9. ***Bidārikā*** like a bulbous root, hard, and hot.
10. ***Bridadi*** is a kind of abscess.

These various forms of eruptions may be produced by the derangements of fat without the presence of *Prameha*; and they are not observable until they have arrived at their full size, as it does not affect the pulse, etc. When they appear about the anus, breast, head, shoulders, back, and other sensible or vital parts, and if accompanied with bad symptoms they are dangerous. When boils, are severe, and the internal heat is diminished, the physician is to give the case over as desperate. At the termination of the eruption, when there is thirst, cough, sloughing of the flesh, fainting, hiccough, delirium, slight fever, erysipelas in the temples, and the other sensible parts are very painful, so that the patient cannot be moved, the case will be fatal. Females are not liable to these diseases, as by the monthly discharge the body and humours are purified.

मेदोनिदानम्

अव्यायाम-दिवास्वप्न-श्लेष्मलाद्धारसेविनः।
मधुरोऽम्लरसः प्राय स्नेहाम्मेदः, प्रवर्द्धयेत्।।
मेदसावृतमार्गत्वात् पुष्यान्त्यन्ये न धावतः।
मेदस्तु चीयते तस्मादसक्तः सर्व्वकर्म्मसु।
क्षुद्रश्वास तृषा मोह स्वप्न क्रथनसादनैः।।
युक्तः क्षुत्स्वेददुर्गन्धै रल्पप्राणोऽल्पमैथुनः।
मेदस्तु सर्व्वभूताना मुदरेऽन्वस्थिसंस्थितम्।।
अतएवोदरे बृद्धिः प्रायो मेदस्विनी भवेत्।।

Samarogā or ***Bahumutra,*** is a disease only mentioned in modern books, most probably by its being classified as a variety of *Prameha.* Some manuscripts state that it is a disease peculiar to woman and is probably mistaken for Lucoreah, although generally considered to be Diabetes.[7]

It is produced by excessive venery, grief, much exertion, and poison. In this disease all the humours are deranged, and pass through the vessels of the urinary passages; and are discharged copiously, without pain, and pure like water. The woman becomes weak suddenly, and the discharge of urine becomes involuntary. The patient becomes uneasy with giddiness, and the mouth and palate become dry, followed by fainting and delirium. The skin is dry and rough, with great thirst.

GREAT FATNESS (*Medah.*)

Cause. When persons remain without exercise, sleep during the day, take too much ghee, milk, and preparations of sweetmeats, rice, and different kinds of indigestable cakes, the chyle becomes oily, and sweeter than natural, and as it circulates it produces fatness. It is accompanied by the following symptoms: – The person feels a difficulty of breathing, thirst, is not sensitive, is always sleepy and uneasy, and cannot excite the

मेदसावृतमार्गत्वाद्वायुकोष्ठे विशेषतः।
चरन् सम्बुक्षयत्यग्नि माहारं शेषयत्यपि॥
तस्मात् सशीघ्रं जरयत्याहार मभिकाङ्क्षति
विकारांश्चाप्नुते घोरान् कांश्रित् कालव्यतिक्रमात्।
एतातुपद्रव करौ विशेषादग्निमारुतौ॥
एतौ तु दहतः स्थूलं वनदावो वनं यथा।
मेदस्यतीव संवृद्धे सहसैवानिलादयः।
विकारान् दारुणान् कृत्वा नाशयत्याशु जीवितम्॥
मेदोमांसातिवृद्धत्वाच्चलस्फिगुदरस्तनः।
अयथोपचयोत्साहो नरोऽतिस्थूल उच्यते॥

उदरनिदानम्

रोगाः सर्व्वेऽपि मन्देग्नौ सुतरामुदराणि च।
अजीर्णन्मलिनैश्चान्नै र्जायन्ते मलसञ्चयात्॥
रुद्धा स्वेदाम्बुवाहीनि दोषाः स्त्रोतांसि सञ्चिताः॥

body or work; such a person has always a good appetite, has perspiration has a disagreeable smell, he has less inclination for women. He speaks indistinctly; and the other essential parts of the body are not nourished. The fat is alone inflamed, and such a person usually dies of diabetis, carbuncle, fever, fistula-in-ano, or large internal abscesses. He is also subject to disease of the air (bāyu), and the diseases he may contract are always severe.

ENLARGEMENT OF THE ABDOMEN (*Udara*)

This disease is divided into eight varieties, three of these are produced by derangements of the air, bile, and phlegm, and one by the combination of the three. The fifth is accompanied by enlargement of the spleen; the sixth is called *Baddaguda,* concretions; the seventh *Parisrābyudara,* or *Agantuka,* or accidental; and the eighth *Dakodara,* or Asitis.

प्राणग्न्यपानान् संदूष्य जनयन्त्युदरं नृणाम्॥
आध्मानं गमने शक्ति दौर्व्वल्यं दुर्व्वलाग्निता।
शोथः सदनमङ्गानां सङ्गो वातपुरीषयोः॥
दाहस्तन्द्रा च सव्वेषु जठरेषु भवन्ति हि।
पृथग्दोषैः समस्तैश्च प्लीहवद्धक्षतोदकैः।
सम्भावन्त्युदराण्यष्टौ तेषां लिङ्गं पृथक् शृणु॥
तत्र वातोदरे शोथः पाणिपान्नाभिकुक्षिषु।
कुक्षिपाश्र्वोदरकटीपृष्ठरुक्पर्व्वभेदनम्।
शुष्ककासोऽङ्गमर्द्दोऽधो गुरुता मलसंग्रहः।
श्यावारुणत्वगादित्वामकस्माद्वृद्धिह्रासवत्॥

This disease (*Udara*) is produced by eating bad food without an appetite; eating dry putrid food, and the improper administration of purgatives, emetics, and other active medicines by which the air, bile, and phlegm are deranged in the abdomen. The first symptoms of this disease resemble *Gulma;* followed by swelling of the abdomen. It is produced by the taking up of the fluid part of chyle, which is conveyed by air into the surface, and produces swelling under the skin, and enlargement of the abdomen.

The disease is ushered in by weakness, unhealthy colour of the skin, languor, and want of appetite. There are no wrinkles on the abdomen, which swells, while the rest of the body is thin, and prominent veins appear over the surface of the abdomen. He has pain in the pelvis; fulness in the abdomen, with burning; the feet swell, and the person is weak and cannot walk. By degrees the body swells, the air and dejections are stopped, the body is hot, and the person complains of faintness. The forms of this disease, called *Busrabi,* and *baddaguda* are incurable; the other forms are cured with much difficulty. In the latter stages of this diesease manual assistance or operations are sometimes required for the cure of the disease.

सतोदभेद मुदरं तनुकृष्णशिराततम्
आध्मातदृतिवच्छब्द माहतं प्रकरोति च।
वायुश्चात्र सरुक्शब्दो विचरेत् सर्व्वतो गतिः॥
पित्तोदरे ज्वरो मूर्च्छा दाहस्तृट् कटुकास्यता।
भ्रमोऽतीसारः पीतत्वं त्वगादावुदरं हरित्॥
पीतताम्रशिरानद्धं सस्वेदं सोष्म दह्यते।
धूमायते मृदुस्पर्श क्षिप्रपाकं प्रदूयते॥
श्लेष्मोदरेऽङ्गसदनं स्वाप-श्वयथु-गौरवम्।
निद्रोतक्लेशोऽरुचिः श्वासः कासः शुक्लत्वगादिता॥
उदरं स्तिमितं स्निग्धं शुक्लराजीततं महत्।
चिराभिवृद्धं कटिनं शीतस्पर्शं गुरुस्थिरम्॥

1. When diseased *air* produces this disease, the hands, feet, and abdomen are swelled, with pain in the sides of the abdomen, pit of the stomach, loins, and back, with pain in the joints as if they were broken. He complains of cough without expectoration, stretching and heaviness about the loins, the dejections and urine are constipated, the skin and eyes are of a dark yellow colour. The swelling is not always the same; sometimes it increases, and at other times decreases, with severe pain 'in, and over the abdomen. Dark coloured vessels are prominent over the abdomen, which is swelled like a leather bottle, and makes a noise like it when it is struck.

2. ***Bile.*** The symptoms of this variety are fever, faintness, burning thirst, and an acid taste in the mouth; the head swings round, looseness is produced, the eyes and skin are of yellow colour, the abdomen is of a green colour, and small yellow vessels appear upon the surface, with much perspiration; the body burns, there is a feeling as if smoke was rising in his throat, and the symptoms of bilious diseases; as well as the peculiar symptoms of this disease are quickly developed.

स्त्रियोऽन्नपानं नखलोममूत्र-विड़ार्त्तवैर्युक्त मसाधुवृत्ताः।
यस्मै प्रयच्छन्त्यरयो गरांश्च दुष्टाम्बुदूषी विषसेवनाद्वा॥
तेनाशु रक्तं कुपिताश्च दोषाः कुर्य्यु सुघोरं जठरं त्रिलिङ्गम्।
तच्छीतवाते भृशदुर्द्दिने च विशेषतः कुन्यति दह्यते च॥
स चातुरो मुह्यति हि प्रसक्तं पाण्डुः कृशः शुष्यति तृष्णया च॥
दूष्योदरं कीर्त्तितमेतदेव प्लीहोदरं कीर्त्तयतो निबोध।
विदाह्यभिष्यन्दिरतस्य जन्तोः प्रदुष्टमत्तर्य मसृक् कफश्च।
प्लीहातिवृद्धिं कुरुतः प्रवृद्धौ प्लीहोत्ममेतज्चठरं वदन्ति।
तद्वामपार्श्वे परिबृद्धिमेति विशेषतः सीदति चातुरोऽत्र।
मन्दज्वराग्निः कफपित्तलिङ्गैः रुपद्रुतः क्षीणबलीतिपाण्डुः॥
सव्यान्यपार्श्वे यकृति प्रवृद्धे ज्ञेयं यकृद्दाल्युदरं तदेव॥

3. ***Phlegm*** (*Shleshmodara*) when much deranged the person cannot work, is always sleepy, the abdomen swells, and there is no feeling in the abdomen, heaviness, sickness, no appetite, difficulty of breathing, cough, the eyes and skin are pale, abdomen cold, and the bowels are constipated; and white vessels appear upon its surface. After many days the swelling is completely formed, and is very difficult to remove. The body feels cold and hard, and the abdomen heavy.

When there is much pain, constipation and swelling of the abdomen, it proves that air is deranged; when faintness, thirst, heat, and fever are present, the bile is deranged; and when there is a sense of weight with no appetite, and hard abdomen, the phlegm is deranged.

4. The derangements of *air*, *bile,* and *phlegm* are said by the moderns to be often caused by enchantment, or by the use of Philters, as of a woman to her husband, or lover. For this purpose the parings of nails, the cuttings of hair, faeces, urine, menstrual blood, etc, are used, on the absurd supposition

उदावर्त्त रुजानाहैर्मोहतृडदद्वन ज्वरैः।
गौरवारुचिकाठिन्यैर्विद्यात्तत्र मलान् क्रमात्॥
यस्यान्तत्रमन्त्रैरुपलेपिभिर्व्वा बालाश्मभिर्वा पिहितं यथावत्।
सञ्चीयते तस्य मलः सदोषः शनैः शनैः शङ्करवच्च नाड्याम्॥
निरुध्यते तस्य गुदे पुरीषं निरेति कृच्छ्रादपि चाल्पमल्पम्।
हृन्नाभिमध्ये परिवृद्धिमेति तस्योदरं वद्धगुदं वदन्ति॥
शल्यं तथान्नोपहितं यदन्त्रं भुक्तं भिनत्यागत मन्यथा वा।
तस्मात् श्युतोऽन्त्रात् सलिलप्रकाशः स्त्रावः स्त्रवेद्वै गुदतन्तु मूयः॥
नाभे रधश्चोदर मेति वृद्धिं निस्तुद्यते दाल्यति चातिमात्रम्।
एतत् परिस्त्राव्युदरं प्रदिष्टं दकोदरं कीर्त्तयतो निबोध॥

of increasing their love towards them. Certain poisons administered by an enemy are said also to produce this disease. These causes not only derange the three humours, but also the blood. This form of disease is increased by cloudy weather, when the abdomen is swelled; and when the air is cold, it is also increased in violence, and the person becomes faint, the body yellow, the person very thin and dry, and he complains of thirst. This form of disease is called *Dakodara.*

5. ***Plihodara (spleen).*** This is a swelling of the abdomen with an enlargement of the spleen. It is produced by eating indigestable food, or of a heavy nature, as also articles which produce cold; as curdled milk, and articles which increase phlegm. These substances when frequently eaten derange blood and cough, and swell the spleen. In this disease there is languor, loss of appetite, and symptoms of deranged phlegm, etc. The person becomes very weak, and the body of a yellow colour. When the liver is swelled it is called *Jakrit Udara.* In this form the air, bile, and phlegm are deranged, and the disease is severe.

6. ***Baddaguda.*** This form is produced by the accumulation

यः स्नैहपीतो पन्युवासितो वा वान्तो विरिक्तोऽप्ययवा निरूढ़ः।
पिवेज्वलं शीतलमाशु तस्य स्त्रोतांसि दूष्यन्ति हि तद्वहानि॥
स्नेहो पलिप्तेष्वथवापि तेषु दकोदरं पूर्व्ववदभ्युपैति॥
स्निग्धं महत्तत् परिवृत्तनाभि समाततं पूर्णमिवाम्बुना च।
यथा दृतिः क्षुभ्यति कम्पते च शब्दायते चापि दकोदरं तत्॥
जन्मनैवोदरं सर्व्वं प्रायः कृच्छ्रतमं मतम्।
वलिन स्तदजाताम्बु यत्नसाध्यं नवोत्थितम्॥
पक्षाद्बद्धगुदं तूर्द्धं सर्व्वं जातोदकं तथा॥
प्रायो भवत्यभावाय छिद्रान्त्रं चोदरं नृणाम्॥
शूनाक्षं कुटिलोपस्थ मुपक्लिन्नतनुत्वचम्॥

of indigestable matter with the food, such as hair, gravel, etc. These form balls which produce constipation, and swelling occurs between the chest and umbiliacus. The person has stercoral vomiting, as a drain is stopped by an accumulation of filth. The air, bile, and phlegm are deranged at the obstructed part, and the faeces is confined. The stools are in small quantities, and are evacuated with great pain, the umbiliacus, and breast are much swelled.

7. ***Parisrābyudara*** is produced by sharp substances, such as fish bones, portions of wood, etc. being taken with the food, and wounding the canal. A watery discharge is evacuated by the anus, proceeding from the wounded surface. The abdomen increases in size under the umbiliacus with much pain and burning. It is to be treated as the last; but both are generally incurable. The other forms are cured with difficulty.

8. ***Asitis,*** (Jalodara, or Dakodara) When a person has taken a large quantity of prepared ghee, or has had frequent enemas, or after emetics or purgatives he drinks large quantities of cold water, they stop the absorbent vessels, and produce this

बलशोणितमांसाग्नि परिक्षीणञ्च वर्ज्जयेत्।
पाश्र्वभङ्गान्नविद्वेषः शोथातिसारपीड़ितम्।।
विरिक्तञ्चयप्युदरिणं पूर्य्यमानं विवर्ज्जयेत्।।

शोथनिदानम्

रक्त-पित्त-कफान् वायु र्दुष्टादुष्टान् वहिः शिराः।
नीत्वा रुद्धगति स्तैर्हि कुर्यऽत्वं मांससंश्रयम्।
उत्सेधं संहतं शोथं तमाहु र्निचयादतः।।
सर्व्वं हेतुविशेषैस्तु रूपभेदान्नवात्मकम्।

disease. In this case the abdomen becomes large, the umbiliacus prominent, and appears shining as of anointed and full of water, and like it moves about, and gives a sound like a leather bag.

In all these forms of diseases there is swelling, weakness, loss of appetite, languor, and swelling of different parts of the body, constipation, burning, and great thirst. When with these symptoms water collects, the disease is incurable.

SWELLINGS (*Shotha)*

Under this head is considered swellings of different kinds. When air is deranged, and mixes with the diseased blood, bile, and phlegm, it conveys them to the external parts of the body, stops the air-vessels, and their contents, which accumulate, and produce swellings.

This disease is caused by great fatigue in walking, with fasting; by eating much indigestable cakes, sour articles of food, vegetables, or clay; by salt, which debilitates the humours and by other indigestable, or unhealthy articles of food and mixtures. In other cases it is produced by leading a sedentary life, personal neglect of medicines. Uncleanness, injuries to

दोषैः पृथगद्वयैः सर्व्वै रभिघाताद्विषादपि॥
तत्पूर्वरूपं दवथुः शिराथामङ्गगौरवम्॥
शुद्ध्यामयाभुक्त-कृषाबलानां क्षाराम्लतीक्ष्णोष्ण गुरूपसेवा।
दध्याम मृच्छाकविरोधि दुष्ट गरोपसृष्टान्ननिषेवणञ्च।
अर्शांस्य चेष्टा न च देहशुद्धि र्मर्म्मोपघातो विषमा प्रसूतिः।
मित्थ्योप चारः प्रतिकर्म्मणाञ्च निजस्य हेतुः श्वयथोः प्रदिष्टः॥
सगौरवं स्यादनवस्थितत्वं सोत्रोधमुष्माथ शिरातनुत्वम्।
सलोमहर्षश्च विवर्णता च सामान्यलिङ्गं श्वयथोः प्रदिष्टम्॥
चलस्तनुत्वक् परुषोऽरुणोऽसितः सुसुप्तिहर्षार्त्तियुतोनिमित्ततः॥

vital parts, untimely parturition, the improper use of emetics and purgatives, and piles. These cause a swelling of the body, which is accompanied with pain and heaviness, restlessness, heat and discolouration of the body.

According to *Charaka* there are nine varieties of *Shotha,* three being produced by air, bile, and phlegm, when affected separately; three when two humours are deranged; one when three are deranged at the same time; one when caused by an injury, and one by poison. *Sushruta* does not allow that three varieties are produced by the combination of two diseased humours; and consequently considers this disease as having only five varieties produced by general, and one by a local, or accidental cause.

1. When *air* is deranged the swelling passes from one part to another, the skin is thin, the surface dry and soft, of a red or black colour, with dullness of feeling. The parts when pressed pit, but they recover the level on the pressure being removed. The symptoms increase in the day time.

2. When the swelling is produced by deranged *bile* the swelling is moist, and has a bad smell, is of yellow,

प्रशाम्यति प्रोन्नमति प्रपीड़ितो दिवाबली च श्वयथुः समीरणात्।
मृदुः सुगन्धोऽसितपीतरागवान् भ्रमज्वर-स्वेद-तृषा मदान्वितः।
य उष्यते स्पष्टरुगक्षिरागकृत् सपित्तशोथो भृशदाहपाकवान्॥
गुरुः स्थिरः पाण्डुरोचकान्वितः प्रसेक निद्रा वमिवह्निमान्द्यकृत्।
सकृच्छ्रजन्मप्रशमो निपीड़ितो नचोन्नमेद्रात्रिबली कफात्मकः॥
निदानाकृतिसंसर्गात् श्वयथुः स्याद्द्विदोषजः।
सर्व्वाकृतिः सन्निपाताच्छोथो व्यामिश्रलक्षणः॥
अभिघातेन शस्त्रादि छेदभेदक्षतादिभिः।
हिमानिलोध्यनिलैर्भल्लात-कपिकच्छुजैः॥

red and black colour, produces various kinds of pain, and ripens soon. In such cases the body is soon fatigued, and patient is feverish, perspires much, complains of thirst, and dullness, the pulse is very frequent, his eyes of a red colour, and the pain is severe.

3. *Phlegm. Dropsy* is characterized by always remaining in one place, is of a yellowish pale, and shining colour, is cold and hard, and painfully itchy. The patient has no appetite, and cough is discharged from the mouth and nose, the person is always sleepy, the swelling and the internal heat are diminished, and when the disease occurs it causes much uneasiness to the person, and is cured slowly. Pressure does not diminish this variety, the symptoms of which increase at night.

4,5,6,7. When two of the above humours are deranged, the symptoms of both forms of the two humours, stated above, are present; and when three are deranged, all the symptoms are present in the separate varieties.

8. *Accidental Swellings (Abhighātaja shotha)*, when the body is wounded by a cutting instrument, by injuries;

रसैः शूकैश्च संस्पर्शाच्छ्वयथुः स्याद्वि सर्पवान्।
भृशोष्म लोहिताभासः प्रायसः पित्तलक्षणः॥
विषजः सविषप्राणि परिसर्पणमूत्रणात्।
दंष्ट्रा दन्तनखाघातादविषप्राणिनामपि॥
विन्मूच-शुक्रोपहतमलवद्वस्त्रशङ्करात्॥
विषवृक्षानिलष्पर्शात् गरयोगावचूर्णनात्।
मृदुश्चलोऽवलम्बी च शीघ्रो दाहरुजाकरः॥
दोषा स्वयथु मुर्द्धं कुर्व्वन्त्यमाशयस्थिताः।
पक्काशयस्था मध्ये तु वर्च्चःख्यानगतास्त्वधः॥
कृतस्नदेहमनुप्राप्ता कूर्य्युः सर्व्वसरं तथा।

or when bruises by and accident, brēathing cold air, and the air of the ocean is of much use. The vapour or juice of the marking-nut (*bhallātaka*) applied to the body, or rubbing the part with cowach (*kapikachchhū*) will be of use. These produce swelling, heat, and redness, accompanied with the other symptoms of diseased bile. Bad water, either drank, or with which the body is washed, produces such swellings of parts.

Bishaja-shotha. When the poison of any animal is taken by the mouth, is introduced into the system by a wound, or by contact; when urine is applied to a wound, or the person wears a cloth that is dirty, is covered with excrement, or he breathes air coming from a poisonous tree it produces this form of swelling. The application of the powder of different poisonous articles, or or certain animals walking over the body, produce the same effect. Thus if frogs, etc., discharge their urine upon a part, it swells. The poison is either discharged from the trunk, teeth, or nails of the animal into the wound. By such causes the part swells, becomes pendulous, and is accompanied with pain. These swellings are soft, rise quickly, and are not fixed in one place, but move about. Sometimes they are quickly produced, and increase downwards (*distid*); and are very hot, and painful.

यो मध्येदेशे श्वयथुः स कष्टः मर्व्वगश्च यः।
अर्द्धाङ्गे रिष्ट भुतः स्याद यश्चोर्द्धं परिसर्पति॥
श्वासः पिपासा छर्द्दिश्च दौर्व्वल्यं ज्वर एवच।
यस्य चान्ने रुचिर्नास्ति श्वयथुतं विवर्ज्जयेत्॥
अन्येपद्वकृतः शोथः पादसमुत्थितः॥
पुरुषं हन्ति नारीञ्च मुखजो गुदजो द्वयम्।
नवोऽनुपद्रवः शोथः साध्योऽसाध्यः पुरोरितः।

When air, bile, and phlegm are deranged in the stomach (*āmāsiya*), the swelling occurs in the head and upper extremities, when deranges in the small intestines (*paukashaya*), the swelling will occur in the trunk, and when in the rectum (*andaka*), the swelling will occur in the lower extremities. When air, bile, and phlegm are deranged over the body, it will swell the whole body, and pass from one part to another.

When the swelling occurs in the trunk of the body it will be cured with difficulty, and also when the swelling is over the body. When the upper or lower half of the body is affected the disease is dangerous, or when the swelling proceeds proximated from the part first affected.

The swelling will not be cured when the person breathes with noise and difficulty, when accompanied with thirst, vomiting, weakness, hiccough and fever, and when he has no appetite, and is affected with diarrhoea and severe pain (*sul*). Such a diseased person will die. When the swelling commences in the feet of the male, or in the face of the female, both are very dangerous. It is also very dangerous in both sexes, when the swelling is about the anus.

When the swelling is recent, with no bad symptoms, it will be cured. When the throat and vital parts are swelled with much pain; or when it attack and vital parts are swelled with much pain; or when it attack infants, or old persons, or very weak persons, the disease will be fatal.

विवर्ज्जयेत् कुक्षुयदराश्रितञ्च तथा गले मर्म्मणि संश्रितञ्च स्त्यूलः
खरश्चापि भवेद्विवर्ज्जयो यश्चापि बालस्थविराबलानाम्।।

वृद्धिनिदानम्

क्रुद्धोऽनुद्धर्योगतिर्वायुः शोथशूलकरश्चरन्।
मुष्कौ वङ्क्षणतः प्राप्य फलकोषाभिवाहिनीः।।
प्रपीड्य धमनीर्वृद्धिं करोति फलकोषयोः।
दोषस्त्रमेदोमूत्रान्त्रैः स वृद्धिः सप्तधा गदः।
मूत्रान्त्रजानन्यनिलाद्धेतुभेदस्तु कैवलम्।।

SHLIPADA (*Elephantiasis.*)

In the *Mādhab Nidān* it is stated that the partient's groin first swells, and become very painful, with fever. The swelling then slowly descends to the foot, producing this disease. In other books, it is stated that the same disease may occur in the hands, ears, eye-lids, nose, lips, and penis. When it occurs in the groin, and descends to the leg and foot, or when situated in the hand it is produced by bad flesh and fat; and the parts affected become hard and rough.

When air produces this disease the swelling is of a black colour, rough dry, with cracks and small sores. This form is very painful, and occurs suddenly, with much fever.

When produced by diseased bile it is of a yellowish colour, hot, soft, and accompanied with fever.

When produced by diseased phlegm, the skin is shining, of white or grey colour, the part is very heavy, hard, fixed to one place, and has the appearance of large white-ant's hill, of an irregular sharp-pointed appearance. This form is difficult to cure after it has been present a year, when very large, when it discharges continually, is itchy, and when all the above symptoms are present, as this indicates that air, bile, and phlegm are diseased.

Elephantiasis is most frequent in those countries where

वापूर्णदृतिस्प्रर्शो रुक्षो वातादहेतु रुक्।
पक्कोडुम्बरसंकाशः पित्ताद्दाहोसम्पाकवान्॥
कफाच्छ्रोतो गुरुः स्निग्धः कण्ठमाच कठिनोऽल्परुक्।
कृष्णास्फोठावृतः पित्तः वृद्धिलिङ्गश्च रक्तजः।
कफ वन्मेदसा वृद्धि मृदुस्तालफलोपमः॥
मूत्रधारणशीलस्य मूत्रजः स तु गच्छतः।
अम्भोभिः पूर्णदृतिवत् क्षोभं यति सरुङ् मृदुः।
मूत्रकृच्छ्रमधः स्याच्च चलयन् फलकोषयोः॥
वातकोपिभि राहारैः शीततोयावगाहनैः।
धारने रणभाराध्व-विषमाङ्गप्रवर्त्तणैः॥
क्षोभनैः क्षुभितोऽऽन्यैश्च क्षुद्रान्त्रावयवं
यदा पवनो विगुणीकृत्य स्वनिवेशादधो नयेत्॥

there is much stagnant water, and in cold damp situations, such as Rungpore, Farridpore, etc.

In the above description the marked accessions and remissions are not mentioned, but it is stated that the damp and cold situations produce this disease, that it attacks different parts of the body, and that it is incurable, after it has remained upwards of a year, or is very large. It is also observed that it is incurable, when the skin is much affected, as indicated by the continual discharge, the itchy or painful nature of the swelling, and its discolouration.

DISEASES OF THE MALE ORGANS OF GENERATION

Diseases of the Scrotum, (Briddhi)

There are seven varieties of swelling of the scrotum produced by air, bile, phlegm, blood, fat, urine, and by the descent of the intestine. Any of those deranged humours may produce the swelling of the scrotum, or the testicle. The bowel, only causes the swelling of the scrotum. The preceding symptoms are pains in the loins, pelvic region, and penis, followed by the swelling of the scrotum.

कुर्य्याद्वङ्क्षणसन्धिख्यो ग्रन्थामं श्वयथुं तथा।
उपेक्ष्यमाणस्यच मुष्कवृद्धि माध्मानरुक् स्तम्भवतीं सवायुः।
प्रपीड़ितोऽन्तः स्वनवान् प्रयाति प्रध्मापयन्नेति पुनश्च मुक्तम्।
अन्त्रबुद्धिरसाध्योऽयं वातवृद्धिसमाकृतिः॥

गलगण्डगण्डमालापचीग्रन्थ्यर्व्वुदनिदानम्

निबद्धः श्वयथुर्य्यस्य मुष्कवल्लम्बते गले।
महान् वा यदि वा ह्रस्वो गलगण्डं तमादिशेत्॥
वातः कफश्चापि गले प्रदुष्टो मन्ये च सश्रित्य तथैव मेदः।
कुर्व्वन्ति गण्डं क्रमशः स्वलिङ्गैः समन्वितं तं गलगण्डमाहुः॥
तोदान्वितः कृष्णशिरावनद्धः श्यावोऽरुणो वा पवनात्मकस्तु।
पारुर्ष्ययुक्तश्चिरवृद्धपाको यदृच्छया पाकमियात् कदाचित्॥
वैरस्यमास्यस्य च तस्य जन्तो र्भवेत्तथा तालुगलप्रशोषः।
स्थिरः सवर्णो गुरुरुग्रकण्डुः शीतो महांश्चापि कफात्मकस्तु॥
चिराभिवृद्धिं भजते चिराञ्चा प्रपञ्चते मदरुजः कदाचित्।
माधुर्य्यमास्यस्य च तस्य जन्तोर्भवेत्तथा तालुगलप्रलेपः॥
स्निग्धोः गुरु पाण्डुरनिष्टगन्धो मेदोभवः कण्डुयुतोऽल्परुक् च।
प्रलम्वतेऽलावुवदल्पमूलो देहानुरुपक्षयवृद्धियुक्तः॥
स्निग्धास्यता तस्य भवेच्च जन्तो र्गलेनु शब्दं कुरुते च नित्यम्।

Symptoms. When the swelling is produced by deranged air the scrotum is extended as a bag of air, the surface is rough, and the peculiar pain produced by air is felt in the scrotum.

When produced by bile the swelling is red like the red fig, has a burning sensation and is accompanied with fever. In this form suppuration soon takes place.

When caused by diseased *phlegm,* the swelling is hard, is not painful, the surface is cool, it is itchy, and is not accompanied with fever.

कृच्छ्राच्छसन्तं मृदु सर्व्वगात्रं संवत्सरातीत मरोचकार्त्तम्।।
क्षौणञ्च वैद्यो गलगण्डयुक्त्वं भिन्नस्वरञ्चापि विवर्ज्जयेच्च।।
कर्कन्धुकोलामलकैः प्रमाणैः कक्षांस-मन्या-गलवङ्क्षणेषु।
मेदः कफाम्यां चिरमन्दपाकैः स्याद्धण्डमाला बहुभिश्च गण्डैः।।
ते ग्रन्थैयः केचिदवाप्तपाकाः स्त्रवन्ति नस्यन्ति भवन्ति चान्ये।
कालानुवद्धं चिरमादधाति सैवापचीति प्रवदन्ति तज्ज्ञाः।।
साध्याः स्मृताः पीनस-पार्श्वशूल-कास-ज्वरच्छर्द्दियुता स्त्वसाध्याः।
वातादयो मांस-मसृक्-प्रदुष्टाः संदुष्य मेदश्च तथा शिराश्च।
वृंत्तोन्नतं विग्रथितञ्च शोघं कुर्व्वन्त्यतो ग्रन्थिरिति प्रदिष्टः।।
आयम्यते बृश्चति तुद्यते च प्रत्यस्यते मथ्यति भिद्यते च।
कृष्णो मृदुवस्तिरिवाततश्च भिन्नः स्त्रजेच्चानिलजास्त्र मच्छम्।।
दंदह्यते धुप्यपि वृश्चते च पापच्यते प्रज्वलतीव चापि।।
रक्तः स पीतोऽप्याथ्वापि पित्तात् भिन्नं स्त्रवेदुष्णा मतीव चास्त्रम्।
शीतो विवर्णोऽल्परुजोऽतिकण्डुः पाषाणवत् संहननोपपन्नः।।
चिराभिवृद्धिश्च.कफप्रकोपाद्भिन्नस्त्रवेछुक्लघनञ्च पूयम्।
शरीरवृद्धि क्षयवृद्धि हानिः स्निग्धो महान् कण्डुयुतो रुजश्च।।
मेदः कृतो गच्छति चात्र भिन्ने पिण्याक सर्पिः-प्रतिमं तु मेदः।
व्यायामजातै रवलस्य तैस्तैराक्षिप्य वायुस्तु शिराप्रतानम्।।
संकुच्य संपीड्य विशोष्य चापि ग्रन्थिं करोत्युन्नतमाशु वृत्तम्।

Produced by *blood* the swellling is surrounded with black tubercles, and is accompanied with the symptoms of bile.

Fat produces the disease which is characterized by softness, shining, itchiness, and little pain. It becomes like the fruit of the palm tree; that is rough and tuberculated.

The form produced by *urine* (yellow serum), collected between the testicle and its external covering, moves like a bag of water.

The last form is herina which is produced by carrying

ग्रन्थिः शिराजः स तु कृच्छसाध्यो मवेद् यदि स्यात् सरुजश्चलश्च।
सचारुजश्चाप्यचलो महांश्च मर्म्मोत्थितश्चापि विवर्ज्जनीयः।।
गात्रप्रदेशे क्वचिदेव दोषाः संमूर्च्छिता मांस भसृक् प्रदूष्य।
वृत्तं स्थिरं मन्दरुजं महान्त मनल्पमूलं चिरवृद्ध्यपाकम्।।
कुर्व्वन्ति मांसोच्छ्रयमत्यगाधं तदर्व्वुदं
शास्त्रविदो वदन्ति वातेन पित्तेन कफेन
ज्चापि रक्त्वेन मांसेन च मेदसा वा तज्जायते
तस्य च लक्षणानि ग्रन्थेः समानानि तदा भवन्ति।
दोषः प्रदुष्टो रुधिरं शिराश्च संकूच्य संपीड्य ततस्तपाकम्।।
सास्त्रवमुन्नह्यति मांसपिण्डं मांसाङ्कुरै राचित माशु वृद्धिम्।।
करोत्यजस्त्र रुधिराप्रवृत्ति समाध्य मेतद्रुधिरात्मकन्तु।
रक्तक्षयोपद्रव-पीड़ितत्वात् पाण्डुर्भवेदर्ब्वुद पीड़ितस्तु।।
मुष्टिहारादिभिरर्द्दितेऽङ्गे मांसं प्रदुष्टं जनयेद्धिशोथम्।
अवेदनं स्निग्धमनन्यवर्णं मपाकश्मोप मप्रचाल्यम्।।

heavy weights, by fighting with strong persons, falling or jumping, and the like. By such causes air is deranged, which propels the intestine downwards, it remains in the groin, and if not treated for some days it descends still lower, and produces a swelling of the scrotum. The tumor is oblong, and when pressed it passes upwards with a peculiar noise, and again descends when the pressure is removed.

Antrabriddhi (Hernia) is incurable, unless when it is recent and situated in the groin.

Brishanakachchhū, (itchiness of the scrotum *pruzigo*). This is a common and troublesome disease. Medical authors say that it is produced by not attending cleanliness, by which the perspiration is accumulated, which irritates and produces an eruption on the part. This sometimes degenerate into sores.

प्रदुष्ठमांसस्य नरस्य गाढ़ मेतद्भवेन्मांसपरायणस्य।
मांसार्व्वुदं ते तदसाध्यमुक्त्वं साध्येध्वपीमानि तु वर्ज्जयेच्च
संप्रश्रुतं मर्म्मणि यच्च यातं स्त्रोतःमु वा यच्च भेवदचाल्यम्।
यज्जाययेऽन्यत्, खलु पूर्नवृते ज्ञेयं तदध्यर्व्वू दमर्व्व् दज्ञैः॥
यद्दन्द्वजातं युगपत् क्रमाद्वा द्विरव्वुदं तच्च भवेदसाध्यम्।
न पाकमायाण्डि कफाधिकत्वात् मेदो बहुत्वाच्च विशेषवस्तु॥
दोषस्थिरत्वात् ग्रहणाच्च तेषां सर्व्वासर्व्वु दान्तेव निसर्गतस्तु।

श्लीपदनिदानम्

यः सज्वरो वङ्कणजो भृशार्त्तः शोथो नृणां पादगतः क्रमेण।
तत् श्लीपदं स्यात् करकर्णनेत्र शिनश्निौष्ठनासास्वपि केचिदाहुः॥
वातजं कृष्णरुक्षञ्च स्फुटितं तीव्रवेदनम्।
अनिमित्तरुजं तस्य बहुशो ज्वर एवच॥

SCROFULOUS SWELLINGS (*Gandamālā)*

When many small tumors like plums appear in the axilla, neck, back, and groins, they are produced by diseased fat, and phlegm. They suppurate slowly, and continue to appear and suppurate for a long period, when it is called *Apachi*. When not attended by any bad constitutional disease it is curable, but when accompanied with *Coriza,* with pain in the sides, cough fever, and vomiting, it is incurable.

GOITRE (*Galaganda)*

The swelling of the throat, whether it be small or large, is called by this name. It is of an oblong form like the scrotum. It is produced when air and phlegm are diseased in the throat, and diseased fat slowly produces it.

When air is diseased there is pain in the throat, and black veins spread over it. The swelling is of green or red colour, dull and irregular. This form increases slowly and rarely suppurates; but, when it does it is without any apparent cause.

पित्तजं पीतसङ्काशं दाहज्वरयुतं मृदु।
श्लैष्मिकं स्निग्धवर्णञ्च श्वेतं पाण्डु गुरु स्थिरम्।
वल्मीकमिव संजातं कण्ठकै रूपचीयते॥
अब्दात्मकं महत्तच्च वर्ज्जनीयं विशेषतः।
त्रीण्यप्येतानि जानीयात् श्लीपदानि कफोच्छ्रयात्॥
गुरुत्वञ्च महत्वञ्च यस्मान्नास्ति कफं बिना।
पुरानोदकमूयिष्ठाः सर्व्वर्त्तुषु च शीतलाः॥
ये देशास्तेषु जायन्ते श्लीपदानि विशेषतः।
सास्त्रवमत्युन्नतसर्व्वलिङ्गं सकण्डुरं श्लेष्मयुतं विवर्ज्यम्॥

विद्रधिनिदानम्

त्वग्रक्तमांसमेदांसि संदूष्यास्थि-समाश्रिताः।
दोषाः शोथं शनैर्घोरं जनयन्त्युच्छ्रिता मृसम्॥
महामूलं रुजावन्तं वृत्तं वाप्यथवायतम्।

The person has a bad taste in his mouth, with dryness of the palate and throat.

Phlegm. In this variety the swelling is hard, fixed, cold, and the colour is not altered. It increases slowly, is heavy, itchy, and large, and sometimes suppurates. The taste of the mouth is sweetish, and the palate and throat is as if covered with some matter.

When produced by diseased *fat* it is slow in its increase, and suppurates with little pain, and is of the shape of a pumpkin (*kadu*), with a small root. The swelling increases, and diminishes with changes in the size of the body. The face is shining as if anointed. The swelling is heavy, of a yellowish colour, and of a bad smell. It is itchy and painful, accompanied with a peculiar change in the voice. The unfavourable symptoms are difficulty in breathing, softness of the part, and after it has continued for one year, it is accompanied with dyspepsia, and hoarseness. When the person is thin and weak he will die.

स विद्रधिरिति ख्यातो विज्ञेयः षड्विधश्च सः॥
पृथग्दोषैः समस्तैश्च क्षतेनाप्यसृजा तथा।
षणामपि हि तेषान्तु लक्षणं संप्रचक्ष्यते॥
कृष्णोऽरुणो वा विषमो भृशमत्यर्थवेदनः।
चित्रोत्थान-प्रपाकश्च विद्रधि र्वातसम्भवः॥
पक्कोडम्बरसङ्काशः श्यावो वा ज्वरदाहवान्।
क्षिप्रोत्थान-प्रपाकश्र विद्रधिः पित्तसम्भवः॥
शरावसदृशः पाण्डुः शीतः स्निग्धोऽल्प-वेदनः।
चिरोत्थानप्रपाकश्च विद्रधिः कफसन्धवः॥
तनुपीतासिताश्चैषा मास्त्रावाः क्रमशः स्मृताः।
नानावर्णो रुजास्त्रावो घाटालो विषमो महान्॥
विषमं पच्यते चापि विद्रधिः सान्निपातिकः।
तै स्तै र्भावै रभिहते क्षते वा पथ्यकारिणः।
क्षतोष्मावायु विसृतः सरक्तं पित्तमीरयेत्॥
ज्वर स्त्रष्णा च दाहश्च जायते तस्य देहिनः।
आगन्तुविद्रधि ह्येष पित्तविद्रधिलक्षणः॥
कृष्णाष्फोटावृतः श्याव स्तीव्रदाह रुजाकरः
पित्तविद्रधिलिङ्गस्तु रक्तविद्रधिरुच्यते।
पृथक् सम्भूय वा दोषाः कुपिता गुल्मरूपिणम्।
वल्मीकवत् समुन्नद्ध मन्तः कुर्व्वन्ति विद्रधिम्
गुदे वस्तिमुखे नाभ्यां कुक्षौ षङ्क्षणायोस्तथा।
वृक्कयोः प्लीह्नि यकृति हृदि वा क्लोम्लि वाप्यथ॥
तेषामुक्तानि लिङ्गानि वाह्यविद्रधिलक्षणैः
अधिष्ठानविशेषेण लिङ्गं श्रृणु विशेषतः॥
गुदे वातनिरोधश्च वस्तौ कृच्छ्राल्पमूत्रता॥
नाभ्यां हिक्का तथाटोपः कुक्षौ मारुतकोपनम्॥
कटीपृष्ठग्रहस्तीव्रो वङ्क्षणोत्थे तु विद्रधौ।
वृक्कयोः पार्श्वसंकोचः प्लीह्युच्छासावरोधनम्॥

सर्व्वाङ्ग-प्रग्रहस्तीव्री हृदि कामश्च जायते।
श्वासो यकृति हिक्का च क्लोम्नि पेपीयते पयः।
नाभेरुपरिजाः पक्का यान्तूर्द्ध मितरे त्वध्यः।
अधःश्रुतेषु जीवेत्तुश्श्रुतेवर्द्धं न जीवति॥
हृन्नाभिवस्तिवर्प्या ये तेषु भिन्नेषु वाह्यतः।
जीबेत् कदाचित् पुरुषो नेतरेषु कदाचन॥
साध्य विद्रधयः पञ्च विर्वज्ज्यः सान्निपातिकः।
आमपक्व विदग्धत्वं तेषां शोथवदादिशेत्॥
आध्मातं वद्धनिष्यन्दं छर्द्दिहिक्कातृषान्नितम्।
रुजाश्वाससमायुक्तं विद्रधिर्नाशयेन्नरम्॥

व्रणशोथनिदानम्

एकदेशोत्थितः शोथो व्रणानां पूर्व्वलक्षणन्।
षड्विधः स्यात् पृथक् सर्व्व रक्तजागन्तुजस्तस्तथा॥
शोथाः षड़ेते विज्ञेयाः प्रागुक्तैः शोथलक्षणैः।
विशेषः कथ्यते चैषां पक्वापक्वादिनिश्चये॥
विषमं पच्यते वातात् पित्तोत्थश्चाचिराच्चिरम्।
कफजः पित्तवच्छोथो रक्तागन्तुसमुद्भवः॥
मन्दोष्मताल्पशोथत्वं काठिन्यं त्वक् सवर्णता।
मन्दवेदनता चैतत् शोथानामामलक्षणम्।
दह्यते दहनेनेव क्षारेणैव च पच्यते।
पिपीलिकागणेनेव दश्यते छिद्यते तथा॥
भिद्यते चेव शस्त्रेण दण्डेनेव च ताड्यते।
पीड्यते पाणिनेवान्तः सूचीभिरिव तुद्यते॥
सोषाचोषो विवर्णः स्यात् अङ्गुल्येव्यावघट्यते।
आसने शयने स्थाने शान्तिं वृश्चिकविद्धवत्॥
न गच्छेदाततः शोथो भवेदाध्मातवस्तिवत्।

ज्वरस्तृष्णारुचिश्चैवं पच्यमानस्य लक्षणम्।
वेदनोपशमः शोथो लोहिताल्पो न चोन्नतः।
प्रादुर्भावो बलीनाञ्च तोदः कण्डू र्मुहुर्मूहुः॥
उपद्रवाणां प्रशमो निम्नता पुठनं त्वचाम्।
वस्ताविवाम्ब सञ्चारः स्याच्छोथेऽङ्गुलिपीड़िते॥
पूयस्य पीड़यत्येक मन्तमन्ते च पीड़िते।
भक्त्वाकाङ्क्षा भवेच्चैच्दोथानां पक्कलक्षणम्॥
नर्त्तेऽनिलाद्रुग्न विना च पित्तं, पाकः कफञ्चापि विना न पूयः।
तस्माद्धि सर्व्वं परिपाककाले पचन्ति शोथा स्त्रिभिरेव दोषैः॥
कक्षं समाश्रिता यथैव वह्निः वान्यीरितः संदहति प्रसह्य।
तथैव पुयो ह्यविनिःसृतो हि मांसं शिरा स्नायु च खादतीह॥
यश्छिनत्त्यममज्ञानात् यो वा पक्क मुपेक्षते।
श्वपचाविव मन्तव्यौ तावनिश्चितकारिणौ।
आमं विदह्यमानञ्च सम्यकं पक्कञ्च यो भिषक्।
जानीयात् स भवेद्वैद्यः शेषा स्तस्करवृत्तयः॥

शारीरव्रणनिदानम्

द्विधा व्रणः स विज्ञेयः शारीरागन्तुभेदतः।
दोषै राद्यस्तयोरन्यः शास्त्रदिक्षतसम्भवः॥
स्तब्धः कठिनसंस्पर्शो मन्दस्रावो महारुजः।
तुद्यते स्फुरति श्यावो व्रणो मारुतसम्भवः॥
तृष्णा मोहज्वरक्लेद-दाह-दुष्टऽवदारुणैः।
व्रणं पित्तकृतं विद्यात् गन्धैः स्त्रावैश्च पूतिकैः
बहुपिच्छो गुरुः स्निग्धः स्तिमितो मन्दवेदनः॥
पाण्डुवर्णोऽल्पसंक्लेद श्चिरपाकी कफव्रणः।
रक्तो रक्तश्रुतीरक्ताद्द्विवत्रिजः स्यात्तदन्वयैः॥
त्वङ्न्यासजः सुखे देशे तरुणस्यानुंपद्रवः।
धीमतोऽभिनवः काले सुखेः साध्यः सुखं व्रणः॥

गुणैरन्यतमैर्हीनस्ततः कृच्छ्रो व्रणः स्मृतः।
सर्व्वैर्विहीनो विज्ञेय स्त्वसाध्यो भूर्युवपद्रवः॥
पूतिः पूयातिदुष्टासृक् स्त्राव्युत्सङ्गी चिरस्थितिः।
दुष्टो व्रणोऽति दुर्गन्धः शुद्धलिङ्गो विपर्य्ययः॥
जिह्वातलामृदु श्लक्ष्णः स्निग्धो विगतवेदनः।
सुव्यवस्थो निरास्त्रावः शुद्धो व्रण इति स्मृतः॥
कपोतवर्णप्रतिमा यस्यान्ता क्लेदवर्ज्जिताः।
स्थिराश्च पिड़कावन्तो रोहतीति तमादिशेत्॥
रूढ़वर्त्मानमग्रन्थि मशूलमरुजं व्रणम्।
त्वक्सवर्णं समतलं सम्यगूढ़ं विनिद्रिशेत्॥
कुष्ठिनां विषयुष्टानां शोषिणां मधुमेहिनाम्।
व्रणाः कृच्छ्रेण सिध्यन्ति येषाञ्चापि व्रणे व्रणाः॥
वसां भेदोऽथ मज्जानां मस्तुलुङ्गञ्च यः स्त्रवेत्।
आगन्तुजो व्रणः सिद्धेत् न सिद्धेद्दोषसम्भवः॥
मद्यगुर्व्वाज्यसुमनः पद्मचन्दनचम्पकैः।
सगन्धा दिव्यगन्धाश्च मूमूर्षुणां क्रणाः स्मृताः॥
ये च मर्म्मसु सम्भूता भवन्त्यत्यर्थ भेदना।
दह्यते चान्तरत्यर्थं वहिः शीताश्च ये व्रणाः।
दह्यते वहिरत्यर्थं भवन्त्यन्तश्च शीतलाः॥
प्राणमांसक्षयंश्वासकामारोचकपीड़िताः॥
प्रबृद्धपूयरुधिरा व्रणा षेषाञ्च मर्म्मसु॥
क्रियाभिः सम्यगारब्धा न सिद्ध्यन्ति च ये व्रणाः।
वर्ज्जयेदपि तान् वैद्यः संरक्षन्नात्मनो यशः॥

सद्योव्रण-निदानम्

नानाधारामुखैः शस्त्रै र्नानास्थान-निपातितैः।
भवन्त्यि नानाकृतयो व्रणस्तां स्तान्निबोध मे॥

छिन्नं भिन्नं तथा विद्ध क्षतं पिच्छिलमेव वा।
घष्ठमाहु स्तथा षष्ठं तेषां वक्ष्यामि लक्षणम्॥
तिर्य्यक् छिन्नमृजुर्वापि यो व्रणस्त्वायतो भवेत्।
गात्रस्य पातनं तद्धि छिन्नमित्यभिधीयते॥
शक्तिदन्तेषु खड्गाग्रविषाणै राशयोहतः।
यत् किञ्चित् प्रस्त्रवेत्तद्धि भिन्नलक्षणमुच्यते॥
स्थानान्यमग्निपक्कानां मूत्रस्य रुधिरस्य च।
हृदुण्डुकफुप्फुसश्च कोष्ठ इत्यभिधीयते॥
तस्मिन् भिन्ने रक्तपूर्णे ज्वरो दाहश्च जायते।
मूत्रमार्ग्गगुदास्येभ्यो रक्तं घ्राणाच्च गच्छति।
मूर्च्छा श्वास तृषाध्मात मभक्तच्छून्द्र एव च॥
विण्मूत्रवातसङ्गश्च स्वेदास्त्रावोऽक्षिरक्ता।
लोहगन्धित्वमास्यस्य गात्रदौर्गन्धमेव च॥
हृच्छलं पार्श्वयोश्चापि विशेषञ्चात्र मे शृणु।
आमाशयस्थे रुधिरे रुधिरं छर्द्दयत्यपि॥
आध्वानमपिमात्रञ्च शुलञ्च मृशदारुणम्।
पक्काशयगते चापि रुजाः गौरवमेव च॥
अधःकाय विशेषेण शीततो च भवेदिह।
मूक्ष्मास्य शल्याभितं यदङ्कस्त्वाशयं विनां
उत्तण्डितं निर्गतं वा तद्विद्ध मितिनिर्द्दिशेत।
नातिच्छिन्नं नातिभिन्नं उभयोर्लक्षणान्वितम्॥
विषमं ग्रणमङ्गेयत् तत्क्षन्त्वभिधीयते।
प्रहारपिड़नाभ्यान्तु यदङ्गं पृथुतां गतम्॥
सास्थि तत् पिच्छितं विद्यात् मज्जरक्त-परिप्लुतम्॥
घर्षणादभिघातादद्वा यदङ्कं विगतत्वंचम्।
उषास्त्रावान्वितं तच्च घृष्ठमिथ्यभिधीयते॥
श्यावं सशोथं पिड़काचितञ्च मुहुर्मूहुः शोणितवाहिनञ्च।

मुहुद्‌गतं बुद्बुदतुल्यमासं व्रणं सशल्यं सरुजं वदन्ति॥
त्वचोऽतित्य शिरादीनि भित्वा वा परिहृत्व्यं वा।
कोष्ठे प्रतिष्ठितं शल्यं कुर्य्याद्वक्त्वानुपद्रवान्।
तत्रान्तर्लोहितं पाण्डु शीतपादकराननं
शीतोच्छासं रक्तनेत्रमामद्धञ्च विवर्ज्जयेत्।
भ्रमः प्रलापः पतनं प्रमेहो विचेष्टणं ग्लानिरधोष्णता च।
स्त्रस्ताङ्गता मूच्र्छनमुर्द्धवात स्तीव्रा रुजो वातकृताश्च तास्ताः॥
मांसोदकाभं रुधिरञ्च गच्छेत् सर्व्वेन्द्रियार्थोपरमस्तथैव।
दशार्द्धसंख्येष्वथ विक्षतेषु सामान्यतो मर्म्मसु लिङ्गमुक्तम्॥
सुरेन्द्रगोपप्रतिम् प्रभुतं रक्तं स्त्रवेत्तत्क्षतजश्च वायुः।
करोति रोगान् विविधान् यथोक्तान् शिरासु छिन्नास्वथ वाक्षतासु॥
कोञ्जं शरीरावयवावसादः क्रियास्वसाक्तिस्तमूला रुजश्च।
चिरादूव्रणो रोहति। यस्यचापि तं स्नायुविद्धं पुरुषं व्यवस्येत्॥
शोषाभिवृद्धिस्तमूला रुजाश्च बलक्षयः सर्व्वत एव शोथः।
क्षतेषु सन्धिष्वचलाचलेषु स्यात् सर्व्वकर्म्मोपरमश्च लिङ्गम्॥
घोरा रुजो यस्य निशादिनेषु सर्व्वास्यवस्थासु च नैति शान्तिम्।
भिषग्विपश्चिद्विदितार्थसूत्र स्तन्तस्यिविद्धं पुरुसं व्यवश्वेत्॥
यथास्वमेतानि विभावयेच्च लिङ्गानि नर्म्मस्वभिताड़ितेषु।
पाण्डुविवर्णः स्पर्शनं न वेत्ति यो मांसमर्म्मण्यभिपीड़ितः स्यात्॥
विसर्पपक्षघातश्च शिरास्तम्नोऽपतानकः।
मोहोन्मादव्रणरुजो ज्वरः-स्तृष्णाऽनुग्रहः॥
कांसश्छर्द्दिरतीसारो हिक्का श्वासः सवेपथः।
षोड़शोपद्रवाः प्रोक्ता व्रणानां व्रणचिन्तकैः॥

भग्ननिदानम्

भग्नं सनसाद्विविधिं हुताभ काण्डे च सन्धौ च हि तत्र सन्धौ।
उत्पिष्ट विश्लिष्ट विवर्त्तितञ्च तिर्षग्गतं क्षिप्त मधश्च षट् च।

प्रसारणाकुञ्चनवर्त्तनोग्रा रुक्स्प्रर्शविद्वेशण मेतदुक्तम्॥
सामान्यतः सन्धिगतस्य लिङ्गमुत्पिष्टसन्धे श्वयथुः समन्तात्॥
विशेषतो रात्रि भवारुजा च विश्लिष्टजे तौ च रुजा च नित्यम्।
विवर्त्तिवे पार्श्वरुजश्च तीव्राः तिर्षवगते तीव्ररुजो भवन्ति॥
क्षिप्तेऽतिशूलं विषमत्वमस्थ्नोः क्षिप्ते त्वधोरुग्विधठश्च सन्धेः।
काण्डे ततः कर्कठकाश्वकर्ण-
विचूर्णितं पिच्छितमस्थि छल्लिकौ।
काण्डे च भग्नं क्ष्यतिपातितञ्च
मज्जागतञ्च स्फुठितञ्च वक्रम्॥
छिन्नं द्विधा द्वादशधापि काण्डे
स्त्रस्ताङ्गता शोथ रुजाति वृद्धिः।
संपीड्यमाने भवतीह शब्दः
स्तर्शासिह स्प्रन्दन वोद मूलाः॥
सर्व्वास्ववस्थासु न शम्नालाभो
भग्नस्य काण्डे खलु चिह्नमेतत्।
भग्नन्तु काण्डे बहुषाः प्रयाति
समासतो नामभिरेव तुल्यम्॥
अल्पाशिनो नात्यवती जन्तीर्वातात्मकस्य च।
उपद्रतैर्वा जुष्टस्य भग्नं कृच्छ्रेण सिद्धति।
भिन्नं कपालं कटयान्तु सन्धियुक्तं तथा चुतम्॥
जयनं प्रतिपिष्टञ्च वर्ज्जयेद्धि विचक्षणः।
असंश्लिष्ट कपालञ्च ललाटे चूर्णितञ्च यत्।
भग्नं स्तनान्तरे पृष्ठे शङ्के मूर्द्धि च वर्ज्जयेत्॥
सम्यक् सन्धितमपऽस्ति दुर्निक्षेपनिवन्धनात्।
संक्षोभाद्वापि यद्गच्छेद्विक्रियां तच्च वर्ज्जयेत्॥
तरुनास्थीति नाम्यन्ते भिद्यन्ते तलकानि च।
कपालानि विभज्यन्ते स्फुटन्ति रुचकानि च॥

नाड़ीव्रणनिदानम्

यः शोथमाममिति पक्कमुपेक्षतेऽज्ञो यो
वा व्रणं प्रचुर पूयमसाधुवृत्य।
अभ्यन्तरं प्रविशति प्रतिदार्य्य तस्य
स्थानानि पूर्व्वविहितानि ततः सपूयः॥
तस्यतिमात्रगमनाद्गतिरिष्यते तु नाड़ीव
यद्वहति तेन मता तु नाड़ी।
दोषैस्त्रिभिर्भवति सा पृथगेकशश्च
संमूच्छितैरपि च सल्यनिमित्ततोऽन्या॥
तत्रानिलात् परुषसूक्ष्ममुखी सशूला
फेनानुविद्धमधिकं स्त्रवति क्षपासु।
पित्तातृधाज्वरकरी परिदाहयुक्ता पीतं
स्त्रवत्याधिक मुष्णमहःसु चापि॥
ज्ञेयो कफाद्बहु घनार्ज्जुनपिच्छिलास्त्रा
स्तब्धा सकण्डुररुजा रजनीप्रवृद्धा॥
दाहज्वरश्वसनमूर्च्छवक्त्रशोषा यस्यां
भवन्त्यभिहितानि च लक्षणानि।
तामादिशेत् पवनपित्तकफोप्रकोपाद्
धोरामसंक्षयकरीमिव कालरात्रिम्॥
नष्ठं कथञ्चदनुमार्गमुदीरितेषु स्थानेषु
शल्यमचिरेण गतिं करोति।
सा फेनिलं मथित मूष्णमसृग्विमिश्रं
स्त्रावं करोति सहसा सरुजा च नित्यम्॥
नाड़ी त्रिदोषप्रभवा न सिद्धेच्छ्रेषाश्च
तिस्त्रः खलु यत्नसाध्याः॥

भगन्दरनिदानम्

गुदस्य द्व्यङ्गुले क्षेत्रे पार्श्वतः पिडकार्त्तिकृत्।
भिन्नो भगन्दरो ज्ञेयः स च पञ्चविधो मतः॥
कषाय रुक्षैस्त्वतिकोपितेऽनिल स्त्वपानदेशे पिड़कं करोति याम्।
उथेक्षणात् पाकमुपैति दारुणं रुजा च भिन्नारुण-फेनवाहिनी॥
तत्रागमो मूत्र-पुरिष रेतस्यं व्रणैरनेकैः शतपोनकं वदेत्॥
प्रकोपनैः पित्तमति प्रकोषितं करोति रक्तां पिड़कां गुदाश्रिताम्।
तदाशुपाका हिमपूतिवाहिनीं भगन्दरन्तूष्ट्रशिरोधरं वदेत्॥

FISTULA-IN-ANO (Bhagandara)

This disease is called *Bhagandara,* because the anus, vagina, bladder, and its surrounding parts, are affected.

It is produced by deranged air, bile, and phlegm and by their combinations, and by external injuries: thus five varieties of this disease are produced.

The symptoms of this disease are ushered in by pain in the loins of an intching nature, and by a swelling near the anus.

1. ***Satapanaka.*** This variety is produced by deranged air, from living on bad food, when accompanied by a bad temper. The swelling usually takes place a finger breadth from the anus, by the air deranging the flesh, and producing swelling and pain of different kinds. When not properly treated the swelling suppurates, and is perforated by many holes, through which a copious discharge of matter with air takes place. Sometimes the pain is as if the part was torn, or needles were thrust into it. Towards the termination air, urine, faeces, and semen is discharged from the opening.

2. ***Utragraba*** is produced by deranged bile, which affects the part, and produces a large red swelling resembling

कण्डुयनो घनस्त्रावी कठीनी मन्दवेदनः।
श्वेतावभासः कफजः परिस्त्रावी भगन्दरः॥
बहुवर्णरुजास्त्रावा पीड़का गोस्तनोपमा।
शम्बकावर्त्तवन्नाड़ी शम्बुकावर्त्तको मतः॥
क्षताद्गति पायुगता विवर्द्धते ह्यपेक्षणात् स्युः क्रिमयो विदार्यते।
प्रकुर्व्वते मार्गमनेकधा मुखै र्व्रणैस्तुदुन्मार्गि भगन्दरं वदेत्॥

the shape of the neck of camel. It produces a burning and painful sensation, like those produced by deranged bile. When neglected it suppurates, and terminates in ulcers. The parts feel burning, as if it was burnt with fire or caustics, and it discharges a foetid and hot fluid. If neglected in this state the air, urine, faeces and semen are discharged.

3. ***Parisrābi*** is produced by diseased *phlegm*. It is characterized by a white, hard, and itchy swelling near the anus, with the peculiar pain characteristic of diseased phlegm. If not properly treated it suppurates, and passes to ulceration. This is hard, itchy, and discharges freely a mucilaginous matter, followed by a discharge of air, urine faeces, and semen.

4. ***Sambūkābarta*** is produced by the combination of these three humours. It appears first in the form of a swelling, like the great toe, and is accompanied with different kinds of pains. It ulcerates, as in the other kinds, and discharges different coloured fluids.

5. ***Unmārga*** or the accidental form of fistula-in ano. When an ignorant person eats the bones with fish, or anima-flesh, they are carried to the rectum with thc hard faeces, and should they be in a transverse direction in the gut, the bones injure the parts, and produce inflammation, and ulceration. Matter is then discharged mixed with blood. When this variety is not properly cleaned, worms form in it, and various openings are formed, and the air, faeces, urine and semen are discharged from these openings. Sometimes an eruption forms rounds the

घोराः सा यावतु दुखाः सर्व्वं एव भगन्दराः।
तेष्वसाध्यः त्रिदोषोत्थः शतजश्च विषेशतः॥
वातमूत्रपुरीषाणि क्रिमयः शुक्रमेव च।
भगन्दरात् स्त्रवन्तस्तु नाशयन्तु तमातुरम्॥

उपदंशनिदानम्

हस्ताभिघातान्नखदन्तपाता दधावनादतुप्यसेवनाद्वा।
योनिप्रदोषाच्च्वं भवन्ति शिश्ने पञ्चोपदंशा विविधापचारैः॥
सतोदभेदस्फुरणः सकृष्णौः स्फोटैर्व्यवस्येत् पवनोपदंशम्।
पीतैर्बहुक्लेदयुतैः सदाहरपित्तेन रक्तात् पिशितावभासैः॥
स्फोटैः सकृष्णौ रुधिरस्त्रवन्त रक्तात्मकं पित्तसमानलिङ्गम्।

anus which is not fistulous. The pain is slight in this disease, and is spontaneously cured. In fistula-in-ano there is much pain accompanied with fever, and the patient feels much inconvenience in walking, or riding, and at the time of the evacuations. He complains likewise of pains in the loins.

All the forms of fistula-in-ano are cured. With difficulty, more particularly when produced by a derangement of the three humours, and by accidents, as by the gut being transfixed by bones, or the like.

SORES ON THE GENITAL ORGANS, (*Upadangsha.*)[8]

These diseases are supposed to be produced by mechanical injuries of the part, want of cleanliness, and washing with impure water, after sexual intercourse. It is also produced by impure connexion, excessive venery, and the stimulants sometimes employed to enlarge the penis. There are five different forms of these sores, which are distinguished from each other by their colour, and the nature of the discharge. These are:

1. ***Bātika,*** characterised by the black colour of the

सकण्डुरैः शोथयुतैर्महद्भिः शुक्लै धनस्त्रावयुतैः कफेन।।
नानाविधस्त्रावरुजोपपन्न मसाध्यमाहु स्त्रिमलोपदंशम्।
विशीर्णमांसं क्रिमिभिः प्रजग्धं मुष्कावशेषां परिवर्ज्जयेच्च।
संजातमात्रेन करोति मुढः क्रियां नरो यो विषये प्रसक्तः।।
कालेन शोथक्रिमिदाहपाकै र्विशीर्णशिश्नो म्रियते स तेन।
अङ्कुरैरिव संघातैरुपर्युपरि संस्थितैः।
क्रमेण यायते वर्त्ति स्ताम्रचूड़शिखोपमा।।

pustules (primary), by the lancinating pain, and white discharge.

2. ***Paittika*** is distinguished by the redness of pustules, by the burning pain, and bloody discharge from the part.
3. ***Shleshmika***. In this form the pustules is larger, and are attended with an itching sensation. The discharge is white, and thick.
4. ***Sannipātika.*** This is a complicated form of the disease, in which the above symptoms appear. It is considered incurable.
5. ***Agantuka, or accidental injuries*** of the organs of generation. In this description no secondary symptoms of syphilis are mentioned. The description is confined entirely to primary sores. The unfavourable symptoms of this oca disease is confined to the suppuration, sloughing, and destruction of the penis, and to the generations of worms in the sores. In such cases the disease was supposed to be incurable.

It is stated that these sores should be treated by an ignorant person, or should the person continue to have intercourse with women, he will die; from the of slonghing the parts, and the irritative fever which accompanies it.

कोषस्याभ्यन्तरे सन्धौ पर्व्वसन्धिगतापि वा।
अवेदना पिच्छिला च दुश्चिकित्सा त्रिदोषजा॥
लिङ्गार्त्तिरभिख्याता लिङ्गार्श इति चापरे।

शूकदोषनिदानम्

अक्रमाच्छेफसो वृद्धिं योभिवाञ्छति मूढ़धीः।
व्याधय स्तस्य जायन्ते दश चाष्टौ च शूकजाः॥
गैरसर्षसंस्थाना शूकदुर्भुग्नहेतुका।

Another local disease of the genitals is named *Mingubarti* (warts) and consists in excrescences near the vagina, between the scrotum and penis, or corona glandis. They appear crop after crop, and resemble a cock's comb; they are without pain, and are cured with difficulty.

HISTORY OF SYPHILIS (*Shukdosh*)

The history of Syphilis is so peculiar, and various opinions as to its origin has produced so much discussion that I shall here add a few remarks on the subject.

From the above account of these diseases of the genital organs, as given in the ancient Sanskrit writings, it appears that there were only five, or rather six, varieties of local sores to which they were liable. These are stated to have been produced by injuries, or other causes of irritation, such as want of cleanliness, etc; which are quite sufficient to account for the varieties of these sores, and resemble those recorded by the Jews. They are quite different from the peculiar disease known by the name of syphilis, or the venereal disease. The history of this disease in Europe affords the explanation of these peculiarities.

The venereal disease, as it now appears in its characteristic local and general features, seems to have been unknown before the return of Columbus to Spain, after the discovery of America (1494), when the sailors introduced the disease into Spain

पिड़का श्लेष्मवाताभ्यां ज्ञेया सर्षपिका तु सा,
कठिनै र्विषमैर्भुग्नै र्वायूनाष्ठीलिका भवेत्॥
शुकैर्यत् पूरितं शश्वदग्रथितं नाम तत् कफात्।

Astruc asseris, on the authority of Oviedo, the historian, and of many contemporary physicians, who flourished a short time after the period, that the disease was communicated to the Spaniards by the Indian women of Hispaniola, when Columbus first arrived in that country; and they, in their turn, communicated it to their country-women.

In the course of a year or two afterwards (1495) Ferdinand, king of Spain, sent an army under the command of the great Gonsalva de Cordova to the assistance of the Neapolitans, at that time engaged in a war with the French. The Spaniards infected the Neapolitans, who communicated the disease to the French. As they had not had the disease before they attributed it to the climate, and called it the "Mal de Naples." The Neapolitans, as much astonished as the French, and treating them as the hostile power, imagined that they had brought it to the country, and called it the French disease.

During such an age we can easily understand how the disease should be rapidly propagated over Europe when introduced into an army of mercinary soldiers, composed of nearly every nation of Europe, who thus conveyed the infection with them on their return to their respective homes; and explains many circumstances related of its progress in different countries. It was from the great intercourse at that time subsisting between the French and Scots that the disease first appeared in Scotland, and it was not until a year afterwards that it appeared in England. Astruc assigns another cause in the licentious manners of the age, for the rapid spreading of the venereal disease, on its first appearance in Europe.

Soon after the appearance of the disease in Europe its ravages extended over a considerable part of Asia and Africa, as well as Europe. This is stated by Fracastorio, who flourished

कुम्भिका रक्तपित्तोत्था जाम्ववास्थिनिभा शुभा
तुल्यजास्तु लजीं विद्याद् यथाप्रोक्तां विचक्षण:॥
मृदितं पीड़ितं यच्च संरब्धं वातकोपत:।
पाणिभ्यां भृशसंमूढे संमूढपिड़का भवेत्॥

at the close of the fifteenth century, was an eye witness of the extnsive progress of the disease; and from his high medical reputation, and residence almost on the spot of its first appearance, and more largely engaged in the cure of it than any physician in his day, had the best opportunities of judging of the nature of the disease. He says, that the disease first appeared in central Europe and extended its revages from France to Great Britain, where it got the name of the French disease; and still approaching towards the East, at was called chuḍāmani danaḥ;" from which country it extended to Persia, where Mir Bahaū Daula Nur Baxsh was said to have been the first who described and treated the disease. From Persia it advanced into Hindustan, where it is still known by its Persian name; Nār Fārsi, Persian pox; or Jumra, blotches; or from its peculiar symptoms A, tshak, nocturnal fire; disease of foreigners, strangers, more especially of Europeans. Soon after (A.H. 950) in the time of Timur Lang, emperor of Persia, Amīr Imāmdin Muhammad Shirāzī wrote a short treatise on the venereal disease; in which he declares it to have been of recent origin, and, with the exception of Nur Baxsh is stated to have been the first who wrote correctly on the subject.

The same evidence is afforded by the Hindu writers. We have seen that the early writers gave minute and characteristic descriptions of the usual local diseases of these organs; and what is remarkable, syphilis has not got a Sanskrit name, but is named from the Europeans, who first visited these shores. This was more readily adopted, as the presence of the disease conveyed a feeling of disgust and reproach. It is in the modern Sanskrit compilations, such as *Bhābaprakāsa*, where the disease is named the "*Faringī Roga*," or Portuguese disease.

दीर्घा वह्वश्च पिड़का दीर्घन्ते मध्यतस्तु याः॥
सोऽधि सन्थः कफासृग्भ्यां वेदना रोमहर्षकृत्।
पिड़काचिता या पिड़का पित्तशोनितसम्भवा।

In this work the disease is characterized by all the symptoms of secondary syphilis, as detailed by European authors; such as cutaneous eruptions, and affections of the bones, particularly those of the nose and palate. In these modern works syphilis is divided into three varieties; one of which is characterized by the appearance of cutaneous eruptions, the second by diseases of the bones; and in the third variety both the skin and bones are affected. The disease is attributed to connection with Portuguese, whether male or female, and it was supposed that it could only by cured by the use of mercury. The same author likewise states that after the mercurial treatment has been completed, *Topchinī*, or China-root, must be administered to complete the cure.

We have thus a disease presenting characteristic appearances, and of peculiar virulence, without a Sanskrit name not even mentioned by the ancient Hindu medical writer; and still called by the name of the people who first visit these shores from Europe. But as the disease was also introduced into Hindustan from the south-east by the Portuguese, is was called the Portuguese or European *(faringhī)* disease; and likewise from Persia in the north-west, when the disease was named the "Persian pox." It was only after the disease was introduced from the north and south of Hindustan, that an account is recorded of the characteristic disease, by modern compilers, including both the local and constitutional symptoms. Hence it would appear that this disease was introduced from America to Europe and Asia, as the small-pox and measles seem to have first appeared in Asia, from whence they spread, and committed such ravages in Africa, Europe, and America.

The following proofs may be thus adduced of the venereal disease having been brought from America:—

पद्मकर्यिकसंस्थाना ज्ञेया पुष्करिका तु मा।
स्पर्शहानिस्तु जनयेच्छोनितं शूकदूषितम्।
मुद्‍गमाधोपमा रक्ता रक्तपित्तोद्भवा तु या।
वशधिरेषोत्तमा नाम शूकाजीर्ण निमित्ततः।

Ist. The opinion of ancient authors who have left us minute descriptions of disease, such as *Moses, Charaka, Sushruta, Hippocrates, Celsus,* etc.,not having mentioned the venereal disease. Local sores on the genitals, and even the occurrence of buboes, etc. beings no proof of the presence of this disease, without its specific secondary symptoms. Any irritating cause applied to the genitals would produce local sores, and if not properly attended to would inflame the inguinal glands; as sores on the feet are often found to produce the same swellings.

2nd. The consternation into which all Europe was thrown by the rapid progress of this fearful disease. Like all new diseases, soon after its introduction into Europe, by the followers of Columbus, it spread in the most alarming manner; or like that leprosy from the east, which at one time filled the Lazarhouses of Europe with its victims. Masses, prayers, and alms, were offered up to avert the anger of offended heaven; as the superstitious notions of the age made people believe that it was a dispensation from God, to correct the licentious, and wicked manners of the times. The severity of a new disease when it occurs in a country is seen in the visits of the small-pox, to islands, and distant countries; as occurred in Mauritius, and committted such dreadful ravages at first, and slowly appeared to wear itself out. Such was the case with Syphilis when it first appeared in Europe, compared with the mitigated symptoms of the present times. This is certainly in part owing to our following a better plan of treatment, but still more to this disease being of a less virulent nature than before.

3rd. The progress of the syphilitic disease indicates that it was first brought to Spain, from whence it spread over Europe, Africa, and Asia.

छिद्रैरनुमुखैर्लिङ्ग चितं यस्य समन्ततः॥
वातशोस्मितजो व्याधिः स ज्ञेयः शतपोणकः॥
वातपित्तकृतो ज्ञेय स्त्वक्पाको ज्वरदाहकृत्।
कृष्णैः स्फोटैःसरक्ताभिः पिड़काभिर्निपीड़ितम्।
यस्य वास्त रुजश्चोग्रा ज्ञेयं तच्छ्रोणिताव्र्वूदम्॥
मांसदोषेण जानीयादर्व्वुदं मांससम्भवम्।

4th. The analogy of other diseases prove that new diseases may so appear, and spread as the small-pox, measles, etc. from Asia; and perhaps to croup and sweating sickness of Britain, etc.

Paribarttika— Phymosis. This disease is produced by pressure, or external injuries, by which the prepuce is swollen by the diseased air, and covers the glans. When it remains swollen, hard, and very painful, the inflammation sometimes passes to suppuration.

Abapātika— Pariphymosis. When much force is used during connection with a young girl, or when the prepuce is forced back with force, it remains there, and is followed with much swelling and pain.

Another variety of the above disease is called *Nirudda-prakasha,* or stricture, or diminution of the urethra. In some cases this is produced by an adhesion of the prepuce to the glans, impeding the passage of the urine, which in some cases only passes in drops.

Shūkadosha, inflammation of the penis, is produced by the pernicious habit of applying stimulants to enlarge the organ. There are eighteen forms of this disease, *Sarshāpikā, Ashithilikā, Grathita, Kumbhikā, Aladi, Mridita, Sammūr-hapiraka, Abamantha, Pushakarikā Sparshahāni, Uttami, Shatāpānaka, Twakapāka, Sanitārbuda, Mangsapaka, Bidradhi, Tilakālaka, Māngsārbuda,* etc.

Sarshāpikā are small pimples, like mustard seed round

शीर्य्यन्ते यस्य मांसानि यस्य सर्व्वाश्च वेदनाः।
विद्यात्तं मांसपाकन्तु सर्व्वदोषाकृतिं भिषक्॥
विद्रधिं सन्निपातेन यथोक्तमपि निद्रिशेत्।
कृष्णानि चित्राण्यथवा सूकानि सविषाणि वा॥
पाचितानि पचन्त्याशु मेढ्रं निरवशेषतः।
कालानि भूत्वा मांसानि शीर्य्यन्ते यस्य देहिनः॥
सन्निपातसमुत्थांस्तु तान् विद्यात्तिलकालकान्।
तत्र मांसार्व्वुदं यच्च मांसपाकश्च यः स्मृतः॥
विद्रधिश्च न सिद्धन्ति ये च सुद्ध सुस्तलकालकाः॥

कुष्ठनिदानम्

विरोधीन्यन्नपानानि द्रवस्निग्धगुरुणि च।
भजता भागतां छर्द्दि वेगां श्चान्यन् प्रतिघ्नताम्॥
व्यायामभतिसन्ताप मतिभूक्त्वा निषेविणाम्।
घर्म्मश्रमभयार्त्तानां द्रुतं शीताम्बुसेविणाम्॥

the penis, which are produced by the presence of a kind of insect, which is sometimes applied to the part with the intention of increasing the size of the organ.

The other forms of inflammation are produced by the application of other stimulants which cause inflammation of a chronic or acute form. Sometimes abscess and mortification of the part occur so as sometimes to destroy the penis. The other varieties are merely modifications of these inflammations, and their terminations.

LEPROSY (*Kushtha or Kuth*)

This disease is the most aggravated of all that afflict the body, and when a person dies with it the Hindus believe that the person will be afflicted with it in the next life, unless he performs the *prāschitta,* penance. This penance consists of abstinence for a day, shaving the whole hair off the head,

अजीर्णाध्यभिनाञ्चैव पञ्चकर्म्मापचारिणाम्।।
नवान्नदधि मत्स्याति-लवणाश्च निशेविनाम्।
माघमूलकपिष्टान्नतिल क्षीर-गुड़ाशिनाम्।
व्यचाय्ययञ्चाप्यजीर्णेऽन्ने निद्राञ्च भजतां दिवा।।
विप्रान् गुरुन् धर्षयतां पापं कर्म्म न कुर्व्वताम्।
वातादय स्त्रयो दृष्टा स्तग्रक्तं मांसमम्बुचं।
दूषयन्ति स कुष्ठानां सप्तको द्रव्यसंग्रहः
अतः कुष्ठानि जायन्ते सप्त चैकादशैव च।
कुष्टानि सप्तधा दोषैः पृथग् द्वन्दैः समागतैः।।
सर्व्वेष्वपि त्रिदोषेषु व्यपदेशोऽधिकस्ततः।
अति श्लक्ष्मक्षरस्पर्शस्वेदास्येद विवर्णताः।।

persents of a certain number of cowries and other articles to the brahmans, who perform certain prayers, and to whom the person confesses his sins. This ceremony is now generally performed before entering upon the treatment of any supposed dangerous disease.

The Hindus distinguish three kinds of Leprosy, the black, white, and red varieties, which are produced by various causes. Sometimes the disease is caused by bad air, and drink; eating substances which do not assimilate, as milk and fish, food of a rancid, salt, and indigestable nature; or thin oleaginous food: when the person eats immoderately of such food, for some time, it will produce this disease. In other cases irregularity in eating and fasting, mental agitation, violent exercise, exposure to fatigue, or too great heat, especially after a full meal; watching with exposure to the night air, using new rice, milk, curds, fish, and the too frequent use of pulse, radishes, sesaman and treacle, produce leprosy. In others it is produced by checking natural evacuations, or suppressing them when artificially excited; such as vomiting or the expulsion of air, urine or dejections or the irregularity and alternate use of hot and cold applications. Sometimes it is produced from eating

दाहः कण्डु स्त्वचिख्यापस्तोदः कोठोऽरतिर्भ्रमः।
व्रणनामधिकं शूलं शीघ्रोत्पत्तिश्चिरस्थितिः॥
रूढ़ानामपि रुक्षत्वं निमित्तेऽल्पिति कोपनम्।
रोमहर्षोऽसृजः कार्ष्ण्यं कुष्ठलक्षणमग्रजम्॥
कृषारुणकपालाभं यदुक्षं परुषं तनु।
कापालं तोदवह्वलं तत् कुष्ठं विषमं स्मृतम्॥
रुग्दाहरागकण्डुभिः परीतं रोमपिञ्जरम्।
उड़्ग्वरफलाभासं कुष्ठमौडुम्बरं वदेत्॥
श्वेतं रक्तं स्थिरं स्त्यानं स्निग्धमुत्मन्नमण्ठलम्।
कृच्छ्रमन्योन्यसंयुक्तं कुष्ठं मण्डलमुच्यते॥
कर्कशं रक्तपर्य्यन्तमन्तः श्याबं सवेदनम्।

hot or cold articles of food, first, at dinner, or after fasting, when the usual food is not eaten, after much perspiration, fatigue, or fear, or when the person bathes or drinks cold water at improper times. In other cases the disease is produced when the food is not digested, or when time has not been given for this purpose, before more is taken into the stomach; when after the use of emetics and purgatives, the usual simple food, etc. is not employed; when the person sleeps during the day with a loaded stomach; or when he visits his wife before the food is digested. The blood and seminal secretions of parents when tainted by leprosy, affects their offspring. Lepers in one life, are born again with the complaint; and the disease is supposed to be communicable by contact, by breathing the same air, by eating together, by wearing the clothes, or ornaments, of a person labouring under the disease. Whoever speaks disrespectfully or does any other improper action, or commits sins against his *guru* or *bipra* (pandit brahman); such as, committing adultery with a brahman's wife, killing a good man, and robbing a person of his estate, will be liable to be afficted with this disease. Such causes derange air, bile, and phlegm, by which the skin, blood, flesh, and watery

यद्दृष्यजिह्वसंस्थानमृष्यजिह्वं तदुच्यते॥
सश्वेतं रक्तपर्य्यन्त पुण्डरीकदलोपमम्।
सोत्सेधञ्च सरागञ्च पण्डरीक तदुच्यते।
श्येत ताम्रं तनु च यद्रजोघृष्ठं विमुञ्चति।
प्रायश्चोरसि तत् सिध्ममलावुकुसुमोपमम्॥
यत् काकणान्तिकावर्णं सपाकं तीव्रवेदनम्।
त्रिदोषलिङ्ग तत् कुष्ठ काकणंनैव सिध्यति।
स्वेदनं महावास्तु यन्मत्स्यशकलोपमम्।

parts of the blood (*ambu)* are deranged, and produce the eighteen forms of leprosy: of these seven are severe, and eleven are mild.

Before leprosy appears the skin becomes glossy, thin, and rough, and of an unnatural colour; there is much perspiration, or a suppression, of it, itchiness and occasional horripilation; the body feels hot, parts of the surface become insensible, and the blood in the veins becomes blacker than usual, while other parts of the suface become discoloured,painful, swell quickly, remain so for a long time, and slowly heal. In such a person any injury turns to a sore, is very painful, heals with great difficulty, and a rough cicatrix is left. The person has fits of giddiness, with impaired, or an irregular state of the appetite. The seven severe forms of leprosy are produced by deranged air, bile, or phlegm: they are thus described.

1. *Sidhma,* is produced by deranged phlegm and air, and is characterized by small, white, coppery, or red spots, which spread over large surfaces accompanied with a thin mealy dust. This is the Lepra Vulgaris, or L. Alphos.

2. *Audumbarā.* In this form the blothces are livid, and resemble the ripe fig, or Ficus glomerata. This form is accompanied with much pain, and burning on the surface. The hair becomes tawny; and the morbid humour is bile.

तदेककुष्ठं चर्म्माख्य बहुलं हस्तिचर्म्मवत्।
श्यावं किण-खरस्वर्ग परुषं किटिमं स्मृतम्।
वैपादिकं पाणिपादस्फुटनं तीव्रवेदनम्
कण्डुमद्भिः सरागैश्च गण्डैरलमकं चितम्।
सकण्डरागापिड़कं दद्रुमण्डलमुद्गतम्।
रक्तं सशूलं कण्डुमत् सस्फोट यद् गल्त्यपि।
तच्चर्म्मदलमाख्यातं संस्पर्शासह मुच्यते।
सूक्ष्मावह्वः पिड़काः स्त्राववत्यः पामेत्युक्ताः कण्डुमत्य सदाहाः।
सैव स्फीटस्तौव्रदाहै रूपेता ज्ञेया पाण्योः कच्छुरुग्रा स्फिचोश्च॥

3. *Rishwajihwa;* the patches of tubercles, are shaped like the tongue of a bear; hard and red round their edges, dark in the centre and are accompanied with sever pain. This form is produced by a derangement of the air, and bile.

4. *Kapala;* is covered with black and purplish patches resembling the broken pieces of a black earthen vessel. These blotches are irregular, hard, and dry, and are accompanied with pricking and pain. The *air* is the humour principally affected.

5. *Kākanaka,* resembles the seed of *kunch* (Abrus precatorious), with red and black spots in the centre. The blotches are extremely painful, and often terminate in suppuration. The three humours are deranged in this variety; which is incurable.

6. *Pundarika.* The patches in this variety are pale red in the centre, with dark dull red edges, and resemble the petals of the lotus when exposed to the sun. this variety is produced by derangements of the phlegm and bile.

7. *Dadrukushtha.* The patches in this variety are elevated, black, round, and spreading; there are many sorts,

स्फोठाः श्यवारुणाभासा विस्फोटाः स्युस्तनुत्वचः।
रक्तं श्यावं सदाहार्त्तिः शताः स्याद्वहुव्रनम्।
सकण्डुपिड़काः श्यावा वहुस्रावा विचर्च्चिका॥
खरं श्यवारुणं रुक्षं वातकुष्ठं सवेदनम्।
पित्तात् प्रकुपितं दाहरागस्रावान्वितं मतम्॥
कफात् क्लेदिघनं स्निग्धं सकण्डु शैत्यगौरवम्।
द्विलिङ्गं द्वन्दजं कुष्ठं त्रिलिङ्गं सान्निपातिकम्।
त्वकस्त्ये वैवर्ण्यमङ्गेषु कुष्ठे रौक्षञ्च जायते।
त्रक्स्वापो रोमहर्षश्च खेदस्यातिप्रवर्त्तनम्।

which are accompanied with much itching, burning,and pain; and are produced by derangements of the phlegm, and bile. These are the general symptoms of the severe forms of leprosy.

The slighter varieties of leprosy, *Kshudra*, are according to *Sushruta* as follows:

1. *Sthalāruska.*	2. *Mahākushtha.*	3. *Ekshyukushtha.*
4. *Charmadala*	5. *Bisarpa.*	6. *Parisarpa.*
7. *Sidhma*	8. *Bicharchikā.*	9. *Kitima.*
10. *Pāmā.*	11. *Rakashā.*	

Charaka has the following arrangement.

1. When there is no perspitation, and patches are very large, and of a dark brown colour, and oblong, like the scales of fish, and rough like an elephant's skin, it is called *ekakushtha*, (Ichthyasis).
2. When it has patches of a dark yellow colour, like the cicatrices of healed ulcers, with a hardness and roughness of the part, it is called *kitima.*
3. When sores and chaps form in the hands and feet about the nails, accompanied with small tubercles of red colour, much pain, and itching, it is called *vaipādikā.*

कण्डु विपुयकश्चैव कुष्ठे शोणितसंश्रिते।
वाहल्य वाक्त्वशोषश्च कार्कश्यं पिड़कोद्गमः।
तोदः स्फोटः स्थिरत्वञ्च कुष्ठे मांससमाश्रिते।
कौण्यं गतिक्षयोऽङ्गानां संभेदः क्षतसर्पणम्।
भेदःस्थानगते लिङ्ग प्रागुक्तानि तथैव च।
नासाभङ्गोऽक्षिरागश्च क्षतेषु क्रिमिसम्भवः।
स्वरोपघातश्च भवेदस्थिमज्जसमाश्रिते।
दम्पत्योः कुष्ठवाहुल्याद् दुष्ट शोणितशुक्रयोः।
यदपत्यं तयोर्ज्यातं ज्ञेयं तदपि कुष्ठितम्॥
साध्यं त्वग्रक्तमांसस्थं वात श्लेष्माधिकञ्च यत्।

4. When the tubercles are large, of a red colour, and very itchy, they are called *ālāsaka*.
5. Should the patches be of slightly dark redish colour, itchy, spreading, and elevated into tubercles, it is called *dadrumanala*.
6. When the spots are of a red colour, with severe pain, and itchiness, the blotches are very sensible, ripen soon, and much matter is discharged, it is called *charmadala*.
7. Small tubercles in great numbers, of a black or purplish hue, with a copious bloody discharge, accompanied with burning, and itching, it is called *pāmā*.
8. When the eruptions are merely larger than the last, and are accompanied with much pain in the palms of the hands, or buttocks, it is called *kachchhū*.
9. When the eruptions are of a dark yellow or red colour, and the skin is dry and thin, the variety is called *bishphotha*.
10. Another form has yellow, or dark redish coloured

भेदसि द्वन्द्वजं याप्यं वर्ज्जं मज्जास्थिसंश्रितम्।
क्रिमितृड् दाहमन्दाग्निसंयुक्तं यत् त्रिदोषजम्।
प्रभिन्नं प्रस्त्रुताङ्कञ्च रक्तनेत्रं हतस्वरम्।
पञ्चकर्म्मगुणातीतं कुष्ठं हन्तीह मानवम्।
वातेन कुष्ठं कापालं पित्तेनौडम्बरं कफात्।
मण्डलाख्यं विवर्च्चीं च ऋष्यख्यं वातपित्तजं।
चर्मैककुष्ठं किठिमं सिध्मालम विपाद्रिकाः।

blotches, accompanied with much heat and pain, and numerous itchy tubercles: it is called *Sotārush*.

11. When the tubercles are small numerous and itchy, of a dark yellow colour, and discharge much ichor, blood, etc., the variety is called *bicharchikā*. The four first varieties are supposed to be produced by derangements of the *air* and *phlegm;* and the seven last by derangements of the *bile and* phlegm.

When leprosy is in the *skin,* its colour is unnatural, rough, dry, and insensible; and the hairs on the body are generally erected, and the person perspires freely. When *blood* is deranged the body becomes itchy with fetor, and the skin is hard, pus is discharged.

When *flesh* is diseased it is called *gajacharma* (Ichthyasis Simplex), the mouth is often parched, perspiration is defective the surface of the body is rough, is like the scales of fish, and eruptions form over the body, with pain. Patches of vesicles sometimes, form and terminate in ulcers, which remain for long periods.

When *fat* is affected the hands and feet become stiff, immovable, and ulcerated, and drop off, with severe pain; the sores pass from one part of the body to another, and the symptoms of diseased flesh appear also in this form.

When the *bones* and *marrow* are leprous, the nose falls in, the eyes become red, and worms breed in the sores. The

वात श्लेष्मोद्भावाः श्लेष्मपित्तादद्रु शतारुषी।
पुण्डरीकं सविस्फोठं पामाचर्म्मदलं तथा॥
सर्व्वैः स्यात् काकणं पूर्व्वत्रिकं दद्रुसकाकणम्
पुण्डरीकर्ष्यजिह्वा च महाकुष्ठानि सप्त तु॥
कुष्ठैकसम्भवं श्वित्रं किलासं वारुणं भवेत्।
निर्द्दिष्टम परिश्राविं त्रिधातुद्भवसंश्रयम्।
वाताद्रुक्षारुणं पित्तातामं कमलपत्रवत्।
सदाहं रोमविध्वंसि कफाच्छ्रेत घनं गुरु
सकण्डुरं क्रमाद्रुक्तमांसमेदःसु चादिशेत्।

voice becomes unnatural, and hoarse. When the leprosy is in the skin, blood, or flesh, or in the air or phlegm, it may be cured. When in the fat, with two of the humours deranged, as air and phlegm, or air and bile, the person will not be cured, nor will it soon destroy the individual. When the bones and marrow are affected and two or three humours are viciated, one of them being the bile, it is incurable.

Fatal symptoms of leprosy occur with worms in the sores, or with the painful disease of the heart (Angina pectoris); with dyspepsia, or with symptoms of diseased air, bile, and phlegm; with sores which discharge copiously; with inflamed eyes, the voice hoarse, and altered, and with weakness of that the person is not able to bear the employment of the five forms of medicine, as purgatives emetics, etc.

The white, and the red leprosy (*shitra and kilāsa*), are distinguished from the black leprosy by their not being accompanied with any discharge, and only affecting the skin, *charaka* adds, that they sometimes affect the *skin, blood, phlegm,* and *fat*.

When the white leprosy is not produced by burns, and when the hair is not white but remains of the natural colour over the white patches; when the patches are not large and do

वणनवेट्टगुभयं कृच्छ्रं तच्चोत्तरोत्तरम्।
अशुक्लरोमबहुल मसंश्लिष्टं मिथो नवम्।
अनग्निदद्धजं साध्यं श्वित्रं वर्ज्जमतोन्यथा।
गुह्यपाणितलौष्ठेषु जातमन्यचिरन्तनम्।
वर्ज्जनीयं विशेषेण किलासं सिद्धिमिच्छता।
प्रसङ्गाद्गात्रसंस्पर्शान्निःश्वासात् सह भोजनात्।
एकशय्यसनाच्चैव वस्त्रमाल्यानुलेपनात्।
कुष्ठं ज्वरश्च शोषश्च नेत्राभिष्यद्य एव च।
औपसर्गिकरोगाश्च संक्रामन्ति नरान्नरम्।

शीतपित्तोदर्द्दकोठनिदानम्

शीतमारुतसंस्पर्शात् प्रदुष्टौ कफमारूतौ।
पित्तेन सह सम्भुय वहिरन्तर्विसर्पतः।

not join each other, and when recent, the disease may be cured. When produced by burns, and the above symptoms are absent, these kinds of white leprosy are incurable.

When situated about the external genitals, palms of the hands, or lips, the white leprosy is incurable although recent.

The leprosy, with fever, and the drying up or emaciation of the body, and other symptoms of pulmonary consumption (*shosha*); a variety of Ophthalmia (*Netrābhishyanda),* and those disease produced by the influence of the planets, such as small-pox, etc. are contagious.

URTICARIA ? (*Sitapita*)

This disease is called *Sitapita* or *Udordah*, and another form is named *Khatah*. The disease is produced by cold air applied to the body, which deranges the *phlegm, air and bile.* These move about on the surface, and within the body, producing thirst, redness of the eyes, nausea, and cause loss of appetite. The body becomes heavy, and the person incapable

पिपासारुचिहृल्लामदेहसादाङ्गगौरवं।
रक्तलोचनता तेषां पूर्व्वरुपस्य लक्षणम्।
वरटीदंष्टंसस्थान:शोथः संजायते वहिः।
सकण्डुतोदवहृलच्छर्द्दिज्वर विदाहवान्।
उदर्द्दमिति तं विद्याच्छीतपित्त मथापरे।
वाताधिकं शीतपित्तमुदर्द्दश्च कफाधिकः।
सोतसङ्गैश्च सरागैश्च कण्डुमद्भिश्च मण्डलैः।
शैशिरः कफजो व्याधि रूदर्द्द इति कीर्त्तितः।
असम्यग्वमनोदीर्णपित्तश्लेष्मान्ननिग्रहैः।
मण्डलानि सकण्डुनि रागवन्ति वहुनि च।
उतकोठः सानुवन्धश्च कोठ इत्यभिधीयते।

of work. The disease appears with slight swellings in different parts of the body; like the sting of the wasp. The part is at first itchy and then very painful, with vomiting, fever, and heat of the body. When the air is much diseased, beyond the other humours it is called *Sitapita;* and when phlegm is much deranged, producing red circles, accompanied with itching, it is called *Udoradah*.

It is called *Khata,* when the stomach is deranged. This is more liable to occur if at the commencement the stomach has not been properly cleared by emetics, and when bile and phlegm are deranged. If in such a case an ignorant person does not promote vomiting, but endeavours to cure to deranged *bile* and *phlegm,* the disease will be aggravated. In such cases the body is covered with large and small circular patches which are itchy, elevated, and have a red colour. They appear and disappear on different parts of the body. This form of the disease will also be produced by repressing vomiting when nature is endeavouring to relieve herself of the contents of the stomach.

अम्लपित्तनिदानम्

विरुद्धदुष्टाम्लविदाहि पित्तप्रकोपि पानान्नभुजो विदग्धम्।
पित्तं स्वहेतुपचितं पुरा मत्तदम्लपित्तं प्रवदन्ति सन्तः।
अविपाक क्लमोत् क्लेशतिक्ताम्लोद्गारगौरवैः।
हृत्कण्ठदाहारूचिभिश्चाम्ल पित्तं वदेद्भिषक्।
तृड्‌ दाहमूर्च्छा भ्रममोहकारि प्रयात्यधो वा विविधप्रकारम्।
हृल्लासकोठानलसादहर्ष-स्वेदाङ्गपीतत्वकरं कदाचित्।
वान्तं हरित् पीतकनीलकृष्णमारक्तरक्ताभमतीव चाम्लं
मांसोदकाभं त्वतिपिच्छलाच्छं श्लेस्मानुजातं विविधं रसेन।
भुक्ते विदग्धे त्वथवाप्यभुक्ते करोति तिक्ताम्लवमिं कदाचित्।
उद्‌गारमेवं विधमेव कण्ठहृत् कुक्षिदाहं शिरसो रूजं वा।
करचरणदाहमौष्णं महतीमरूचिं ज्वरञ्च।
कफपित्तं जनयति कण्डुमण्डल
पिड़काशतनिचितगात्ररोगनिचयम्।

ACIDITY OF STOMACH, VOMITING OF BILE (*Amlapitta*)

This disease is produced by improper mixtures of food, by bad water, or articles that derange the bile, which is collected, and is discharged producing this disease. It is characterized by dyspepsia, languor, nausea, sour and bitter eructations, and the body is heavy, with burning of the breast and throat. The person has no appetite, is thirsty, complains of syncopy, and the head turns round. A dullness of the intellect may be observed, and the faeces are various in appearance, and hot. The internal heat and pain of body diminishes, and the person sometimes vomits green, yellow, and blue matter. Sometimes it is like blood, and is very sour; sometimes it is like phlegm, or the washings of flesh, or has mucilaginous appearance. In other cases jaundice is produced with free perspiration, and the body is of a yellow colour. When phlegm and bile are

रोगोऽयमम्लपित्ताख्यो यत्नात् संसाध्यते नवः।
चिरोत्थितो भवेत्द्याप्यः कृच्छ्रसाध्यः स कस्यचित्।
सानिलं सानिलकफं सकफ तच्च लक्षयेत्।
दोषलिङ्गेन मतिमान् भिषङ्मोहकरं हि तत्॥
कम्पप्रलापमूर्च्छा चिमिचिमिगात्रावसादशूलानि।
तमसो दर्शन विभ्रमो प्रमोह हर्षाण्यनिलकोपात्॥
कफनिष्ठीवन गौरवः जड़तारूचि शीतसाद वमिलेपाः॥
दहनवलसाद कण्डु निद्राचिह्नं कफानुगते।
उभय मिद मेव चिह्नं मारुतकफसम्भवे भवत्यम्ले॥

diseased, the abdomen is very hot when any thing is eaten, and if nothing is taken, the vomited matter and eructations are bitter and sour. The neck, chest, and sides are hot; there is head-ache, and the hands and feet are burning. The person has a disgust for food, is feverish, and itchy eruptions, and patches appear over the body.

If this disease be recent it may be cured with difficulty; and if old, it will often be incurable. There are three forms of the disease: when air or phlem are deranged; when air and phlegm; or when phlegm alone is deranged, which will be distinguished by the experienced physician.

When *air* is diseased the person speaks foolishly, is affected with syncopy, and his body is languid, with slight uneasiness and pain. The room he is in appears dark; in other cases he is still, is always forgetting, and complains of severe pain of the body.

Phlegm. In this form phlegm is always discharged from the mouth, the body feels heavy, the person is languid, has no appetite, the body is cold, and the person is lazy and vomits. The surface of the body feels as if it was rubbed with something, it is itchy, the patient looses his appetite, and he takes much sleep.

तिक्ताम्ल कटुकोद्गार हृत् कुक्षि कण्ठदाहकृत्।
भ्रममूर्च्छारुचिच्छर्द्दि रालस्यञ्च शिरोरुजा।
प्रसेको मुखमाधुर्य्य श्लेष्मपित्तस्य लक्षणम्।।

विसर्पनिदानम्

लवणाम्लकटुष्णादिसंसेवाद्दोषकोपतः।
विसर्पः सप्तधा ज्ञेयः सर्व्वतः परिसर्पनात्।
पृथक् त्रयस्त्रिभिश्चैको विसर्पा द्वन्द्रजास्त्रयः।
वातिकः पैत्तिकश्चैव कफजः सान्निपातिकः।
चत्वार एते विसर्पा वक्ष्यन्ते इन्द्रजास्त्रयः।
आग्नेयो वातपित्ताभ्यां ग्रन्थ्याख्याः कफ वातजः।
यस्तु कर्द्दमको घोरः स पित्तकफसम्भवः।
रक्तं लसीका त्वङमासं दूष्यं दोषास्त्रयो मलाः।
विसर्पाणां समुत्पत्तौ विज्ञेयाः सप्त धातवः।
तत्र वातात् स विसर्पो वातज्वरसमव्यथः।
शोफस्फुरणनिस्तोद भेदायासार्त्ति हर्षवान्।
पित्ताद् द्रुतगतिः पित्रज्वरलिङ्गोऽतिलोहितः।

When air and phlegm are deranged in one place, the sumptoms of the two above forms of disease are present.

ERYSIPELAS, CARBUNCLE ? (*Bisharpa*)

When *air, bile, and phlegm* are all deranged in the skin, flesh, or blood, they produce a slight swelling of the whole body, which passes from one part to another. When produced by air, the part becomes black, soft, and unequal; accompanied with pain, as if needles were thrust into the part, and the fever produced by deranged air. When surrounded with vesications it is incurable.

When the disease is produced by bile it spreads quickly, and is accompanied with inflammatory fever. This form is

कफात् कण्डुयुतः स्निग्धः कफज्वरसमानरुक्।
सन्निपातसमुत्थश्च सर्व्वलिङ्गसमन्वितः।
वातपित्ताज्वरच्छर्द्दिमूर्च्छातीसारतृड्भ्रमैः।
ग्रन्थिभेदाग्नि सदनतमकारोचकैर्युतः।
करोति सर्व्वमङ्गञ्च दीप्ताङ्गारावकीर्णवत्।
यं यं देशं विसर्पश्च विसर्पति भवेत् स स।
शान्ताङ्गारासितो नीलो रक्तो वाशु च चीयते।
अग्निदग्ध इव स्फोटैः शीघ्रगत्या दुतं स च।
मर्म्मानुसारी विसर्पः स्याद्वातोऽतिबलस्ततः।
व्यथेताङ्गं हरेत् संज्ञां निद्राञ्च श्वासमीरयेत्।
हिक्काञ्च सगतोऽवस्थामीदृशीं लभते न ना।
क्कचिच्छर्म्मारतिग्रस्तो भूमिशय्याशनादिषु।
चेष्टमान स्ततः क्लिष्टो मनोदेहसमुद्भवान्।
दुष्प्रवोधोऽश्नु ते निद्रां सोऽग्निवीसर्प उच्यते।
कफेन रूद्धः पवनो भिन्नं तं बहुधा कफम्।
रक्तं वा वृद्धरक्तस्य त्वक्शिरास्नायुमांसगम्।
दूषयित्वा तु दीर्घानुवृत्त स्यूलखरात्मनाम्।
ग्रन्थीनां कुरुते मालां सरक्तां तीव्ररूग्ज्वरम्।

accompained with redness, and vesications. When the inflamation is deep, the flesh and vessels are destroyed, and it discharges a matter like a mixture of water and clay. Such cases are incurable.

When produced by *phlegm* it spreads slowly, has an oily appearance, and is white. There is little pain in such cases, with considerable itching. When produced by the derangement of the three humours the symptoms are of a mixed nature. When this disease passes to suppuration it is incurable. When produced by sharp instruments, or such like injuries, the bile and blood are deranged and produces a swelling of the part;

श्वासकासातीसारस्य शोषहिक्कावमिभ्रमैः।
मोहवैवर्ण्य मुच्छाङ्गभङ्गिग्निसदनैर्युताम्।
इत्ययं ग्रन्थिवीसर्पः कफमारूतकोपजः॥
कफपित्ताज्वरस्तम्भोनिद्रातन्द्राशिरोरूजा।
अङ्गावसादविक्षेपौ प्रलेपारोचक भ्रमाः।
मूर्च्छाग्निहानिर्भेदास्थ्रां पिपासेन्द्रिय गौरवम्।
द्यामोपवेशनं लेपः स्त्रोतसांस च सर्पति।
प्रायेणामाशयं गृद्गन्नेकदेशं न चातिरूक्।
पीड़कै रवकीर्णीतिपीत लोहितपाण्डुरैः।
स्निग्धोऽसितो मेचकाभो मलिनः शोथवान् गुरुः।
गम्भीरपाकोप्राह्योष्मापृष्टः क्लिन्नोऽवदीर्य्यति।
पङ्कवच्छ्रीर्णमासंश्च स्प्रष्टस्नायुशिरागणः।
शवगन्धी च वीसर्पः कर्द्दमाख्य मुशन्तितम्।
वाह्यहेतोः क्षतात् क्रुद्धः सरक्तं पित्तमीरयन्।
विसर्प मारूतः कुर्य्यात् कुलत्थसदृसैश्चितम्।
स्फोटैः शोथज्वररुजादाहाद्यं श्यावशोणितम्।
ज्वरातीसारौवमथुस्त्वङ् मांसदरणंक्लमाः।
आरोचका विपाकौ च विसर्पाणा मुपद्रवाः।
सिद्धन्ति वातकफ पित्तकृता विसर्पाः
सर्व्वात्मकः क्षतकृतश्च न सिद्धिभेति।
पित्तात्मकोऽङ्गन वपुश्च भवेदसाध्यः
कृच्छ्राश्च मर्ग्मसु भवन्ति हि सर्व्व एव।

which becomes black and red, and is accompanied with violent inflammatory fever. The affected part is surrounded by a black edge, and eruptions like peas.

The first three forms of this disease are curable, and the two last are incurable.

विस्फोटनिदानम्

कटुम्लतीक्ष्मोष्ण-विदाहिरूक्ष-क्षारैरजीर्णध्यशनातपैश्च।
तथर्त्तुदोषेण विपर्य्ययेण कुप्यन्तिः दोषाः पवनादयस्तु।
त्वच्यमाश्रित ते रक्तमांसास्थीनि प्रदुध्य च।
घोरान् कुर्व्वन्ति विस्फोटान् सर्व्वान् ज्वर पुरःसरान्।
अग्निदग्धनिभाः स्फोटाः सज्वरारक्तपिजजाः।
क्वचित् सर्व्वत्र वा देहे विष्फोटक इति स्मृतः।
शिरोरूक् शूल भूयिष्ठं ज्वर स्तट् पर्व्वभेदनम्।
सकृष्ण वर्णता चेति वातविष्फोटलक्षणम्।
ज्वरदाहरूजास्त्रावपाकतृष्णाभिरन्वितम्।
पोतलोहितवर्णश्च पित्तविष्फोटलक्षणम्।
छर्द्यरोचकजाड्यानि कण्डुकाठिन्यपाण्डुताः।
आवेदनश्चिरात् पाकी स विष्फोठः कफात्मकः।
वातपित्तकृतो यस्तु कुरूते तीव्र वेदनाम्।

BOILS, PUSTULES, ERYSIPELAS ? *(Bishphotaka)*

The causes of this form of disease are using too much heating, sour, or acid substances; - heavy and indigestable or salt food; – eating too freely, and exposure to the sun – or to too sudden alterations of the weather. By such cause, *air, bile,* and *phlegm* are deranged, which affect the blood, flesh, bones, and skin; and produce large bullae, accompanied with fever. This part appears as if burnt. Sometimes these bullae appear over all the body, and in other cases they are confined to particular parts. When the air is much deranged in this disease it is accompanied with head-ache, fever, thirst, pain in the joints, and the bullae become black, accompanied with much pain. When produced by deranged bile there is much fever, burning of the body, and a large discharge of fluid from the bullae. They then become red, or yellow.

कण्डुस्तैमित्य गुरुभिर्जानीयात् कफवातिकम्।
कण्डुर्दाहोज्वरश्छर्द्दिरेतैस्तु कफपैत्तिकः।
मेध्य निम्नोन्नतोऽन्ते च कठिनोऽल्प प्रपाकवान्।
दाहरागतृषामोह श्छर्द्दिमूर्च्छारूजा ज्वरः।
प्रलापीवेपथुस्तन्द्रा सोऽसाध्यः स्यात् त्रिदोषजः।
रक्ता रक्तसमुत्थाना गुञ्जाविद्रुमसन्निभाः।
वेदिव्यास्तु रक्तेन पैत्तिकेन च हेतुना।
नते सिद्धिं समायान्ति सिन्धै र्योगशतैरपि।
एकदोषात्थितः साध्यः कृच्छ्रसाध्यो द्विदोषजः।
सर्व्वदोषोत्थितो घोरस्त्वासाध्ये भूयुर्फप्यद्रवः।

मसूरिकानिदानम्

कट्वम्लवणक्षार-विरुद्धाध्यशनाशनैः॥
दुष्टनिष्पावशाकाद्यैः प्रदुष्टपवनोदकैः।

When produced by deranged phlegm it is accompanied with vomiting, dyspepsia, languor, and the affected parts become itchy, hard, and white, without pain. Suppuration often takes place, and continues for a long time.

When the three humours are deranged the disease is incurable; and also when the bullae are depressed in the centre and hard. The patient in such cases complains of a burning sensation, thirst, fainting, vomiting, fever, delirium, rigors, and drowsiness. These are unfavourable symptoms, as also when the bullae become red.

When the disease is produced by blood, the tubercles are like the seed of the *gunja;* (that is red with a black spot). This form is incurable (*Charaka*).

SMALL -POX (*Masurikā*)[9]

Stimulating and heating substances produce this disease; as also pungent, acid, or saline substances and improper

क्रुरग्रहेक्षणाच्चापि देहे दोषाः समुद्धताः।
जनयन्ति शरीरेऽस्मिन् दुष्टरक्तेन सङ्गताः।
मसूराकृतिसंस्थानाः पिड़काः सुर्म्यसूरिकाः।
मासां पूर्व्वज्वरः कण्डुर्गात्रभङ्गोऽरतिर्भ्रमः।
त्वचिशोथः सर्ववर्णो नेत्ररागश्च जायते।
क्षोटाः श्यवारुणारूक्षास्तीव्रवेदनयान्विताः।
कठिनाश्चिरपाकाश्च भवन्त्यनिलसम्भवाः।
सन्ध्यस्थिपर्व्वणां भेदः कासः कम्पोऽरतिःक्लमः।
शोषस्ताल्वोष्ठजिह्वानां तृष्णा चारुचिस्युंता।
रक्ताःपीताः सिताः स्फोटाः सदाहा स्तीव्रवेदनाः।

mixtures of food; eating before the former food has been digested: unwholesome meats, and certain roots or fruits; bad air or water; and the influence of a bad planet. These causes derange air, bile, and phlegm, etc., which with the bad blood produces an eruption like the *masūra*.

Before small-pox appears, fever occurs, with pain over the body, but particularly in the back; and itching, lassitude, stretching, restlessness, redness of the face and eyes, with cough. The skin swells slightly, and is of an unusually red colour.

When air is much deranged in this disease the pustules are of a dark-green, and red colour; or dull, hard, and rough, and are accompanied with severe pain. This variety ripens slowly.

When bile is deranged, in this disease, severe pain is felt in the large and small joints, with cough, shaking, listlessness and langour; the palate, lips and tongue are dry with thirst, and no appetite. The pustules are red, yellow, and white, and they are accompanied with burning pain. This form soon ripens.

When produced by diseased *phlegm* the pustules are large,

भवन्त्यचिर चिरपाकश्च पित्तकोपसमुद्भवाः।
विड्भेदश्चाङ्गमर्दश्च दाहतृष्णा रूचिस्तथा।
मुखपाकोऽक्षिरागश्च ज्वरस्तीव्रः सुदारूणः।
रक्तजायां भवन्त्येते विकाराः पित्तलक्षणाः।
कफप्रसेकः स्तैमित्यं शिरौरूगगात्रगौरवं।
हल्लासः सारूचिर्निद्रा तम्नालस्य समन्विताः।
श्वेताः स्निग्धाभृशं स्थूला कण्डुरा मन्दवेदनाः।
मसूरिकाः कफोत्थाय चिरपाकाः प्रकीर्त्तिताः।
नीलाश्चिपिटविस्तीर्णा मध्ये निम्ना महारुजाः।
चिरुपाकाः पूतिस्त्रावाः प्रभुताः सर्व्वदोषजाः।

white, and shining, with much itching, and less pain than the former kind. They ripen slowly. In this form, some of the general symptoms of small-pox are aggravated. There is catarrh with chilliness, head-ache, fever, heaviness of the body, nausea, loss of the appetite, languor, drowsiness, and the patient sleeps much.

When blood is deranged diarrhoea, lassitude, and stretching occur; with thirst, laziness, want of appetite, burning over the surface, and the mouth becomes ulcerated. The eyes are red, strong fever is present, with the symptoms already enumerated under deranged bile.

When air, bile and phlegm are thus deranged the patient is always dozing, he has no appetite, breathes with difficulty, and is drowsy, restless and delirious. This form is cured with much difficulty, and it is called *Charma* or fatal form.

The folowing are other varieties of Small-pox:—

1. *Measles (Romāntikā, Hām, B.)* is produced by vitiated phlegm and bile, and the symptoms are fever followed by an eruption of small red papellae, like the roots of hairs; these appear over the body, accompanied with loss of appetite and cough.

कण्ठरोधारूचिस्तम्भ प्रलापारतिसङ्गताः।
दुश्चिकित्स्याः समुद्दिष्टाः पीड़काश्चर्म्मसंज्ञिताः।
रोमकूपोन्नतिसमारागिण्यः कफपित्तजाः।
कासारोचकसंयुक्ता रोमात्योयेज्वरपूर्व्विकाः।
तोयवुद्बुदसङ्काशा त्वग्‌गतास्तु मसूरिकाः।
स्वल्पदोषाः प्रजायन्ते भिन्ना स्तोयं सवन्ति च
रक्तख्या लोहिताकाराः शीघ्रपाका स्तनु त्वचः।
साध्यनात्यर्थदुष्टाश्च भिन्ना रक्तं स्त्रवन्ति च।
मांसस्थाः काठिनाः श्निग्धा श्चिरपाका घनत्वचः।

Water-pox (*Togotoh, Masūrikā, Pāni-Basanta, B.*) The pustules are large, and full of water. In this form the skin is alone affected.

When the blood is particularly affected in small-pox, the pustules are of a redder colour, have a thinner cuticle than usual, and quickly ripen. They may generally be cured, but on being opened should blood be discharged, the disease is incurable.

When the pustules proceed from *flesh* they are hard and shining, they ripen slowly, and the skin covering the part is thick. The pain over the body is severe, with listlessness, itchiness of the skin, thirst, and fever.

When the disease is produced by diseased *fat,* the pustules are large, soft, round, and slightly elevated, with severe fever and pain. This form is very dangerous, and is accompanied with loss of sense, laziness and stupor. Some strong persons may be cured of this disease.

When the *marrow* is particularly diseased, the pustules are very small, flat, and slightly elevated and dry. The person is insensibile, with severe pain of a gnawing kind in the vital parts. This form quickly destroys the person.

When the *bones* are particularly affected in this disease; they feel pained, as if bored by an insect. The pustules appear

गात्रशूलतृषा कण्डुज्ज्ववारतिसमन्विताः।
मेदोजा मण्डलाकारा मृदवः किञ्चिदुन्नताः।
घोरज्वरपरीताश्च ख्यूलाः श्निग्धाः सवेदनाः।
समोहा रतिसन्तापाः कश्चिदाभ्यो विनिस्तरेत्।
क्षुद्रा गात्रसमा रूक्षा श्चिपिटाः किञ्चिदुन्नताः।
भज्जवोत्था तृशसंमोहवेदनारतिसंयुताः।
छिन्दति मर्म्मधामानि प्राणनाशु हरन्तिहि।
भ्रमरेणेव विद्धानि कृर्व्वन्त्यस्थीनि सर्व्वतः।
पक्काभाः पिड़काः स्निग्धाः सूक्ष्णाश्चात्यर्थवेदनाः।

as if ripe, small, shining and very tender. The person feels chilly, restless, and delirium occurs, with a burning feeling.

When *semen* is affected in this disease, the symptoms are the same as when the bones are affected; and this form it so fatal that as soon as a person is affected with it he dies, so that there is no time for the pustules appearing.

These different forms will be known by an experienced physician. When small-pox is caused by derangements in the skin, blood, bile, or phlegm; or phlegm and bile, it will be quickly cured. When air or bile; or phlegm and air; and when the air, the bile, and phlegm are deranged the disease is incurable. Of the latter kind the eruptions are sometimes like coral, or like rose-apple (Jam), oval, like the iron weight of a fishing net, or like a grain of linseed. The colour of this dangerous form of small-pox varies according to the strength of the individual. The other bad symptoms are cough, hicchough, coma, fever of a severe kind, delirium, listlessness, and thirst. The body remains very hot, blood flows from the mouth, eyes and nose, and there is a gurgling (*gharghari*) noise in the throat, with difficult and sonorous respiration. Such cases of small-pox are incurrable; as also those in which great thirst is accompanied with difficulty in breathing, which is performed through the mouth.

स्तैमित्यारतिसंमोहदाहोम्नादसमन्विताः।
शुक्रजायां मसूर्य्यान्तु लक्षणानि भवन्ति हि।
निर्द्दिष्टं केवलं चिह्नं दृश्यते न तु जीवितम्।
दोषमिश्रास्तु सप्तैता द्रष्टव्य दोषलक्षणैः।
त्वग्गता रक्तजाश्चैव पित्तजाः श्लेष्मजा स्तथा।
श्लेष्मपित्तञ्चजाश्चैव सुखसाध्या मसूरिकाः॥
वातजा वातपित्तोत्थाः श्लेष्मवात कृताश्च वाः।
कृच्छ्रसाध्या मता स्तस्मात् यत्नादेता उपाचरेत॥
असाध्याः सन्निपातोत्था स्तासां वक्ष्यामि लक्षणम्।
प्रवालसदृशः काश्चित् काश्चिज्जम्बुफलोपमाः॥

Should the elbow, wrists, or axilla swell after the small-pox, the person will be cured with difficulty.

It appears that the Chinese as well as the Hindus were familiar with small-pox many centuries before the Arabian physicians described it. It was probably conveyed westward by the Persian conquerors of Hindustan; which seems to be a further confirmation of the country from which it originally came, and the manner in which it gradually approached and eventually reached Europe. The distance and the hot deserts through which the only intercourse for so long a period was held, prevented for a time its progress westward; but, as navigation extended, ships from India would frequently touch at the Arabian ports of the Persian Gulf, and Red Sea. Where it seems first to have appeared, A.D.900.

The description of the small-pox by Rhazes,[10] the distinguished Arabian physician, first drew the attention of the European physicians to the disease.

Some say it was introduced into Arabia in 572, the year that gave birth to Mohammad; other testimonies seems to accord with the statement that it was at the siege of Mecca (A.D. 569), by Abraham that the Arabians were first affected with the disease.

The conquests of the followers of Mohammad conveyed

लोहजालसमाः काश्चिदतसीफलसन्निभाः।
आसां बहुविध्यवर्णा जायन्ते दोषभेदतः॥
कासोहिक्का प्रमोहश्च ज्वरस्तीव्रः सुदारुणः।
प्रलापश्चारतिर्मूच्छातृष्णा दाहोतिघुर्णता॥
मुखेन प्रस्त्रवेद्रक्तं तथा घ्राणेन चक्षुषा।
कण्ठे घुर्घूरकं कृत्वा श्वासित्यत्यर्थवेदनम्॥
मसूरिकाभिभुतस्य यस्यैतानि भिषग्वरैः॥
लक्षणानि च दृश्यन्ते न दद्यात्तत्र भेषजम्।
मसूरिकाभिभूतो यो भृशं घ्राणेन निश्वसेत्॥
सभृशं त्यजति प्राणान् तृष्णार्त्तो वायुदूषितः।
मसूरिकान्ते शोथः स्वात् कुर्परेमणिवम्वके।
तथांसफलके चापि दुश्चिकित्साः सुदारुणः॥

the disease to Persia, Syria, and Egypt; and the successful stand made by the inhabitants of Constantinople, for some time prevented the spread of the disease beyond the Hellespont. So completely does this appear to have been the case, that Honus, a resident physician in that city in the tenth century, states that neither the small-pox nor measles were known in his time in Constantinople.

The whole of the southern coast of the Mediterranean sea had been subdued by the Arabians; but, it was not till the commencement of the eight century that the disease was introduced into Spain by the Moors. The Victorious Saracens overran Spain crossed the Pyrenese mountains, and inundated the southern provinces of France. They were driven back by Charles Martel; but they left the small-pox and measles with the conquerors. From this source the disease quickly spread over Europe.

The Spaniards in their invasion of Hispaniola and Mexico conveyed the same diseases to these countries, where it committed the most extensive ravages. It would thus appear that the small-pox as well as the measles commenced in Asia, and extended to Africa, Europe, and the new World.

क्षुद्ररोगनिदानम्

१. स्निग्धाः सवर्णा ग्रथिता नीरुजा मुद्गसन्निभाः।
कफवातोत्थिता ज्ञेया बालानामजगल्लिकाः॥

२. यवाकारा सुकठिना ग्रथिता मांससंहृता।
पीड़का कफवाताभ्यां यवप्रख्येति सोच्यते॥

३. घनामवक्रां पिड़कामुन्नतां परिमण्डलाम्।
अन्त्रालजी मल्पमूयां तां विद्यात् कफवातजाम्॥

४. विवृत्तास्यां महादाहां पक्कोडुम्बरसन्निभाम्।
परिमण्डलां पित्तकृतां विवृतां नाम तां विदुः॥

५. ग्रथिताः पञ्च वा षड् वा दारुणाः कच्छपोपमाः।
कफानिलाभ्यां पिड़का ज्ञेया कच्छपिका बुधैः॥

६. ग्रीवांसकक्षा करपाददेशे सन्धो गले वा वा त्रिभिरेव दोषैः।
ग्रन्थिः सवल्मीकवदक्रियाणां जातः क्रमेणैव गतः प्रवृद्धिम्॥

Small diseases are arranged under the following heads :

(Locales) (Kshudra)

1. ***Ajagallikā***—Small tuberculous eruption of the form of peas. It occurs in children.
2. ***Jabaprakhia,*** are hard fleshy eruptions, like the grains of barley. They are produced by diseased phlegm and air.
3. ***Andālajī***—Round elevated pimples containing matter, produced by diseased phlegm and air.
4. ***Bibritā***—An eruption like the ripe fig with inflammation.
5. ***Kachhapikā***—Five or six tumors of the shape of turtles; produced by diseased phlegm and air.
6. ***Balmikī,*** are tumors in the soles of the feet or palms of the hand, or in a joint, or in the neck, axilla, and other parts. They increase by degrees, like the hills of

मुखैरनेकैः श्रुतितोदवद्भि र्बिसर्पवत् सर्पति चोन्नताग्रैः।
वल्मीकमाहुर्भिषजो विकारं निष्प्रत्यनीकं चिरजं विशेषात्॥

७. पद्मकर्णिकवन्मध्ये पीड़काभिः समाचिताम्।
इन्द्रविद्धां तु तां विद्यद्वातपित्तोत्थितां भिषक्॥

८. मण्डलं वृत्तमुत्सन्नं सरक्तं पीड़काचितं
रुजाकरी गर्द्दभिकां तां विद्यद्वातपित्तजाम्॥

९. वात श्लेष्मसमुद्भुतः श्वयथु र्हनुसद्धिजः।
स्विरो मन्दरुजः स्निग्धो ज्ञेयः पाषाणगर्द्दभः॥

१०. कर्णस्याभ्यन्तरे जातां पीड़का मुग्रवेदनाम्।
स्थिरां पनसिका तान्तु विद्यादन्तः प्रपाकिनीम्॥

११. विसर्पवत् सर्पति यः शोथस्तनुरपाकवान्।
दाहज्वरकरः पित्तात् स ज्ञेयो जालगर्द्दभः॥

१२. पीड़का मुत्तमाङ्गस्थां वृत्तामुग्ररुजां जराम्।
सर्व्वात्मिकां सर्व्वलिङ्गां जानीयादिरिवेल्लिकाम्॥

white ants; and are surrounded with painful and itchy ulcers, and accompanied with a discharge.

7. ***Indrabriddhā***—Tumors surrounded by small eruptions, like the inside of a water-iily.

8. ***Gardhabikā***—Elevations surrounded by small eruptions with many openings.

9. ***Pāsānāgar dabhā***—is a hard swelling below the ear, or in the articulation of the lower jaw. It is produced by diseased phlegm, and is hard, painful, and shining.

10. ***Panāsikā***—An eruption in the inside of the ear, which suppurates.

11. ***Jalagordaba***—A slight swelling which spreads rapidly, without passing to suppuration. It is accompanied with a strong inflammatory fever.

12. ***Jrebillikā***—A painful eruption over the head, accompanied with much pain and fever.

१३. बाहुपार्श्वांसकक्षेषु कृष्णस्फोटां सवेदनाम्।
पित्तप्रकोपसम्भूतां कक्षामित्यभिनिर्द्दिशेत्॥
१४. एकामेतादृशां दृष्ट्वा पीड़कां स्फोटसन्निभाम्।
त्वग्गतां पित्तकोपेन गन्धमालां प्रचक्ष्यते॥
१५. कक्षभागेषु ये स्फोटा जायन्ते मांसदारुणाः।
अन्तर्द्दाहज्वरकरा दीप्तपावकसन्निभाः॥
सप्ताहाद्वा दशहाद्वा पक्षाद्वाघ्नन्ति मानवम्।
तामग्निरोहिणीं विद्यादसाध्यां सर्व्वदोषजाम्॥
१६. नखमांसमधिष्ठाय वायुः पित्तञ्च देहिनाम्।
कुर्व्वते दाहपाकौ च तं व्याधिं चिप्पमादिशेत्॥
१७. तदेवाल्पतरै दोषैः परुषं कुनखं वदेत्।
१८. गम्भीरामल्पसंरम्भां सवर्णा मुपरि स्थिताम्।
पादस्यानुशयीं तान्तु विद्यादन्तः प्रपाकिनीम्॥
१९. विदारीकन्दवृद्वत्तां कक्षावङ्क्षणासन्धिषु।
विदारिकेति तां विद्यात् सर्व्वजां सर्व्वलक्षणम्॥
२०. प्राप्यं मांसशिरास्नायुः श्लेष्मा मेद स्तथानिलः।
ग्रन्थिं करोत्यसौ भिन्नेमधुसर्पिर्वसानिभं॥

13. *Kakhia*—Swellings of the glands in the axilla.

14. *Gundanama*—Pustules over the body, like the last.

15. *Agnihini*—A hard inflammatory swelling in the axilla, with strong fever, and other severe symptoms. It is a dangerous disease when not treated in the first stage.

16. *Chippa*—Ulceration destroying the nails, (see before).

17. *Kunakha*—Discolouration of the nails, which drop off.

18. *Pādānusoie*—Small scrofulous tumors in the feet.

19. *Bidarikā*—Large swellings in the axilla and groin.

20. *Shakārārbuda*—Are bleeding tumors, (see before).

स्त्रवत्यास्त्र्यवमनिल स्ता वृद्धिं पुनर्गतः॥
मांसं संशोष्य ग्रथितां शर्करां जनयेत्ततः।
दुर्गन्धि क्लिन्नमित्यर्थं नानावर्ण ततः शिराः।
स्त्रवन्ति रक्तं सहसा तं विद्याच्छर्करार्व्वुदम्॥

२१. परिक्रमणशीलस्य वायुरत्यर्थरुक्षयोः।
पादयोः कुरुते दारीं पाददारीं तमादिशेत्॥

२२. शर्करोन्मथिते पादे क्षते वा कण्ठकादिभिः।
ग्रन्थिः कोलवदुत्पन्नो जायते कदरं हि तत्॥

२३. क्लिन्नाङ्गुल्यन्तरौ पादौ कण्डुदाहरुजान्वितौ।
दुष्ट कर्द्दमसंस्पर्शादलसं तं विभावयेत्॥

२४. रोमकूपानुगं पित्रं वातेन सह मूच्छितम्।
प्रच्यावववति रोमाणि ततः श्लेष्मा सशोणितः॥
रुणद्धि रोमकूपांस्तु ततोऽन्येषामसम्भवः।
तदिन्द्रलुप्तं खालित्यं रुह्येति च विभाव्यते॥

२५. दारुणा कण्डुरा रुक्षा केशभूमिः प्रपाट्यते।
कफ मारुतकोपेन विद्याद्दारुणकन्तु तम्।

२६. अरुंषि बहुवक्त्राणि बहुक्लेदीनि मूर्द्धितु।
कफासृक् क्रिमिकोपेन नृनां विद्यादरुंषिकाम्॥

21. *Cadara*—Hard swellings like the seeds of the plum in the soles of the feet, produced by external injuries.
22. *Alasa*—Sores beteween the toes.
23. *Indralupta*—Baldness.
24. *Darunaka*—Scaley eruptions in the roots of the hairs of the head.
25. *Arunsīkā*—Small pustules in the head, which discharge.
26. *Palīta*—Gray hair.

२७. क्रोधशोकश्रमकृतः शरीरोष्मा शिरोगतः।
पित्तञ्च केशान् पचति पलितं तेन-जायते॥
२८. शाल्मलीकण्ठकप्रख्याः कफमारुतरक्तजाः।
युवान पीड़कां धुनां विज्ञेया मुखदूषिकाः॥
२९. कण्टके रोचितं वृत्तं मण्डलं पाण्डु कण्डूरम्।
पद्मिनी कण्टकप्रख्यं तदाख्यं कफवातजम्॥
३०. सममुत्सन्नमरुजं मण्डलं कफरक्तजम्।
सहजं लक्ष्म चेकैषां लक्षी जतुमणिस्तु सः॥
३१. अवेदनं स्थिरञ्चैव यस्मिन् गात्रे प्रदृश्यते।
माषवत् कृष्णमुत्सन्नमनिलान्माषकन्तु तम्॥
३२. कृष्णानि तिलभात्रानि नीरुजानि समानि च।
वातपित्तकफोद्रेकात् तान् विद्यात्तिलकालकान्॥
३३. महद्वा यदि वा चाल्मं श्यावं वा यदि वासितम्।
नीरुजं मण्डलं गात्रे न्यच्छमित्यभिधयीते॥

27. *Mukhadusīkā*-Small eruptions appearing in the face, at the time or puberty.

28. *Pudīnīkantaka*—Rough circular spots on the surface of the body.

29. *Jatumani*—Black and sometimes red or white spots, in any part of the body.

30. *Masaka*—Blackish spots like the figure of *māskalāi*, (a kind of pea).

31. *Tīlakālaka*—Very black spots over the body. These are not accompanied with pain, and are like *til* seed.

32. *Nayachchhu*—Spots of grey or dark colour, sometimes covering most parts of the body. These are indolent, and without pain.

33. *Byanga*—Small circular spots in the face.

३४. क्रोधायास प्रकुपितो वायुः पित्तेन
संयुतः मुखमामाद्य सहसा मण्डलं विसृजत्यतः।
नीरुजं तनुकं श्यावं मुखेव्यङ्गं तमादिशेत्॥
३५. कृष्णमेवं गुणं गात्रे मुखे वा नीलिकां विदुः॥
३६. मर्द्दनात् पीड़नाद्वाति तथैवाप्यभिघाततः।
मेढ्रचर्म्मयदा वायुर्भजते सर्व्वतश्चरन्॥
तदा वातोपसृष्टत्वात् तच्चर्मं परिवर्त्तते।
मणेरधस्तात् कोषश्च ग्रन्थिरूपेण लम्वते॥
परिवर्त्तिकेति तां विद्यात् सरुजां वातसम्भवाम्।
सकण्डुकठिना वापि सैव श्लेष्मसमुत्थिता॥
३७. अल्पीयः खां यदा हर्षाद्बलादगच्छ्रेत् स्त्रियं नरः।
हस्ताभिघातदथवा चर्म्मणपद्वर्त्तिते बलात्।
यस्यावपाट्यते चर्म्म ता विद्यादवपाटिकाम्॥
३८. वातोपसृष्टे मेढ्रे वै चर्म्म संश्रयते मणिम्।
मणिश्चर्म्मोपनद्धस्तु मूत्रोश्रोतोरुणद्धि च॥
निरुद्धप्रकशे तस्मिन् मन्दधारं संवेदनम्॥
मूत्रं प्रवर्त्तते जन्तो र्मणि र्विव्रियते न च।
निरुद्धप्रकश विद्यात् सरुजं वातसम्भवम्॥

34. *Nilika*—Bluish coloured spots in the face.

35. *Pariburtika*—Swelling of the prepuce, (Phymosis, see before).

36. *Adapātika*—When the prepuce turns backwards, and swells (Paraphymosis, see before).

37. *Nirudhoprokasa*—Strictutre of the urethra, (see before).

38. *Sanniradaguda.*—Stricture of the anus, (see before).

३९. वेगसन्धारणाद्वायु विहितो गुदसंश्रितः।
निरुणद्धि महास्त्रोत सूक्ष्मद्वारं करोति च॥
मार्गस्य सौक्ष्म्यात् कृच्छेण पुरीषं तस्य गच्छति।
सन्निरुद्धगुदं व्याधिं मेतंविद्यात् सुदारुणम्॥

४०. शकृन्मूत्रसमायुक्ते धौतेऽपाने शिशो र्भवेत्।
स्विन्ने वा स्नाप्यमानं वा कण्डुरक्ताकफोद्भवा॥
कण्डुयनात्ततः क्षिप्रं स्फोटः स्त्रावश्च जायते॥
एकीभूतं व्रणं घोरं तं विद्यादहि पूतनं॥

४१. स्नानोत्सादनहीनस्य मलो वृषणसंख्यितः।
यदा प्रक्लिद्यते स्वेदात् कण्डुं जनयते तदा।
कण्डुयनात्ततः क्षिप्रं स्फोटः स्त्रावश्चजायते।
शहुर्वृषणकच्छुंतां श्लेष्मरक्तप्रकोपजाम्।

४२. प्रावाहनातिसाराभ्यां निर्गच्छति गुदं वहि।
रुक्ष दुर्व्वलदेहस्य गुदभ्रंशं तमादिशेत्॥

४३. सदाहो रक्तपर्य्यन्त स्तकपाकी तीव्रवेदन।
कण्डूमान् ज्वरकारी च स स्याच्छूकरदंष्ट्रकः॥

39. *Ahiputana*—Small eruptions round the anus, particularly in children.
40. *Brisanakuchu*—Peculiar itch of the scrotum produced by uncleanness.
41. *Gudabhrunsa*—Prolapsus ani.
42. *Shukarādunstraka*—Swellings with inflammation of the skin.
43. *Grunthi*—Tumors and diseases of glands.
44. *Bisharpa*—Erysipelatous inflammation, (see before).

मुखरोगनिदानम्

औष्ठगतनिदानम्

आनुपपिशितक्षीर-दाध-मत्स्यातिसेवनात्।
मुखमध्ये गदान् कुर्य्युः क्रूद्दादोषा स्त्रय स्तथा॥
कर्कशौ परुषौ स्तब्धौ संप्राप्तानिलवेदनौ।
दाल्येते परिपाट्येते ओष्ठौ मारुतकोपतः।
चीयते पिड़काभिश्च सरुजाभिः समन्ततः।
सदाहपाकपिड़कौ पीताभासौ च पित्ततः।
सवर्णाभिश्च चीयेते पीड़काभि रवेदनौ।
भवतस्तु कफादोष्ठौ पिच्छिलौ शीतलौ गुरु।
सकुत्कृष्णो सकृत् पीतौ सकृतश्वेतौ तयैव च।
सन्निपातेन पिज्ञेयावनेकपिड़काचितौ।

DISEASES OF THE MOUTH (*Mukharoga*)

The diseases of the mouth are sixty-five: viz. Eight diseases of the lips; fifteen of the gums; eight of the teeth; four of the tongue; nine of the palate, seventeen of the throat; and three general diseases.

DISEASES OF THE LIPS (Austha)

By using too much food, such as fish, the flesh of buffaloes, milk, curdled milk, etc. the three humours are deranged producing diseases of the Lips. They become rough, hard, and stiff. When the bile is much deranged they are very painful, and small eruptions appear upon the surface. When bile is deranged, there is much inflammation, the lips become yellow, and the eruptions are painful, and of a yellow colour. When phlegm is deranged the lips are covered with a thin oleaginous looking matter, are cold, stiff, and of a dark yellow, white, or mixed colour. The eruptions are likewise of different colours.

खर्ज्जूरफलवर्णाभिः पिड़काथ र्निपीड़ितौ।
रक्तोपसृष्टौ रुधिर स्त्रवतः शोणितप्रभौ।
गुरु स्थूलौ मांसद्रुष्टौ मांसपिण्डवद्रुदूगदतौ।
जन्तवश्चात्र मूर्च्छन्ति नरस्योभयतो मुखात्॥
सर्पिर्मण्डप्रतीकाशौ मेदसा कण्डुरौ गुरू।
अच्छूं स्फटिकसङ्काशं मास्त्रावं स्त्रवतो भृशम्॥
तयो ब्रणो न संरोहेन्मृदुत्वञ्च न गच्छति।
ओष्ठौ पर्य्यदोर्य्येपाट्येते चभिघाततः।

दन्तवेष्टगतनिदानम्

शोणितं दन्तवेष्टेभ्यो यस्याकस्म्यात् प्रवर्त्तते।
दुर्गन्धीनि सकृष्णानि प्रक्लेदीनि मृदुनि च॥
दन्तमांसानि शीर्य्यन्ते पचन्ति च परस्परम्।
शीतादो नाम स व्याधिः कफशोणितसम्भवः॥

When blood is deranged in the lips they become red, swollen, and very painful. They often bleed. When the flesh is affected they become swollen, heavy, sometimes ulceration takes place, and worms form in it. When fat is affected the lips become glistening, like the surface of ghee. They are also itchy and heavy, and the discharge is like pure water. These ulcers do not heal easily.

DISEASES OF THE GUMS (Dantavestha)

There are fifteen diseases described under this head.

Sitāda is when the gums are black and blood is discharged without any external cause. In such cases the gums are separated from the teeth, soft, and putrid. In other cases they slough. This disease is produced by derangements of phlegm, and blood.

Dantapapataka. This disease is produced by derange-

दन्तयो स्त्रिषु वा यस्य श्वयथु र्जायते महान्।
दन्त पुप्पुटको नाम स व्याधिः कफरक्तजः।
स्त्रवन्ति पूयरुधिरं चला दन्ता भवन्ति च।
दन्तवेष्टः स विज्ञेयो दुष्टशोणित सम्भवः।।
श्वयथु द्रन्तमूलेषु रुजावान् कफरक्तजः।
लालास्त्रावी स विज्ञेयः शैशिरो नाम नामतः।।
दन्ताश्चलन्तिवोष्ठेभ्यः स्तालुश्चाप्यवशोर्य्यते।
यस्मिन् स सर्व्वजो व्याधिर्महाशैशिरसंज्ञितः।।
दन्तमांसानि शीर्य्यन्ते यस्मिन् ष्ठीवति चाप्यसृक्।
पित्तासृक कफजो व्याधि र्ज्ञेयः परिदरो हि सः।।
वोष्ठेषु दाहः पाकश्च ताभ्यां दन्ताश्चलन्ति च।
यस्मिन् सोपकुशो नाम पित्तरक्तकृतो गदः।।

ments of phlegm and blood; and is characterized by painful swelling of the gums, covering two or three of the alveolar processes.

Dantabeshta is produced by deranged blood, and is characterized by a discharge of pus mixed with blood. In this disease the teeth become loose.

Sawesara is characterized by a painful swelling of the gums, which are itchy, and are accompanied with a copious discharge of saliva. This disease is caused by a derangement of phlegm, and blood.

Mahāsansira is produced by the derangement of air, bile and phlegm. In this variety the teeth become loose, with severe pain about the palate. Matter is formed in the gums, and the inside of the mouth is inflamed.

Parīdarah is produced by derangement of bile, blood, and phlegm; and is characterized by blood being discharged from the gums; which are flabby, and separate from the teeth.

Apakusa is produced by derangement of bile and blood.

घृष्टेषु दन्तमांसेषु संरम्भो जायते महान्।
भवन्ति दन्ताश्चपलाः स बैदर्भोऽभिघातजः॥
मारुतेनाधिको दन्तो जायते तीव्रवेदनः॥
खलिवर्द्धनसंज्ञोऽसौ जाते रुक् च प्रशाम्यति॥
शनैः शनैः प्रकुरुते वायुद्रन्तसमाश्रितः।
करालान् विकटान् दन्तान् करालो न स सिद्धति॥
हानव्ये पश्चिमे दन्ते महान् शोथो महारुजः।
लालास्त्रावी कफकृतो विज्ञेयः सोऽधिमांसकः।
दन्तमूलगता नाड्यः पञ्च ज्ञेया यथेरिताः॥

दन्तगतनिदानम्

दीर्य्यमानेष्विव रुजा यस्य दन्तेषु जायते।
दालनो नाम स व्याधिः सदागतिनिमित्तजः॥

In this disease, abscesses form in the gums with little pain; the teeth become loose, and when the gums are touched, they bleed. There is fector of the mouth, and after the discharge of blood from the gums, they again swell.

Baidurba. This disease is caused by external injury, as by cleaning the teeth with too hard a tooth-brush. In this disease the teeth become loose.

Adidanta. When the air is deranged it produces irregularity in the growth of the teeth, with much pain; such teeth should be extracted, apply the actual cautery, and then treat it as of a caries of the tooth.

Adīmānsīka is the swelling round the wisdom-teeth, producing much pain and swelling, with the discharge of saliva. It is produced by diseased phlegm.

DISEASES OF THE TEETH (*Danta*)

Tooth-ache (Dālana), in which the tooth becomes very painful. This is caused by the derangement of air. When there

कृष्णश्छिद्रश्चलः स्रावी संसरम्नो महारुजः।
अनिमित्तरुजो वाताद्विज्ञेयः क्रिभिदन्तकः॥
वक्त्रं वक्रं भवेद्यस्य दन्तभङ्गश्च जायते॥
कफवातकृतो व्याधिः स भञ्जनकसंज्ञितः॥
शीतरुक्षप्रवाताम्ल स्पर्शानामसहा द्विजाः।
पित्तमारुतकोपेन दन्तहर्षः स नामतः।
मलो दन्तगतो यस्तु कफ मारुतशोषितः।
शर्करैव खरस्पर्शा सा ज्ञेया दन्तशर्करा॥
कपालेष्विव जीर्य्यतसु दन्तानां सैव शर्करा।
कापालिकेति विज्ञेया सदा दन्तविनाशिनी॥
असृड्भिश्रेण पित्तेन दग्धो दन्त्वस्वसेषतः॥
श्यावतां नीलतां वापि गतः स श्यावदन्तकः॥

is a small black decayed part of the tooth which is painful, and discharges matter with swelling, and much pain, it is called *Krimidantaka* or warm-eaten tooth.

When the mouth is turned to a side, and the teeth broken, as in spasms, it is produced by phlegm, and is called *Bangana*.

SENSIBLE TEETH (*Dantaharsa*)

In this disease the person cannot bear cold, or hot applications; cool air, and sour articles produce much pain. Diseased bile air produce this form of disease.

When bile and blood are deranged, the teeth become of a dark colour, as if burnt in the fire, and the disease is named *Siābadantaka*.

An when deranged, may produce dislocation of the lower jaw, which is called *Hanamaka,* and the symptoms are the same as the form of the disease named *Ardīta*.

जिह्वागतनिदानम्

जिह्वानिलेन स्फुटिता प्रसुप्ता भवेच्च शाकच्छदनप्रकाशा।
पित्त्येन दह्यत्युपदीयते च दीर्घैः सरक्तैः रपि कण्टककैश्च॥
कफेन गुर्व्वी बहुलाचिता च मांसोच्छ्रयैः शाल्मलिकण्टकाभैः।
जिह्वातले यः स्वयथुः प्रगाढः सोऽलाससंज्ञः कफरक्तमूर्त्तिः॥
जिह्वां स ततु स्तम्मयति प्रवृद्धो मूले च जिह्वा भृशमेति पाकम्।
जिह्वाग्ररूपः स्वयथुहि जिह्वा मुन्नस्य जात कफरक्तमूल॥
लालाकरः कण्डुयुतः सचोष सा तूपजिह्व पठिता भिषग्भिः॥

तालुगतनिदानम्

श्लेष्मासृग्भ्यां तालुमूले प्रवृद्धो दीघः।
शोथाष्मात वस्तिप्रकाशः तृष्णा कास श्वासयुक्तं॥

DISEASES OF THE TONGUE (*Jihva*)

When air is deranged in the tongue the person has no sense of feeling or taste in the organ, which is rough and divided into fissures. *Bile*. In this variety there is great heat, long and red papillae over its surface. When *phlegm* is deranged the tongue becomes heavy, thick, and the papillae over the surface of the tongue enlarge.

Alāsa. This form of disease is produced by deranged phlegm and blood, and is characterized by swelling on the upper surface of the tongue, particularly near its root. In this disease the tongue cannot be moved, and sometimes abscesses form.

Apasiba is produced by diseased phlegm and blood, under the tongue. It is like a second tongue. In this disease there with is a profuse discharge or saliva, accompanied with itchness and burning pain.

DISEASE OF PALATE (*Talu*)

1. When the phlegm and blood are deranged in the soft palate, it becomes large, like a full bladder, and is accompanied thirst, cough and difficulty in breathing.

वदन्ति व्याधिं वैद्यो गलशुण्डीति नाम्ना शाथः।
स्थूल स्तोददाहप्रपाकी प्रागुप्ताभ्या दण्डिकेरी मतातु॥
मन्दः शोथो लोहितो शोणितात्थो
ज्ञेयो ध्रवः सज्वर स्तीव्ररुक् च।
कुर्म्मोन्नतोऽवेदनोऽशीघ्रजन्मा रागा
ज्ञेयः कच्छपः श्लेष्मणा तु॥
पद्म्यकारं तालुमध्ये तु शोथं विद्याद्रक्तादर्व्वूदं प्रोक्तलिङ्गम्।
दुष्ट मांसं नीरुजं तालुमध्ये कफात् प्रोक्तो मांसङ्घात एषः।
अरुक् स्थायी कीलमात्रः कफात् स्थात्
भेदो युक्तात् पुप्पुटस्तालुदेशे। शोषत्यर्थं

This disease is called *Kantasunda* (enlarged tonsils). In other cases the swelling is accompanied with much pain and heat; suppuration being produced by phlegm, and blood. It is called *Tundikari*.

2. When the part is much swelled, hard, and of a red colour, and is produced by diseased blood it is called *Adussah,* which is accompanied with fever and severe pain. When the swelling is of the shape of a turtle, is without pain, is produced slowly, being caused by diseased phlegm, it is called *Kachhapa*.
3. Sometimes the swelling is like a water-lily and in the soft palate is called *Raktabuda,* and is produced by a disease of the blood.
4. When flesh is swelled in the palate, there is no pain; when produced by phlegm, it is called *Mānsa-sangāhāta*.
5. When swelled like a plum, without pain, and remains in one spot, being produced by phlegm, and mixed with fat it is called *Puputah*.
6. *Tālupāka*. Is produced by deranged bile, and is characterized by suppuration in the soft palate.

दीर्य्यते चापि तालुं श्वासश्चोग्रस्तालुशोषोऽनिलाच्च॥
पितं कुर्य्यात् पाकमत्यर्थघोरं तालुन्येवं तालुपाकं वदन्ति॥

कण्ठगतनिदानम्

गलेऽनिलः पित्तकफौ च मूर्च्छितौ प्रदूष्य मांसञ्च तथैव शोणितम्।
गलोपसंरोधकरै स्तथाङ्कुरै र्निहन्त्यसून् व्याधिरियं हि रोहिणी॥
जिह्वा समन्ताद्भृशवेदनास्तु सांसाङ्कराः कण्ठ विरोधिनो ये।
सा रोहिणी वातकृता प्रदिष्टा वातात्मकोपद्रव गाढ़युक्ता॥
क्षिप्रोद्गमा क्षिप्रविदाहपाका तीव्रज्वरा पित्तनिमित्तजा तु।
स्त्रोतोविरोधिन्यचलोद्गता च स्थिराङ्कुरा या कफसम्भवा सा।
गम्भीरपाकिन्यनिवार्य्यवीर्य्या त्रिदोषलिङ्गां त्रितयोत्थिता च।
स्फोटैश्चिता पित्तसमानलिङ्गा साध्या प्रदिष्टा रुधिरात्मिका तु॥

7. *Talushosh*. In this disease the palate is very dry, and is accompanied with difficulty in breathing, and much pain.

DISEASES OF THE NECK

These diseases consist of 1. Diseases of the throat; 2. Hoarseness; 3. Goitre; 4. Scrofulous swellings; and 5. Tumors of the neck.

THROAT (*Kantha*)

There are five forms of diseases of the throat.

When air, bile and phlegm are deranged in the throat separately or combined, or when the blood is diseased they form the five varieties of this disease. These produce a swelling in the throat, which shuts up the wind-pipe, and produces sudden death. It is called *Rahini*.

When the *air* is deranged, in the severe forms all the symptoms of deranged air are produced.

Bile. In this form papillae of flesh quickly enlarge, become hot, and ripen, and severe fever.

कोलास्थिमात्रः कफसम्भवो यो ग्रन्थिर्गले कण्टकशूकभूतः।
स्वरः स्थिरः शस्त्रनिपातसाध्य स्तं कण्ठशालूक मिति ब्रुवन्ति॥
जिह्वाग्ररूपः श्वयथुः कफात्तु जिह्वोपरिष्टादपि रक्तमिश्रात्॥
ज्ञेयोऽधिजिह्वः खलु रोग एष विवर्ज्जयेदागतपाकमेनम्।
वलाश एवायतमुन्नतञ्च शोथं करोत्यन्नगतिं निवार्य्य॥
तं सर्व्वथैवा प्रतिवार्य्य वीर्य्य विवर्ज्जनीयं वलयं वदन्ति॥
गले तु शोथं कुरुतः प्रवृद्धौ श्लेष्मानिलौ श्वासरुजोपपन्नम्।
मर्म्मच्छिदं दुस्तरमेनमाहुर्वलाशसंज्ञं निपुण विकारम्।
वृत्तान्नतोऽन्तः स्वयथुः सदाहः सकण्डुरोऽपाक्यभृद्गुर्गूरुश्च॥
नाम्नैकवृन्दः परिकीर्त्तितोऽसौ व्याधि र्वलासक्षतजप्रसूतः।
ससुन्नतं वृत्तमन्ददाहं तीव्रज्वरं वृन्दं मुदाहरन्ति।
तच्चापि पित्तक्षतजः प्रकोपात् ज्ञेयं सतोदं पवनाताकन्तु॥

Phlegm. The passage of the throat is closed, and the swelling remains long and at length supparates. Fleshy elevations are formed.

When air, bile and phlegm are deranged at the same time, the swelling suppurates to a great depth in the tongue. It is incurable, and the three forms of symptoms of diseased air, bile, and phlegm appear. When blood is deranged many small swellings form upon the tongue, and near its root, accompanied with symptoms of deranged bile, this form may be cured.

When a swelling like a plum is situated in the throat, and produces difficulty in breathing, and a hard and rough swelling, it is caused by phlegm, and is naked *Kantasāluka*. *Adījība* is a swelling at the root of the tongue like a second tongue, (this is probably a swelling of the epiglottis,) and is produced by the phlegm and blood. When it suppurates it is incurable. Various other swellings of the throat which prevents swallowing, and is produced by phlegm. It is incurable. Phlegm and air produce the swelling in the throat, which is accompanied with severe

वर्त्तिर्धना कण्ठनिरोधिनी या चितातिमात्रं पिशितप्ररोहैः।
अनेकरुक् प्राणहरी त्रिदोषात् ज्ञेया शतघ्नी तु शतघ्नीरूपा॥
ग्रन्थि र्गले त्वामलकास्थिमात्रः स्थिरोऽतिरुग् यः कफरक्तमूर्त्तिः।
संलक्ष्यते सक्त मिवाशनञ्च सशस्त्रसाध्यस्तु शिलायुसंज्ञः॥ सर्व्वें
गलं व्याप्य समुत्थितो यः शोथोरुजाः सन्ति च यत्र सर्व्वाः।
स सर्व्व दोषो गलविद्रधिस्तु तस्यैव तुल्यः खलु सर्व्वजस्य॥
शोथो महानन्नजलावरौधी तीव्रज्वरो वायुगते र्निहन्ता॥
कफेन जातो रुधिरान्वितेन गले गलौः परिकीर्त्तते तु।
यस्त्वाम्यमानः श्वशिति प्रसक्तं भिन्नस्वरः शुष्वाविमुक्तकण्ठः॥
कफोपदिग्धेष्वीनलायनेषु ज्ञेयः स रोगः श्वसनात् स्वरघ्नः।

pain, and difficulty in breathing. This is also a very dangerous form of disease.

Diseased phlegm and blood produce a swelling in the throat accompanied with itchiness, and a burning sensation. It is soft, heavy, and does not suppurate. It is called *Ekabrinda.* When it is accompanied with fever, it is called *Brinda*. This is an incurable disease.

A thick swelling of the throat, causing difficulty in breathing, and surrounded by small papulae like piles with much pain, is produced by air, bile and phlegm ; it is called *Satagni,* (or it is like the instrument of this name which at once kills 100 persons :) it is incurable.

Gīlin. The swelling in this disease is like the stone of a plum, not painful, but hard ; and is produced by diseased phlegm, and blood.

Sarungna. (Croup?) when phlegm stops the passage of air, this produces dryness of the throat, hoarseness, difficulty in breathing and great uneasiness. It is incurable.

Mānsatāna, is a swelling in the throat which produces suffocation. It is very dangerous.

प्रतानवान् यः स्वयथुः सुकष्टो गलोपरोधं कुरुते क्रमेण॥
स मांसतानः कथितोऽवलम्वी प्राणप्रणुत् सर्व्वकृतो विकारः।
सदाहतोदं स्वयथुं सुताम्रमन्तर्गले पूतिविशीर्णमांसम्।
पित्तेन विद्याद्वदने विदारीं पार्श्वे विशेषात् स तु येन शेते॥

सर्व्वसरानिदानम्

स्फोटैः सतोदै र्वदनं समन्ताद् यस्याचितं सर्व्वसरः स वातात्।
रक्तैः सदाहै स्तनुभिः सपीतै र्यस्याचितञ्चापि स पित्तकोपात्॥
अवेदनैः कण्डुयुतैः सवर्णै र्यस्याचितञ्चापि स वै कफेन॥
ओष्ठप्रकोपे वर्ज्ज्याः स्यु र्मांसरक्तत्रिदोषजाः।
दन्तमूलेषु वर्ज्जौ च त्रिलिङ्गगतिशौषिरौ॥
दन्तेषु च न सिध्यन्ति श्याव दालनभञ्जनाः॥
जिह्वगतेष्वलासस्तु तालव्येष्वर्ब्बुद स्तथा॥
स्तरघ्नो बलयो वृन्दो बलाशः स विदारिका।
गलौघो मांसतानश्च शतघ्नी रोहिणी गले॥
असाध्याः कीर्त्तिता ह्येते रोगा नव दशैव तु।
तेषु चापि क्रिया वैद्यः प्रत्याखाय समाचरेत्॥

कर्णस्रोतोगतनिदानम्

समीरणः श्रोत्रगतोऽऽन्यथा चरन् समन्ततः शूलमतीव कर्णयोः।
करोति दीषैश्च यथास्वमावृतः स कर्णशूलः कथितो दुराचरः॥

Bidārī. The swelling is accompanied with great pain, redness, followed by sloughing. This is an incurable disease.

Gullagha, is a large swelling in the throat extending over the throat with great pain, and high fever. The patient cannot swallow food nor drink water. It is produced by phlegm and blood, and is considered incurable.

कर्णस्त्रोतः स्थिते वाते शृणोति विविधान् स्वरान्॥
भेरीमृदङ्गोशंखानां कर्णनादः स उच्यते।
यदाशब्दवहं वायुः स्त्रोत आवृत्य तिष्ठति॥
शुद्धः श्लेष्मान्वितोवापि वाधिय्युं तेन जायते॥
वायुः पित्तादिभि र्यक्तो वेणुघोषोपमं स्वनम्॥
करोति कर्णयोः क्षेड़ं कर्णक्ष्वेड़ स उच्यते॥
शिरोऽभिघातदथवा निमज्जतो जले प्रपाकादथवापि विद्रधेः।
स्त्रवेद्धि पूयं श्रवणोऽनिलार्द्दितः सकर्णसंस्त्राव इति प्रदिष्टः।
मारुतः कफसंयुक्तः वार्णकण्डूं करोति च॥
पित्तोष्मशोषितः श्लेष्मा जायते कर्णगूथकः।
स कर्णगूथो द्रवतां गतो यदा विलायितो घ्रानमुखं प्रपद्यते।
तदा स कर्णप्रतिनाह संज्ञितो भवेद्विकारः शिरसूर्द्धभेदकृत्॥
यदा तु मूच्छन्त्यथवापि जन्तवः सृजन्त्यपत्यान्यथवावपि मक्षिकाः।
तद्व्यञ्जनत्वाच्छ्रवणो निरुच्यते भिषग्भिराद्यैः क्रिमिकर्णिको गदः॥
पतङ्गाः शतपद्यश्च कर्णस्त्रोतः प्रविश्य हि।
अरतिं व्याकुलत्वञ्च भृशं कुर्व्वन्ति वेदनाम्॥
कर्णो निस्तुद्यते तस्य तथा फरफरायते॥
कीटे चरति रुक् तीव्रा निस्पन्दे मन्दवेदना।
क्षताभिघातप्रभवस्तु विद्रधि र्भवेत्तथा दोषकृतोऽपरः पुनः।
सरक्तपीतारुणमश्रमाश्रवेत् प्रतोदधूमायनदाहचोषवान्॥
कर्णपाकस्तु पित्तेन कोथविक्लेदकृद्भवेत्॥
कर्णविद्रधिपाकाद्वा जायते चाम्बुपूरणात्॥
पूयं स्त्रवति यः पूति स ज्ञेयः पूतिकर्णकः।
कर्ण शोथ्श्रार्व्वुदार्शांसि जानीयादुक्तलक्षणैः॥

कर्णरोगनिदानम्

नादोतिरुक् कर्णमलस्य शोषः स्त्रावस्तनुश्चाश्रवणञ्च वातात्।
शोथः सरागो दरणं विदाहः सपीत पूतिस्त्रवणञ्च पित्तात्॥
वैश्रुत्य कण्डुस्थिरशोथशुक्लस्निग्धश्रुतः श्लेष्मभवेऽल्परुक् च।
सर्व्वाणि रूपाणि च सन्निपाते स्त्रावश्च तत्राधिक दोषवर्णः॥
सौकुमार्य्याच्चिरोत्सृष्टे सहसातिप्रवर्द्धिते।
कर्णशोथो भवेत् पाल्यां सरुजः परिपोटवान्॥
कृष्णारुणनिभः स्तब्धः स वातात् परिपोटकः।
गुर्ब्बाभरणसंयोगात् ताड़नाद्घर्षणादपि॥

DISEASES OF THE EARS (*Karnaroga*)

The more copious secretion from the external ears, and the most changes of temperature of the air, render diseases of this organ of frequent occurrence in this country. They produce much suffering, and much attention seems to have been paid by the Hindus to their nature and cure.

There are twenty-eight diseases of the ear. The corporeal *air* is the cause of all these diseases. When it is deranged in the ear, and is confined in its passage by the other humours, it produces severe pain in the organ, which is called *Karnashūla*, and is very difficult to cure. When air is deranged in the passages of the ear, several kinds of sounds are heard, like those of certain instruments called *Karnanāda*. When air is deranged with phlegm in the ear passages, and if not treated it will produce defness called *Bādhirjya*.

Fatigue, or eating hot or astringent substances, or the frequent use of errhines produce a derangement of the air in the ear passages called *Karnakshyera*, which consist in a peculiar ringing noise. In others the disease is produced by blows on the ear, by bathing in water during which water enters the ears, or by a boil in the part which suppurates. This disease is called *Karnasangsrāba*.

शोथः पाल्यां भवेच्छ्यावो दाहपाकरुजान्वितः॥
रक्तो वा रक्तपित्ता भ्यामुत्पातः स गदो मतः॥
कर्ण बलाद्वर्द्धयतः पाल्यं वायुः प्रकुप्यति॥
कफं संगृह्य कुरुते शोथं स्तब्धभवेदनम्।
उन्मन्थकः सकण्डुको विकारः कफवातजः॥
संवर्द्धमाने दुर्विद्धे कण्डुदाहरुजान्वितः।
शोथो भवति पाकश्च त्रिदोषो दुःखवर्द्धनः॥
कफासृक् क्रिमयः क्रुद्धाः सर्षपाभाः विसर्पिणः।
कुर्व्वन्ति पाल्यां पिड़काः कण्डुदाहरुजान्विताः॥
कफासृक्-क्रिमिसम्भूतः स विसर्पान्वित स्ततः।
लिहेत् सशष्कुलीं पाली परिलेहीति स स्मृतः॥

When *air* and *phlegm* are deranged in the ear it produces itchiness; and bile being deranged dries up the phlegm, and wax in the ear. This disease is named *Karnagūthaka*. When the wax melts it passes out of the nose (*Susruta*), or mouth *Nidāna*, and the disease is called *Pratināha*, and is accompanied with much pain in the head.

If worms form in the ear by flies depositing their eggs in the ear, the disease is called *Krimikarnaka*.

When the ear is wounded or otherwise injured it is called *Bidradhi*. In other cases there is great pain, burning, and tightness in the part, with a discharge of yellow pus or blood ; it is then called *Karnabidradhi*. By the derangements of bile abscesses are formed, which is called *Karnapāka*.

When *phlegm* is deranged and dried up by the heat of the bile, it melts, and then is discharged from the ear, with a disagreeable smell. It is called *Pritikarnaka*. There are also four kinds of bloody tumors, seven varieties of other tumors, and four kinds of swellings to which the ear is liable.

In defects of the external ear, *Susruta* recommends the surgeon to prepare a new ear, by removing skin from the neighbouring part, leaving a connection to keep up its vitality.

नासारोगनिदानम्

अनह्यते यस्य विशुष्यते च प्रक्लिद्यते धूप्यति चापि नासा।
न वेत्ति यो गन्धरसांश्च जन्तु र्जुष्टं व्यवस्येत्तमपीनसेन।।
तच्चानिल श्लेष्मभवं विकारं ब्रूयात् प्रतिश्याय समानगलिङ्गम्।
दोषै विदग्धैर्गलतालुमूले संमूच्छितो यस्य समीरणस्तु।।
निरेति पूति र्मूखनासिकाभ्यां तं पूतिनस्यं प्रवदन्ति रोगम्।
घ्राणश्रितं पित्तमरुंसि कुर्य्यात् यस्मिन् विकारे बलवांश्च पाकः।।
तं नासिकापाकमिति व्यवस्येद् विक्लेदकोऽथावथवापि यत्र।
दोषै र्विदग्धै रथवापि जन्तो र्ललाटदेशेऽभिहतस्य तैस्तैः।।
नासा स्त्रवेत् पूय मसृग्विमिश्रं तं पूयरक्तं प्रवदन्ति रोगम्।।
घ्राणाश्रितो मर्म्मनि संप्रदुष्टो यस्यानिलो नासिकया निरेति

DISEASES OF THE NOSE

There are thirty-one diseases of the nose. When the nostrils are closed, when one is dry, very dirty, and hot, when matter has formed, and when the patient can neither smell nor taste, the disease is called *Pinasa,* and is produced by a derangement of air and phlegm. When the air is stopped in the palate and nostrils, and there is a bad smell which proceeds from the mouth and nose, the disease is called *Putinaska*.

Bile when deranged in the nose produces small pimples, which quickly suppurate, and are called *Nāsīkāpāka*. In this disease a disagreeable discharge often proceeds from the nose and umbiliacus, for which blood-letting is to be used. When blood flows from the nose it is called *Nāsa-raktapitta,* in which case *air, bile and phlegm* are deranged. When the vital part of the nose is wounded, deranged air, etc. passes through the nostrils producing a bad smelling secretion mixed with blood, it is called *Puerakta*. When stimulating substances are applied to the nostrils, or by regarding the fire, the air is mixed with phlegm and passes from the nostrils with a noise, this is called *Kabuti* or sneezing. If phlegm thickens, as if prepared by fire,

कफानुजातो बहुशोऽतिशब्द स्तं रोगमाहुः क्षवतु र्विधिज्ञाः।
तीक्ष्णीपयोगादभिजिघ्रतों वा भावान् कटूनर्क निरीक्षणाद्वा।
सूत्राड्डिभि र्वा तरुणास्थिमर्ग्मण्युद्घाटितेऽन्यः क्षवतु र्निरेति॥
प्रभ्रश्यते नामिकया तु यस्य सान्द्रो विदग्धो लवणः कफस्तु।
प्राक्सञ्चितो मूर्द्धनि सूर्य्यतप्त स्तं भ्रंशथूं रोग मुदाहरन्ति॥
घ्राणे भृशं दाहसमन्विते तु विनिःसरेद्धूम इबेह वायुः।
नासा प्रदौंप्तेव च यस्य जन्तो र्व्याधिस्तु तं दीप्त मुदाहरन्ति॥
उच्छासमार्गन्तु कफः सवातो रुन्ध्यात् प्रतीनाह मुदाहरेत् तम्॥
घ्रानाद्घनः पीत सीत स्तनुर्व्वा दोषः स्त्रवेत् स्त्राव मुदाहरेत्तम्॥
घ्राणाश्रिते स्त्रोतसि मारुतेन गाढं प्रतप्ते परिशोषिते च॥
कृच्छ्रोच्छसेदूर्द्धमधश्च जन्ततु र्यस्मिन् स नासापरिशोष उक्तः।
शिरोगुरुत्वमरुचि र्नासास्त्राव स्तनुः स्वरः॥
क्षामः ष्ठीवत्यथाभीक्ष्णमामपीनस लक्षणम्।
आमलिङ्गान्वितः श्लेष्मा घनः खेषु निमज्वति॥
स्वरवर्णविशुद्धिश्च परिपक्कस्य लक्षणम्॥

and has a saltish taste, it is called *Bransuti*. If hot air proceeds from the nostrils, and air is discharged like smoke or is very hot, it is called *Dipta*. Phlegm when deranged with air so as to close the nostrils is called *Pratinaha*. When *air, bile, and phlegm* are deranged in the nostrils it dries. When the discharge is thin like water, and passes from the nostrils, particularly at night, it is called *Pāsāparsisrābah*.

When the nose is very hot and dry, and the passage of air gives great uneasiness, it is called *Nāsāparisasah*.

Pīnasa has an acute and chronic form. In the first the head is havey, the patient has no appetite, and the discharge from the nose is thin. The voice becomes altered, with occasional vomiting and weakness of the body. When chronic, the phlegm as it is discharged from the nose, thickens, and the

सन्धारणाजीर्णरजोऽतिभाष्य क्रोधर्त्तु वैषम्यशिरोऽभितापैः।
प्रजागरातिस्वपनाम्बुशीतै रवश्यया मैथुनवास्पधमैः॥
संस्तानदोषे शिरसि प्रवृद्धो वायुः प्रतिश्याय मुदीरयेत्तु।
चयं गता मुर्द्धनि मारुतादयः पृथक् समस्ताश्च तथैव शोणितम्।
प्रकुप्यमाना विविधैः प्रकोपनै स्ततः प्रतीश्यायकरा भवन्ति हि॥
क्षवप्रवृत्तिः शिरसोऽतिपूर्णता स्तम्भोऽङ्गमर्दः परिहृष्टरोमता॥
उपद्रवाश्चाप्यपरे पृथग्विधा नृणां प्रतिश्याय पुरःसराः स्मृताः।
आनद्धा पिहिता नासा तनुस्त्राव प्रसेकिनी।
गलताल्वोष्ठशोषश्च निस्तोदः शङ्ख्यो स्तया।
क्षवप्रवृत्तिरत्यर्थं वक्त्रवैरस्य मेव च॥
भवेत् स्वरोपघातश्च प्रतिश्यायेऽनिलात्मके।
उष्णः सपीतकः स्त्रावो घ्राणात् स्त्रवति पैत्तिके
कृशोऽतिपाण्डुः सन्तप्तो भवेदुष्टाभि पीड़ितः।
मधुममग्निं सहसा वमतीव स मानवः॥

voice becomes natural. The colour of the skin is natural, and the discharged phlegm is thick, and very adhesive.

Pritisyaiah resembles *Apinnasa* and is sometimes produced by the neglect in the calls of nature, by eating indigestable food, and allowing the accumulation of dust in the nostrils; speaking or crying much; frequent fits of anger, unusual and sudden alteration in the seasons, such as want of the accustomed rain, and exposure of the sun, watching or sleeping during the day, being wet with very cold water or dew, and excessive venery produce the diseases of the nose; as also hot tears passing into the nostrils. By thses causes the humours are deranged in the head, producing the usual symptoms of catarrh; the general symptoms of which are sneezing, heaviness of the head, languor and pain, and stiffness over the body (*Guseska*).

When produced by *air* the nostrils become filled up, there is a thin discharge with dryness of the throat, palate, and lips, with severe throbbing pain of the temples, and hoarseness.

घ्राणात् कफकृते शीतः कफः पाण्टुः स्त्रवेद्बहुः॥
शुक्लावभासः शुक्लाक्षो भवेद्गुरुशिरा नरः।
कण्ठताल्वोष्ठशिरसां कण्टूभिरतिपीड़ितः॥
भूत्वा भूत्वा प्रतिश्वायो यस्याकम्मान्निवर्त्तते।
संपक्को वान्य पक्को वा स सर्व्व प्रभवः स्मृतः॥
प्रक्लिद्यते पुनर्नासा पुनश्च परिशुष्यति।
पुनरानह्यति वापि पुनर्विव्रियते तथा॥
निश्वासो वातिदुर्गन्धो नरो गन्धान्न वेत्ति च।
एवं दुष्टप्रतिश्वायं जानीयात् कृच्छ्रसाधनम्॥
रक्तजे तु प्रतिश्वाये रक्तस्त्रावः प्रवर्त्तते।

When *bile* is deranged the symptoms are a hot discharge of a yellow colour, the body is weak, of a gray colour, and hot. There is much thirst, and what is vomited is hot, and like smoke.

When *phlegm* is deranged the discharge is white or grayish and is copious and cold. The body becomes pale, eyelids swollen, head very heavy, and the throat, palate, lips, and head, are itchy.

When *air, bile* and *phlegm* are deranged the symptoms occur rapidly, disappear, and recur again, whether they be acute or chronic. At one time the nose is clean but it again becomes dirty, dry, and closes with foetid breath, and loss of smell. This is the bad form of the disease, and is cured with difficulty. If neglectd this disease passes into *Pinasa*. When it has continued for a long time it produces deafness, blindness, loss of smell, cough, and dyspepsia.

When *blood* is deranged, and is discharged from the nostrils, the eyes are reddish. This form is produced by injuries of the chest, and both the mouth and nostrils have a bad smell. He loses the sense of smell, and worms are produced in the nostril. These worms are small and of a black and white colour. The different forms of *Prahsiāka*, if not seen by the practitioner early, are not curable.

ताम्राक्षश्च भवेज्जन्तुरुरोघात-प्रतीड़ितः।
दुर्गन्धोच्छासवदनो गन्धानपि न वेत्ति सः॥
सर्व्व एव प्रतिश्याया नरस्याप्रतिकारिणः
दुष्ठतां यान्ति कालेन तदास्यध्या भवन्ति हि॥
मूच्छन्ति चात्र क्रिमयः श्वेताः स्निग्धा स्तथाणवः।
क्रिमितो यः शिरोरोग स्तुल्यं तेनास्य लक्षणम्।
वाधिर्य्यमन्ध्यमघ्रत्वं घोरांश्च नयनामयान्॥
शोथाग्निसादकासांश्च वृद्धाः कुर्व्वन्ति पीनसाः॥
अर्व्वूदं सप्तधा शोथा श्चत्वारोऽर्शश्चतुर्विधम्।
चतुर्विधं रक्तपितमुक्तं घ्राणेऽपितद्विदुः।

नेत्ररोगनिदानम्

सर्व्वगतनिदानम्

नव सन्ध्याश्रयास्तेषु वर्त्मजास्तेकविंशतिः।
शुक्लभागे दशैकश्च चत्वारः कृष्णभागजाः।
सर्व्वाश्रयाः सप्तदश दृष्टिजाः द्वादशैव तु॥

There are five forms of *Arbuda,* or tumors attacking the nose, and four of *Sota* (swellings), four kinds of *Arsa* (Polypus), and *Raktapitta* (Hemorrhage).

DISEASES OF THE EYES, (*Akīroga*)

It is related that *Janaka Rājā* of Mithilā or Tirhoot, did not perform the usual ceremonies and prayers to the sun, for which he was afflicted with the diseases of the eye. By abstinence and humiliation before the sun, however he was cured of the disease; and since then, by proper offerings he obtained the favour of, and was instructed by *Surya* concerning these diseases. He afterwards wrote a *Shāstra* on the subject, called *Sātāka Tantra,* which is stated to be "in profundity like the ocean."

बाह्यजौ द्वौ समाख्यातौ रोगौ परमदारुणौ।
भूय एतान् प्रवक्ष्यामि संख्यारूपचिकित्सितैः॥
उष्णाभितप्तस्य जले प्रवेश दुरेक्षणात् स्वप्न्यीपर्य्ययाच्च।
स्वेदाद्रजो धूमनिषेवनाच्च छर्द्दे र्विघाताद्वमनातियोगात्॥
द्रवात्तथान्नान्निशि सेविताच्च विन्मूत्रवातक्रमनिग्रहाच्च॥
प्रमक्तसंरोदन कोपशोकाच्छिरोऽभिघातादतिमद्यपानात्॥
तथा ऋतुनाञ्च विपर्ययेण क्लेशाभिघातादतिभैथुनाच्च।
वाष्पग्रहात् सूक्ष्मनिरीक्षणाच्च नेत्रे विकारान् जनयन्ति दोषाः॥
वातात् पित्तात् कफाद्रक्तादभिष्यन्द श्चतुर्विधः।
प्रायेन जायते घोरः सर्व्वनेत्रामयाकरः।
निस्तोदन-स्तम्भनरोमहर्ष-संहर्ष पारुष्य-शिरोऽभितापाः॥

There are 76 diseases of the eye, of these 10 are air diseases, 10 bile, 13 phlegm, 25 are produced by the derangement of the three humours, 16 by blood, and 2 external diseases. These diseases are again sub-divided into 9 of the joinings of the eye, 21 of the eyelids, 11 of the white part of the eye, 4 of the black part, 17 of the eye in general, 12 diseases of the true organs of vision *(Dristi)*, and two external diseases from injuries.

1. *Description of the eye.* After a description of the size of the eye it is stated that it is formed by a combination of all the elements. the flesh being produced by the earth, blood from the fire, the black part from the air, the white part from the water, and the different canals for the tears are produced by ether or sky. The black part extends over one-third of the eye, and the pupil about one-seventh part of the black part. The tunics are the two eyelids, and of the globe of the eye. The first surrounds the vitreous humour (*Tezajala,* or glistening water), the second is covered with flesh, the third with fat, and the fourth with bone. They distinguish five circles, the eyelashes, eyelids, the white sclerotic coat, the iris, and the pupil. There are five joinings, the eyelashes with the eyelids, the eyelids and

विशुष्कभावः शिशिराश्रुता च वाताभिपन्ने नयने भवन्ति।
दाहप्रपाकौ शिशिराभिनन्दा धूमायनं वाष्पसमुच्छ्रयश्च।
उष्णाश्रुता पीतकनेत्रता पित्ताभिपन्ने नयने भवन्ति।
उष्णाभिनन्दा गुरुताक्षिशोफः कण्डुपदेहावतिशीतता च॥
स्त्रावो मुहुः पिच्छिल एव चापि कफाभिपन्ने नयने भवन्ति।
पित्तस्य लिङ्गानि च यानि तानि रक्ताभिपन्ने नयने भवन्ति।
वृद्धैरेतैरभिष्यन्दै र्नराणामक्रियावताम्॥
तावन्तु स्त्वधिमन्थाः स्युर्नयने तीव्रवेदनाः।
उत्पाट्यत् इवात्यर्थ्यं नेत्रं निर्म्मथ्यते तथा॥
शिरसोऽर्द्धञ्च तं विद्यादधिमन्थं स्वलक्षणैः।
हन्याद्दृष्टिं श्लैष्मिक सप्तरात्रा दधिमन्थो रक्तजः पञ्चरात्रात्॥

white of the eye (sclerotic), the white with the transparent cornea, and this with the pupil, and the corunculo lachrymalis. The humours are carried into the eye by the vessels, and produce many diseases.

The causes of these diseases are bathing when the body is very hot, intensely regarding minute objects, or those at a great distance, or sleeping at irregular periods, frequent crying, grief, anger, external injuries, excessive venery, constipated or sour articles of food, or a kind of pea (*māskalāi*). Irregularities of seasons produce them, retaining the tears in the eye, smoke and dust, profuse vomiting, or stopping it suddenly. These causes with derangements of air, bile and phlegm or blood, produce diseases of the eye. The deranged humours are conveyed into the eye by the vessels, and produce the different diseases in the different parts of the eye. The gereral symptoms of diseases of the eye are its changing its natural colour, pain, redness, a discharge of tears, and there is a burning sensation in the eye as if there was an external body in it. The eyelids feel painful, as if thorns were under the eyelid, and there is intolerance of light.

षड्रात्राद्वा वातिको वै निहन्यान्मिथ्यचारात् पैत्तिकः सद्य एव॥
उदीर्णा वेदनं नेत्रं रोगशोकसमन्वितम्॥
धर्षनिस्तोदशूलाश्रुयुक्त मामान्वितं विदुः।
मन्दवेदनता कण्डुः संरभनाश्रुप्रशान्तता।
प्रशस्तवर्णता चाक्ष्णीः संपक्कदोषमादिशेत्।
कण्डुपदेहाश्रुयुतः पक्कोडुम्बरसन्निभः।
संरम्भी पच्यते यस्तु नेत्रपाल स शोतजः॥
शोथहीनानि लिङ्गानि नेत्रपाके त्वशोथजे।
उपेक्षणादक्षि यदाधिमन्थो वातात्मकः सादयति प्रसह्य॥
रुजाभि रुग्राभि रसाध्य एष हताधिमन्थः खलु नाम रोगः॥
वारं वारञ्च पर्येति श्रुतौ नेत्रे च मारुतः॥

2. *Inflammation.* There are four varieties of inflammation of the eye, produced by derangement in the air, bile, phlegm, and blood. The ten diseases of the air are characterized by severe pain in the eye, which remains immoveable, a feeling of sand in the eye, which is dry, with an inclination to rub it. The patient complains of head-ache, and the tears are cold.

Bile produces inflammation of the eye, which is characterized by burning, with the discharge of blood and pus and cold applications are grateful. The eye seems to be covered with a haze, feels hot, and has a yellow colour. There is likewise a discharge of warm tears.

Cough, when it produces inflammation it is characterized by hot applications being grateful to the eye, which feels heavy, swelled, itchy, and cold. There is also a copious discharge of tears, which arc of an oily nature.

Blood produces inflammation which is characterized by the discharge of a copper colour, the eye is red, and the small vessels of the eye become turgid. Before this appears the peculiar symptoms of bile are present. When this inflammation is

रुजश्च विविधा स्तीव्राः स ज्ञेयो पातपर्य्ययः।
यत् कुणितं दारुणरुक्षवर्त्म संदह्यते चाविलदर्शनं यत्।
सुदारुणं यत् प्रतिबोधने च शुष्काक्षिपाकोपहतं तदक्षि।
यस्यावटुः कर्णशिरोहनुस्थो मन्यागतो वान्यनिलोऽन्यतोषा।
कुर्य्याद्रुजं भुवि लोचने च तमन्यतो वात मुदाहरन्ति॥
श्यावं लोहितपर्य्यन्तं सर्व्वञ्चाक्षि प्रपच्यते॥
सदाहशोथं सास्त्राव मम्लाध्युषमिम्लतः।
अवेदना वापि संवेदना वा यस्याक्षिराज्यो हि भवन्ति ताम्राः।
मुहु र्विरज्यान्ति च या स तादृग्व्याधिः शिरोतपात इति प्रदिष्टः॥
मोहात् शिरोत्पात उपेक्षितास्तु जायेत रोगस्तु शिराप्रहर्षः।
ताभ्राभ मस्त्रं स्त्रवति प्रगाढ़ं तथा न शक्नोत्यभिवीक्षितुञ्च।

neglected, or improperly treated, it produces one of the four varieties of severe ophthalmia (*Adimanta*). This aggravated form has the following symptoms; severe pain, as if the eyes were torn; throbbing, which extends to half of the head, and is characterized by the above symptoms of each variety. When this is produced by phlegm it will destroy the eye in seven days; if blood is diseased it will destroy the organ in five days, if air in six days, and if bile in one day. In the acute stage of this ophthalmia the pain is severe, as if a foreign body was in it, with redness and swelling, and a copious discharge of tears from the eye. When merely chronic the pain is less, with itchiness in the part, the discharge of tears is slight, and the eyelids can be opened, and the globe appears healthy. When the inflammation produced by air is neglected, the accessions recur at intervals, and produce pain of different kinds. The eye swells, suppurates, and is red like a wild fig. It suppurates without swelling, when the other symptoms are the same. The eye in such cases is very painful, and the disease is incurable.

Another form of the disease is named *Bātaparjiya*, in which air is deranged, and the eyebrow and eye are painful, so that the person winks, and brings the eyelids forcibly together.

कृष्णगतनिदानम्

निमग्नरूपन्तु भवेहि कृष्णे सूचीव विद्धं प्रतिभाति यद्वैः।
स्रावं स्रवेदुष्णमतीव यच्च तत् सव्रणं शुक्र मुदाहरन्ति॥
दृष्टैः समीयेन भवेत्तु यच्च न चावगाढ़ं न च संस्रवेद्धि।
अवेदनं वा न च युग्म शुक्लं तत् सिद्धिमायाति कदाचिदेव॥
स्यन्दात्मकं कृष्णगतं सचोषं शङ्खेन्दुकुन्द्यं-प्रतिमावभासम्।
वैहायसाभ्रप्रतिमाप्रकाश मथाव्रणं साध्य मुदाहरन्ति।
गम्भीर जातं बहुलञ्च शुक्लं चिरत्थितञ्चापि वदन्ति कृच्छम्।
विच्छिन्न मध्यं पिशितावृतं वा चलं शिरासूक्ष्मदृष्टिकृच्च।
द्वित्वग् गतं लोहितमन्ततश्च चिरोत्थितञ्चापि विवर्ज्जनीयम्॥

Suskākipāka. When the eyelids are dry, and suppurate, the eye is very painful, the sight is troubled, and the patient cannot shut the eyelids.

Anutāyabāta. When the air of the neck and head, ears, cheeks, or vessels of the back of the neck are deranged, and in other situations, the eyebrow and eye are very painful.

In *Amlādhastia*, the eye is of a green colour with a red circumference, from the colour of the blood in the part. It extends over the eye which is hot, swelled, and tears continually flow. This is produced by sour articles of food.

Sirotpāta. It is accompanied with more or less pain in the eye, which becomes red. When neglected this form is called *Sirāharsa*; when the discharge is of a copper colour, and the person cannot see. These are the general diseases of the eye.

2. *The diseases of the black part of the Eye. Ulcers of the Cornea, (Bruna-sukra.)* in this disease the black part appears spotted, the discharge is very hot, and if it is not near the pupil and there is only one spot, which is without pain and any discharge, it may sometimes be cured.

When the ulcer is of long standing, extensive, and deep-

उष्णाश्रु पातः पिड़का च नेत्रे यस्मिन् भवेत् मुद्गनिभञ्च शुक्लम्।
तदप्यसाध्यं प्रवदन्ति केचिदन्यच्च यत् तित्तिरिपक्षतुल्यम्।
श्वेतं समाक्रामति सर्व्वतो हि दोषेण यस्यासितमण्डलञ्च।
तमक्षिपाकात्थयमक्षिरोगं सर्व्वात्मकं वर्ज्जयितव्यमाहुः।
अजापुरीषप्रतिमो रुजवान् सलोहितो लोहितपिच्छलास्त्रः।
विगृह्य कृष्णं प्रचयोऽभ्युपैति तच्चाजकाजातमिति व्यवस्येत्॥

दृष्टिजनिदानम्

प्रथमे पटले दोषा यस्य दृष्ट्यां व्यवस्थियताः।
अव्यक्तानि स रूपाणि कदाचिदश्च पश्यति।
दृष्टिर्भृशं विह्वलति द्वितीयं पटलं गते।

seated, it is difficult to cure. When depressed in the middle and the margin elevated it will destroy vision. When both coats (cornea and iris) are destroyed by the ulcer, which has a red margin, and has been of long standing, it is incurable.

Abruna-sukra. When the inflammation is in the black part of the eye with a burning sensation, it is very white like the moon, it is curable. If of old standing, is white, large, and deep-seated, it will be cured with difficulty.

Pākātiya, or opacity of the cornea following inflammation.

Ajakāyāta, small tumors like the litter of goats, slightly red, which protrudes through the cornea, from which a bloody discharge proceeds mixed with pus.

The *Dristi* (crystalline lense) is the principal part of the organ of vision. It is like the form of a pea (*masuri*), and is produced by a mixture of the essential parts of the five elements. It resembles the firefly, and it is largely supplied with the eternal fire (*Abaytazi*). It is covered by the external tunic of the eye, and has externally an opening (pupil ?). By cold it is kept in a healthy state. The diseases of this part of the eye are very tedious in their cure.

मक्षिकामशकांश्चापि जालकानि च पश्यति॥
मण्डलानि पताकांश्च मरीचिं कुण्डलानि च॥
परिप्लवांश्च वर्षमभ्रं तमांसि च॥
दूरस्थानि च रूपाणि मन्यते स समीपतः।
समीपस्थानि दूरे च दृष्टेगोचरविभ्रमात्।
यत्नवानपि चात्यर्थं सूचीपाशं न पश्यति॥
ऊर्द्धं पश्यवि नाधस्तात् तृतीयं पटलं गते।
महान्त्यपिच रूपाणि छादीतानीव चाम्वरैः॥
कर्णनासाक्षिहीनानि विकृतानीव पश्यति।
यथा दोषञ्च रज्येत दृष्टिर्दोष बलीयसी॥
अधस्थिते समीपख्यं दूरस्थं चोपरिस्थते॥
पार्श्यस्थिते तथा दोष पार्श्वस्थं नैव पश्यति॥

3. *Diseases of the membranes of the Eye.* When the first tunic (*Pratarnapatala*) is deranged, the vision is indistinct. When the second tunic is affected the sight is very imperfect, and the person sees an appearance of motes, musquitoes, hairs, and nets. In other cases it is in the form of a circle like spectres, rays, and as everything were indistinct and immersed in water, or like rain, clouds, and darkness. The person cannot distinguish distance, so that near objects seem at a distance.

When the third membrance is deranged he can either see above nor below ; large objects appear covered, and he cannot distinguish the features of a person placed before him. Such a person has often double vision.

Linganāsa. In this form the whole crystalline lens (*Dristi*) is affected, and if not very deep the person can see the moon, star, and lightning. When *air* is much increased the patient sees every object red ; and bile is affected, he can see the sun, the rainbow, and lightning. In other cases every thing appears black, variegated, and like the feather of a peacock. When affected by *phlegm* every object appears as if covered with oil

समन्ततः ख्यिते दोषे महद्रूपञ्च पश्यति।
द्विधा स्थिते द्विधा पश्येद्बहुलञ्चानवस्थिते॥
दोषे दृष्टाश्रिते तिर्यक् स एकं मन्थते द्विधा॥
तिमिराख्यः स वै दोष श्चतुर्थं पटलं गतः।
रुणन्धि सर्व्वतो दृष्टिं लिङ्गनाशमतः परम्॥
अस्मिन्नपि तमो भूते नातिरूढ़े महागदे॥
चन्द्रादित्यै सनक्षत्रावन्तरीक्षे च विद्युतम्।
निर्म्मलानि च तेजांसि भ्राजिष्णून्यथ पश्यति।
स एव लिङ्गनाशस्तु नीलिका काचसंज्ञितः॥
वातेन चापि रूपाणि भ्रमन्तीव च पश्यति।
आविलान्यरुणाभानि व्याविद्धानीव मानवः॥
पित्तेनादित्यस्वद्योतशक्रचापतड़िद्गुणान्॥

and white. When the three humours are deranged, every thing appears spotted as of a mixture of different colours. When *blood* is deranged every object appears red and dark. In *Linganāsa* the colour is made of six different tints.

When the eye is affected with deranged *bile,* it is called *Pittabidagdha dristi,* which is characterized by the yellowness, and images appearing yellow. If it affects the third membrane he cannot see during the day, but can see at night.

When *phlegm* is affected it is called *Sleshmabidagdha dristī* which is characterized by the white appearance, and every thing seems white. When deranged in the three membrance of the eye it is called *Nyctalopia,* or nightblindness. He can see during the day. Grief, fever, vexation, severe diseases of the head, cause this disease of the eye, in which every object appears enveloped in smoke ; hence it is called *Samadarsher*. In other cases the person cannot see small objects during the day, but sees every thing at night. This is called *Rasajāta*.

When air, bile, and phlegm are deranged, and produce a change in the iris like the mungoose eye (which is very red)

नृत्यतश्चैव शिखिनः सर्व्वं नीलञ्च पश्यति।
कफेण पश्येद्रूपाणि स्निग्धानि च सितानि च॥
पश्येदसूक्ष्माणत्यर्थं वभ्रमेवाभ्रसंप्लवम्॥
सलिलप्लावितानीव परिजाड्यानि मानवः।
पश्येद्रक्त्वेन रक्तानि तमांसि विविधानि च॥
स सितान्यपि कृष्णानि पीतान्यपि च मानवः॥
सन्निपातेन चित्राणि विप्लुतानीव पश्यति॥
बहुधा च द्विधा चापि सर्व्वाण्येव समन्ततः।
हीनाधिकाङ्गान्यथवा ज्ज्योतींस्यपि च भूयसः।
पित्तं कुर्य्यात् परिम्लायि मूर्च्छितं पित्ततेजसा॥
पीता दिशस्तु खद्योन् भास्करञ्चापि पश्यति।
विकीर्यमानान् खद्योतै र्वृक्षां स्त्येजोभिरेव वा॥
वक्ष्यामि षड्विधं रागैर्लिङ्गनाशमतः परं।
रागोऽरुणो मारुतजः प्रदिष्टो म्लायी च नीलश्च तथैव पित्तात्।
कफात् सितः शोणितजः सरक्तः समस्तदोषप्रभवो विचित्रः।

everything appears of a mottled appearance during the day. It is named *Nakulāndha*.

Gambirakā. When air is deranged it produces the disease in which the pupil of the eye is contracted, and it diminishes the size of the eye; and is accompanied with great pain.

Linganāsa is of two kinds. The first is called *Sanimita* and the second *Animita*: the first is produced by inflammation of the eye, and the second by the sight of holy sages, by regarding a kind of large snake (*Maharaza*), or luminous objects by which vision is destroyed. The eye in this disease docs not lose its natural appearance.

Abigāta hatadristī is produced by accidents or injuries to the eye, by which the person cannot see; the organ becomes red like coral, and severe pain is felt as if a person was tearing the eye out.

अरुणं मण्डलं दृष्ट्यां स्थूलकाचारुणप्रभम्।
परिम्लायिनि रोगे स्यान्म्लायि नीलञ्च मण्डलम्।
दोषक्षयात् स्वयन्तत्र कदाचित् स्यात्तु दर्शनम्।
अरुणं मण्डलं वातात् चञ्चलं परुषं तथा॥
पित्तान्मण्डलमानीलं कांस्याभं पीतमेव वा।
श्लेष्मनो बहुल पीतं शङ्ख कुन्देन्दुपाण्डुरम्॥
चलत् पद्मपलाशस्थः शुक्लो विन्दु रिवाम्मसः।
नृत्यमाने च नयने मण्डलं तद्विसर्पति।
प्रवालपद्मपत्र्यभं मण्डलं शोणितात्मकम्॥
दृष्टिरागो भवेच्चित्रो लिङ्गनाशे त्रिदोषजे।
यथास्वं दोषलिङ्गानि सर्व्वष्वेव भवन्ति हि॥

DISEASES OF THE WHITE PART OF THE EYE

Prastārījarma. In this disease there is a thin red or dark-coloured memebrance covering the white part of the eye.

Suklārma. The enlargements in this disease are white and soft, and it advances slowly.

Raklārma is characterized by fleshy growths of a red colour.

Adimānsarma (Ptergium) is a liver-coloured thickening of the white part of the eye. It is stationary. Another form is thick, and fleshy, and of a white colour.

Stārjarma is fleshy swelling of the white of the eye.

Sukti, when there are many small spots of a green flesh colour.

Arjana is when there is a red spot.

Pistaka is a round white elevation of the white of the eye like a drop of water.

Jāla. The white part in this case is like a net-work, with hard small vessels of red colour.

षड़्लिङ्गनाशाः षड़िमे च रोगा दृष्ट्यश्रयाः षट् च षड़ेव वाच्याः।
पित्तेन दुष्टेन सदा तु दृष्टिः पीता भवेद् यस्य नरस्य किच्चित्॥
पीतानि रूपानि च तेन पश्येत् स वै नरः पित्त विदब्धदृष्टिः॥
प्राप्ते तृतीयं पटलन्तु दोषे दिवा न पश्येन्निशि चेक्षते सः॥
रात्रौ च शीतानुगृहीतदृष्टिः पित्ताल्पभावादुपि तानि पश्येत्॥
तथा नरः श्लेष्मविदग्धदृष्टिः जान्येव शुक्लानि तु मन्यते सः।
त्रिषु स्थितोऽल्पः पटलेषु दोषो नक्तान्ध्यमापादयति प्रसह्य।
दिवा स सूर्य्यानुगृहीतदृष्टिः पश्येत्तु रूपाणि कफाल्पभावात्॥
शोकज्वरायासशिरोऽभितापै रव्याहता यस्य नरस्य दृष्टिः।
धुम्रांस्तथा पश्यति सर्व्वभावान् स धुमदर्शीतिनरः प्रदिष्टः।
यो ह्रस्वजाड्यो दिवसेषु कृच्छात् ह्रस्वानि रूपाणि च तेन पश्येत्।

Sirāja, in which white pimples appear in the white of the eye, surrounded by enlarged vessels.

Balāsaka is a silvery copper-coloured spot surrounded by vessels.

Disease of the joinings of the eyes:— of the eyeball,

cornea and sclerotica, eyelids, eyelashes, etc.

These diseases are nine in number. The parts sometimes swell, suppurate and are painful; the disease is called *Puyalisa.* Blood and thick pus are discharged in these cases. Another form swells much, but does not suppurate; is itchy, but without pain. It is called *Upanāha.*

When air, bile and phlegm are deranged at the joints, and the passage of the tears are discharged over the eyelids in the form of tears, it is called *Netranāri* (Fistula Lachrymalis), of which there are four varieties according to the nature of their discharges. When pus alone is discharged it is called *Parsāsarba.* when phlegm is alone, diseased, and the joint suppurates without pain, the discharge is of a white colour, thick, and shining like oil: it is then called *Sleshmāsrāba.*

विद्योतते यस्य नरस्य दृष्टि दोषाभिपन्ना नकुलस्य यद्वत्।।
चित्राणि रूपाणि दिवा स पश्येत् स वै विकारो नकुलान्ध्यसंज्ञः।।
दृष्टिर्विरूपा श्वसनोपसृष्टा सङ्कुच्यतेभ्यन्तरतस्तु याति।।
रुजावगाढ़ा च तमक्षिरोगं गम्भीरिकेति प्रवदन्ति तज्ज्ञाः।।
वाह्यो पुनर्द्वाविह संप्रदिष्टो निमित्ततश्चाप्यनिमित्ततश्च।
निमित्तत स्तत्र शिरोभितापात् ज्ञेयस्त्वभिष्यन्दनिदर्शनः सः।
सुरर्षिगन्धर्ब्बमहोरगाणां सन्दर्शने नापि च भास्करस्य।
हन्येत दृष्टिर्मनुजस्य यस्य स लिङ्गनाश स्त्वनिमित्तसंक्षः।
तत्राक्षिविस्पष्ट मिवातिभाति वैदूर्य्यवर्णा विमला च दृष्टिः।

शुक्लजनिदानम्

प्रस्तार्य्यम्मस्तनुस्तीर्णः श्यावं रक्तनिमं सिते।
सश्वेतं मृदु शुक्लार्म्म शुक्ले तद्वर्द्धते चिरात्।।

Diseased blood sometimes produces this disease, and when there is a hot discharge mixed with much blood it is called *Raktasraba*. When bile is diseased, the discharge has a yellow colour, and it is called *Pittatsrāba*.

When small pimples appear at the joints of the eye, of a red colour, they burn and are painful. They are called *Parbānikā*. Sometimes this occurs at the juncture of the cornea and sclerotica, and are accompanied by the same symptoms as the last. They are of a red colour, and are called *Alaghi*.

Krimāgranti. Sometimes worms are produced at the juncture of the eyelids, and eyelashes. They produce much itching; and sometimes they form between the eyelid and the white part of the eye. They are of different colours and forms, and destroy the eye.

DISEASES OF THE EYELIDS

There are twenty-one disease of the eyelids. In this class of diseases, air, bile, and phlegm may be diseased in a combined

पद्माभं मृदु रक्तागर्म यन्मांसं चीयते सिते।
पृथुमुद्वधिमांसार्म्म बहुलञ्च यकृन्निभम्॥
स्थिरं प्रस्तारि मांसाढ्यं शुष्कं स्नायुवर्म्मपञ्चमम्।
श्यावाः स्युः पिशितनिभाश्च विन्दवो।
ये शुक्ताभाः सितनियताः सतशुक्तिसंज्ञः॥
एकोयः शशरुधिरोपमश्च विन्दुः
शुक्रस्थो भवति तमर्ज्जुनं वदन्ति।
श्लेष्मारुतकोपेन शुक्ले पिष्टं समुन्नतम्॥
पिष्टवत् पिष्टकं विद्धि मलाक्तादर्शसन्निभम्॥
जलाभः कठिनशिरो महान् सरक्तः
सन्तानः स्मृत इह जालसंज्ञितः।
शुक्रस्थाः सितपिड़काः शिरावृताया
स्वाब्रूयादसित समीपजाः शिराजाः॥
कांस्यभो मृदुरथ वारिविन्दुकल्पो
विज्ञेयो नयनमिते बलाससंज्ञः॥

सन्धिजनिदानम्

पक्वः शोथाः सन्धिजो यः सतोदः स्त्रवेत् पूयं पूति पूयालसाख्यः।

or separate form. In other cases these derangements affect the vessels of the eye, and the blood and flesh, etc. may separately, or when combines, produce diseases of the eyelids.

Atsangani are small eruptions of the external part of the lower eyelids, they often open internally; and are produced by diseases of the blood.

Kambikā are swellings at the borders of the upper eyelid. When they break, pus and blood are evacuated; and they are like small castor-oil seeds.

Another form of swelling is of the colour of blood; of the size of a mustard seed, hard, and itchy; and water, pus, and

ग्रन्थिर्नाल्पो दृष्टिमन्धावपाकी कण्डुप्रायो नीरुज स्तूपनाहः।।
गत्वा सन्धीनश्रुमार्गेण दोषाः कुर्य्युः स्त्रावान लक्षणैः खैरूपेतान्।
तं हि स्त्रावं नेत्रनाड़ीति केचित्तस्या लिङ्गं कीर्त्तयिष्येचतुर्द्धा।।
पाकात् सग्धौ संस्त्रवेद् यस्तु पूयं पूयस्त्रावोऽसौ गदः सर्व्वजस्तु।
श्वेतं सान्द्रं पिच्छिलं यः स्त्रवेत्तु म्लेष्मास्त्रावीऽसौ विकारो मतस्तु।।
रक्तस्त्रावः शोणितीत्थो विकारः स्त्रवेत् दुष्टं तत्र रक्त्वं प्रभूतम्।
हरिद्राभं पीतमुष्णं जलं वा पित्तास्त्रावः संस्त्रवेत् सन्धिमध्यात्।।
ताम्रा तन्वी दाहोशूलोपपन्ना ज्ञेयावैद्यैः पीड़का पर्व्वणीका जाता
सन्धौ कृष्णशुक्लेऽजलीस्यात्तष्मिन्नेत ख्यापिता पूर्व्वलिङ्गैः।।
क्रिमिघ्नन्थिर्वर्त्मतः पक्ष्वतश्च कण्डुं कूर्य्यूः क्रिमयः सग्धिजाताः।
नानारूपा कर्त्म शुक्कान्तसन्धौ चरन्त्यन्तर्लोचनं दूषयन्तः।।

वर्त्मजनिदानम्

अभ्यन्तरमुखी ताम्रावाह्यतोवर्त्मनश्च या।
स्योत्सद्धोत्सङ्क पीड़का सर्व्वजा ख्यूलकण्डुरा।।

blood are evacuated from them. When painful they are called *Pataki*. When numerous clusters of small eruptions, are rough, elevated, and situated on the inner side of the lid, they are called *Bartasarkara*. Another form are small like melon seeds; have little pain, are situated in the eyelids, are rough to the feel, and are called *Arsabarta or Bartarsi*. When like the new shining germ of plant, the eyelids are long, hard, rough, indolent and irregular, and the patient cannot open the lid, the disease is called *Saskarsa*, or dry hemorrhoidal tumors of the eyelid.

Another form is very hot, painful, and of a copper colour; and is soft, and small, with little pain: it is called *Angannanā-mika*.

Sometimes the eyelids are covered with small eruptions, and all the small swellings have the same appearance and colour and are stationary. They are called *Bahalabarta*.

वर्त्मान्ते पीड़काध्वाता भिद्यन्ते च स्त्रवन्ति च।
कुम्भीकवीजसदृशाः कुम्भीनकाः सन्निपातजाः॥
स्राविण्यः कुण्डरा गुर्व्वो रक्तसर्षपसन्निभाः।
रूजावत्यश्च पीड़काः पोथक्य इति कीर्त्तिताः॥
पीड़का या खरास्थूला मुक्ष्माभिरभि संवृताः।
वर्द्धर्यस्था शर्करा नाम स रोगो वर्त्मदूषकः॥
एव्वांरुवीजप्रतीमाः पीड़का मन्दवेदनाः।
श्लक्ष्णाः खराश्च वर्त्मस्था स्तदर्शीवर्त्म कीर्त्तते॥
दीर्घाङ्कुर खरस्स्तब्धो दारुणोभ्यन्तरोद्भवः
व्याधिरेषोऽभिविख्यातः शुष्कार्शो नाम नामतः।
दाहोतोदवती ताम्रा पीड़का वर्ता सम्भवा॥
मृद्वी मन्दरुजा शूष्मा ज्ञेया साञ्चन नामिका।
वर्त्मापचियते यस्य पीड़काभि समस्ततः॥
सवर्णभिः स्विराभिश्च विद्याद्वहुलवर्तातत्।
कण्डुमताल्पतोदेन वर्ताशेथेनः यो नरः॥
न स संछादयेदक्षि यात्रासौ वर्ताबन्धकः।
भृद्वल्पवेदनं ताम्रं यद्वर्त्म सममेव च।

Another form of swelling is when the lids are swollen, itchy, and painful, the lids being tight over the eye, and the eyelids do not completely cover the globe of the eye. This disease is called *Bartabanda*.

When the internal part of the eyelid is spungy, hot, painful, of a copper colour, and changes quickly to a red colour, it is called *Klishtahbarta*.

If in this disease bile is deranged and affects the blood, much dirty matter is discharged called *Bartahkardama*.

When the swelling of the lids is both external and internal, with burning and itchy pain of a dark yellow colour with a discharge, it is called *Sābabarta*.

अकस्माच्च भवेद्रक्तं क्लिष्टवर्त्मीति तद्विदुः।।
क्लिष्टं पुनः पित्तयुतं शोणितं विदहेद् यदा।।
ततः क्लिन्नत्वमापन्न मुच्यते वर्त्मकर्द्दमः।
यद्वता वाह्यतोऽन्तश्च श्यावं शूनं सवेदनम्।।
तदाहुः शववर्त्मेति वर्त्मरोगविशारदाः।
अरुजं वाह्यतः शूनं वर्त्म यस्य नरस्य हि।।
प्रक्लिन्नवर्त्न तद्विद्यात् क्लिन्नमत्यर्थमन्ततः।।
यस्य धौतान्यधौतानि सम्बह्यन्ते पुनः पुनः।
वर्त्मान्यपरिपक्वानि विद्यादक्लिन्नवर्त्म तत्।
विमुक्तः सन्धिनिथेष्टं वर्त्म यस्य न मील्यते।
एतद्वातहतं वर्त्म जानीयादक्षिचिन्तकः।।
वर्त्मान्तरख्यं विषमं ग्रन्थिभूतमवेदनन्।।
आचक्षितार्व्वुदमिति।
सरक्त मविलम्बितम्।।
निमेषिणीः शिरी वायु प्रविष्टवर्त्म संश्रयाः।
चालयत्यक्षिवर्त्मानि निमेष इति तद्विदुः।।

When the upper lid is externally swollen, of a red, colour, and much matter is discharged in its inner surface, it is called *Prakninabarta*.

When the eyelids are shut, and they cannot be opened without their being previously soaked in water, on account of the secretion, the disease is called *Akhnabarta*.

When the joints of the eyelids become immoveable, and everted it is called *Bātahattabarta (Entropium)*.

When a pendulours swelling forms in the inside of the eyelid without pain, and is caused by blood, it is named *Arbuda*.

When the vessels which move the eyelids are deranged they produce winking, or a continual movement of the eyes, when it is called *Nimassa*.

यः स्थितो त वर्त्म मध्ये तु लोहितो मृदुरङ्कुरः।
तद्रक्तजं शोणिर्थं श्छिन्नं भिन्नं प्रवर्त्तते॥
अपाकौ कठिनो स्त्यूली ग्रन्थिर्वर्त्म भवोरुजः॥
नगणो नाम स व्याधिर्लिङ्गत परिकीर्त्तितः।
त्रयो दोषा वहिः शोथं कूर्यूश्छिद्रानि वर्त्मनोः॥
प्रस्त्रवन्त्यनन्तरुदकं विषवद्विषवर्त्म तत्।
वाताद्या वर्त्म संकोचकं जनयन्ति मला यदा॥
तदा द्रष्टं न शक्नोति कुञ्चनं नाम तद्विदुः।
प्रचालितानि वातेन पक्षान्यक्षि विशन्ति हि।
घृष्यत्यक्षि मुहुस्तानि संरम्नां जनयन्ति च।

When the small fleshy excrescences, situated in the eyelids, are of a red colour, soft, painful, and grow again when removed by the knife, they are produced by diseased blood, and are called *Sunitārsa.* Another form of tumor forms on the eyelids like a plum, hard, soft, moist, and does not suppurte, but becomes large and knotted it is called *Lagannah.*

When air, bile, and phlegm are deranged the swelling appears above the eyelids, breaks, and blood, water and pus are discharged through many openings. The pain is so severe as to resemble poison, and is called *Bishabarta.* In other cases these derangements contract the eyelids so that the person can not see distincly. This disease is called *Kuncharna.*

When air is deranged the eyelashes are turned inwards, and inflame the eye, and the person is always rubbing them. It is called *Pakakapat,* (Entropeon,) and is a difficult disease to cure.

Bile when deranged in the eye produces the fallling off the eyelashes; when the eyelids are itchy and hot, the disease is called *Pakaksāta.*

Besides the seventy-six diseases, which are common both to childdren and to the adult, there is another which is peculiar

असिते सितभागे च मूलकोषात् पतन्त्यपि।
पक्ष्मकोपः स विक्षेपी व्याधिः परमदारुणः।
वर्त्मपक्ष्यपयगतं पित्तं रोमाणि शातयेत्।
कण्टुं दाहञ्च कुरुते पञ्चाशतं तमादिशेत्।

शिरोरोगनिदानम्

शिरोरोगान्तु जायन्ते वातपित्तकफे स्त्रिभिः।
सन्निपातेन रक्तेन क्षयेण क्रिमिभि स्तथा॥
सूर्य्यवर्त्तानस्तवाताद्धर्विभेदक शङ्खकैः॥
यस्या निमित्तं शिरसो रुजश्च भवन्ती तीव्रा निश्चातिमात्रम्।
बन्धोपतापैश्च भवेद्विशेषः शिरोऽभितापः स समीरणेन॥

to the former. This is called *Kukunāka* or purlent ophthalmia. It is caused by the bad milk of the mother, and also by the derangement of phlegm, air, bile or blood, singly, or collectively. It affects the eyelids. The symptoms are the continual rubbing the eye, as well as the nose and forehead; great in tollerance of light, and a copious discharge.

DISEASES OF THE HEAD (Siraroga)

Under this order will be arranged the varieties of Headache, and the diseases of the organs of sense.

Head-ache—There are eleven varieties of head-ache; which are produced by derangements of the air, bile, and phlegm; by the mixture of the three; by diseased blood; by a deranged or diminished state of the humours, by worms, the eighth is named *Sūrjyabārtta,* the ninth, *Anantabāta, tenth, Ardhayabhedaka,* and the eleventh *Sankhaka*.

1. When air is diseased in the head, it is suddenly affected with pain, which is severe at night.
2. *Bile*. In this variety, the head is hot, as if burning charcoal was placed over it, and there is an appearance of smoke proceeding from the mouth.

यस्योष्णमङ्गारचितं यथैवः भवेच्छिरोधुमवतीव नासा॥
शीतेन रात्रौ च भवेद्विशेषः शिरोऽभितापः सतु पित्तकोपात्॥
शिरो भवेद् अस्य कफोपदिग्धं गुरुप्रतिष्ठब्ध मतो हिमञ्च।
शूनाक्षि कुटं वदनञ्च यस्य शिरोभितापः स कफप्रकोपात्।
शिरोऽभितापे तृतयप्रवृत्ते सर्व्वाणि लिङ्गानि समुद्भवन्ति।
रक्तात्मक पित्तसमानलिङ्ग स्पर्शासहत्वं शिरसो भवेच्च॥
असृग्वसा श्लेष्मसमीरणानानां शिरोगतानामिह संक्षयेण।
क्षयप्रवृत्तः शिरोसोऽभिघातापः कष्टो भवेदुगुरुजातिमात्रम्॥
संस्वेदम च्छर्द्दनधूमनस्यै रसृग्विमोक्षैश्च विवृद्धि मेति॥
निस्तुद्यते यस्य शिरोऽतिमात्रं संभक्ष्यमाणं स्फुरतीव चान्तः।
घ्राणाच्च गच्छेद्रुधिरं सपूयं शिरोभितापक्रिमिभिः सघोरः॥

3. *Phlegm.* In this variety the head is heavy and dull, and it cannot be turned about. The head feels cool, and the eyelids and mouth are swollen.
4. When the above three *dhātu* are diseased, the different symptoms are combined.
5. When the blood is deranged, producing this disease, the symptoms are the same as when bile is deranged. The pain in this variety is so severe, that the head cannot be touched, or bent forward.
6. When the disease is produced by a diminution of brain, or fat, phlegm, or blood, in the head, it produces great uneasiness and pain.
7. Worms sometimes produce severe pain in the head, of a kind as if an animal was eating, or tearing the head. A watery red or bloody discharge flows from the nose, and the patient's life is to be considered as in danger.
8. *Sūrjyābartta.* In this variety, when the sun rises the eyes and brow feel painful; and it continues, and

सूर्य्योदयं वा प्रतिमन्दमन्द मक्षिभ्रुवं रुक्समुपैति गाढ़म्।
विवर्द्धते वांशुमता सहैव सूर्य्यापवृत्ती विनिवर्त्तते च।
सर्व्वात्यकं कष्टतमं विकारं सूर्य्यपवर्त्त तमुदाहरन्ति॥
दोषास्तु द्वुष्टास्त्रय एव मन्यां संपीड्यघाटासुरुजां सुतीव्राम् कुर्व्वन्ति
योऽक्षि भ्रुविशङ्कदेशे स्थिति करोत्याशु विशेषतस्तु॥
गण्टस्य पार्श्वे तु करोति कम्पं हनुग्रहं लोचनजाश्च रोगान्॥
अनन्तवातं तमुदाहरन्तिः दोषत्रयोत्थं शिरसो विकारम्।
रुक्षाशनाध्यशन–प्राग्वातावश्यायमैथुनैः॥
वेगसन्धारणायास व्यायामैः कुपितोऽनिलः॥
केवलः सकफोवार्द्ध गृहीत्वा शिरसो बली।
मन्यभ्रूशङ्ककर्ण्यक्षिललाटार्द्धेऽतिवेदनाम्।

increases, while the sun is above the horizon. It diminishes in the evening, and towards night. It is produced by derangement in the air, phlegm, and bile.

9. *Anantabāta*. When air, bile, and phlegm are deranged in the vessels of the neck, they produce great pain, particularly in the eyebrows, temples, and cheeks. It also produces shaking of the head, pain in the lower jaw, and diseases of the eyes (*neuralgia*).

10. *Ardhāyabhedaka, (hemiplegia)*. When much dry food is taken it produces this disease; or eating without an appetite, or too frequent; exposure to the easterly wind, or to dew, and the abuse of venery. When the urine and bowels are constipated, and the person has been subjected to much grief, or severe exertion, he is liable to the attacks of this disease; as also by derangements of air, bile, and phlegm. The attack occurs sometimes every fortnight, in other cases every tenth day, or in other cases every day. The half of the neck, brow, temples, ears, eyes are very painful. When severe, as it often is like that of poison, or as if burnt,

शस्त्ररणिनिभां कुर्यात् तीव्रां सोऽर्द्धावभेदकः॥
नयनं बाथवा श्रोत्रमतिबृद्धो विनाशयेत्।
रक्तपित्तानिला दुष्टाः शङ्कदेशे विमुर्च्छिताः।
तीव्ररुग्दाहरागं हि शोथं कुर्व्वन्ति दारुणम्॥
सशिरो विषवद्वेगी निरुध्याशु गलस्तता।
त्रिरात्राज्जीवितं हन्ति शङ्ककोनामतः परम्।
त्र्यहाज्जीवति भेषज प्रत्याख्याय समाचरेत्॥

स्त्रीरोगनिदानम्

प्रदरनिदानम्

विरुद्धमद्याध्यशनादजीर्णाद्गर्भप्रयातादतिमैथुनाच्च।
यानाध्वशोकादतिकर्षणाच्च भाराभिघाताच्छ्रयनाद्दिवा च॥

and the sight and hearing become imperfect. This disease is very obstinate, and most distressing; so that a thousand physicians cannot sometimes cure it.

11. *Sank-haka.* When air, bile, and phlegm, with blood are deranged, it produces severe pain in the temples, and head, which becomes hot. This form is dangerous, like poison. When the person cannot swallow, he will die in three days.

But if he lives beyond this time, medicines may then be given for the cure.

DISEASES OF THE FEMALE ORGANS OF GENERATION

There are twenty forms of these diseases, which are produced by using bad food, or taking improper exercise. They are also caused by diseased menses, or semen. In other cases they are produced without any apparent causes.

असृद्गरं भवेत् सर्व्वं साद्गमर्द्दं संवेदनम्।
तस्यातिवृद्धौदौर्व्वल्यं भ्रमोमूर्च्छामदस्तषा।
दाहः प्रलापः पाण्डुत्वं तन्द्रारोगाश्च वातजाः।
तं श्लेष्मपित्तानिलसन्निपातैश्चतुः प्रकारं प्रदरं वदन्ति॥
आमं सपिच्छाप्रतिमं सपाण्डु पूलाकतोयप्रतिमं कफात्तु
सपीतनीलासितरक्तमुष्णं पित्तार्त्तियुक्तं भृशवेगि पित्तात्॥
रुक्षारुणं फेनिलमल्पमल्पं वातार्त्ति वातात् पिशितोदकाभम्॥
सक्षौद्रसर्पिहारतालवर्णं मज्ञप्रकाशं कूणपं त्रिदोषात्।
तञ्चाप्य साध्यं प्रवदन्ति तज्ज्ञा न तत्र कूर्व्वीत भिषक् चिकित्साम्॥
सम्वत् स्त्रवन्ती मास्त्रावं तृष्णादाहज्वरान्विताम्।
क्षीणरक्तां दुर्व्वलाञ्च तामसाध्यां विनिर्द्दिशेत्।
मासान्निष्पिच्छदाहार्त्ति पञ्चरात्रानुवन्धि च।
नैवातिबहुलात्यल्प मार्त्तवं शुद्धमादिषेत्॥
शशासृक् प्रतिमं यञ्च यद्वालाक्षा रसोपमम्।
तदार्त्तवं प्रशसंन्ति यच्चप्सु च विरज्ज्यते॥

योनिव्यापन्निदानम्

विंशति र्व्यापदो योनौ निवार्द्दष्टा रोगसंग्रहे।
मिथ्याचारेण ताः स्त्रीणां प्रदुष्टेनार्त्तवेन च।
जायन्ते वीजदोषाच्च दैवाच्च सृणु ताः पृथक्।

1. *Udābertā*. When the menses are discharged with great pain and are frothy.

2. *Bandhyā*. Difficult menstruation, Dismenorrhagaea (*mostartoboh)* where the menses are stopped, by the accumulation of unhealthy humours in the part. When the woman is barren, the disease is called *Bandhya*.

3. *Biplutā*. Continued pain in the genital organs.

4. *Parīplutā*..Severe pain during connection.

सा फेनिलमुदावर्त्ता रजः कृच्छ्रेण सुञ्चति।
वन्ध्या नष्टार्त्तवां विद्याद्विप्लुतां नित्यवेदनाम्॥
परिप्लुतायां भवति ग्राम्यधर्म्मेण रुग् मृशमृ।
वातला कर्कश स्तुब्धा शूलनिस्तोद पीड़िता।
चतसृष्वपि चाद्यासु भवन्त्य निलवेदनाः॥
सदाहं क्षीयते रक्तं यस्यां सा लोहितक्षया।
सवात मुद्ग्रेद्बीजं वामिनी रजसा युतम्॥

5. *Bātalā*. In this disease the vagina is contracted and rough, accompanied with pain. In these five diseases *air* is locally deranged, the parts are hard and swollen, with the various seven varieties of pain produced by diseased air.

6. When the menses are discharged very hot, the disease is named *Sanitakara*. When there is an unusual discharge of a red colour from the vagina, accom-panied with pain, and followed by lassitude, etc. the disease is named *Prodorah* or *Menorrhagia*. This disease is produced by bad food, diet, or milk, or any improper mixture of food, sleeping during the day, by the use of ardent spirits, or hot food, or eating frequently without being hungry; by abortion, or frequent venery, by severe exercise particularly riding and walking, by grief, by carrying heavy weights, and by external injuries. These causes produce the disease which is accompanied with fever, and pain over the body; and after a time the patient becomes weak, is affected with giddiness, fainting, thirst, great heat, delirium, jaundice, and drowsiness. It is also accom-panied with the general symptoms of diseased phlegm, air, and bile separately, or combined.

When *phlegm* is particularly deranged in this disease; the discharge is whitish, mucilaginous, and has the smell of the water in which flesh had been steeped, or of the colour of water in which straw has been immersed.

प्रस्रंसिनी स्रंसते च क्षोभिता दुष्प्रजायिनी।।
स्थितं स्थितं हन्ति गर्भं पुत्रघ्नी रक्तसंक्षयात्।।
अत्यर्थं पित्तला योनिर्दाहपाकज्वरान्विता।
चतसृष्वपि चाद्यासु पित्तलिङ्गोऽश्रयो भवेत्।।
अत्यानन्दा न संतोषं ग्राम्यधर्म्मेण गच्छति।
कर्णिन्यां कर्णिका योनौ श्लेष्मासृग्भ्याञ्च जायते।।

When *bile* is particularly deranged, the discharge is sudden, and is of a yellow or reddish, blue or black colour. It is hot, and the other symptoms of diseases of bile appear.

When *air* is particularly affected the discharge is of a red colour, like the washings of flesh, is frothy, is in smaller quantities than the last variety, and is accom-panied with more pain.

When the three humours are deranged producing this disease, the discharge is of the colour of honey mixed with ghee, or of a yellow colour like marrow, and has a foetid smell. In this form a cure is not be expected, and the practitioner should refuse to attend such a patient.

The unfavourable symptoms of this disease are when it has continued long, is accompanied with a copious discharge, with fever, great thirst, and heat followed by great debility. When the menses occur every month, without pain or burning, are of the natural colour, and neither too copious, not too scanty, it is advantageous to health. When the discharge is red, like the colour of the blood of hare, or like a decoction of lac, and does not permanently discolour cloth when it falls upon it, it is healthy.

7. *Bāmini*. When semen is discharge with the menses.

8. *Srangsinī*. When the blood is discharged, and the parts are diseased, so that it prevents easy delivery.

मैथुनेऽचरणापूर्व्वं पुरुषदतिरिच्यते।
बहुशश्चातिचरणा तयोर्वीजं न विन्दति॥
श्लेष्मला पिच्छिला योनिं कण्डूग्रस्तातिशीतला॥
चतसृष्वपि चाद्यासु श्लेष्मलिङ्गोच्छ्रयो भवेत्।
अनार्त्तवास्तनी षण्डी खरस्पर्श च मैथुने॥

9. *Patraganī*. When the infant has dieα, or abortion has taken place with a great discharge of blood. In all these cases bile is much diseased, and is accompanied with fever.

10. *Pittalā*. When bile is deranged , there is much heat of the part, which suppurates and is accompanied with fever. These five last diseases are the symptoms of bile.

The folowing are the diseases produced by deranged phlegm.

11. *Atyānandā*. When the woman has no pleasure in the embraces of her husband.

12. *Karnīnī*. When phlegm and blood are deranged in the vagina, small granulations form, like the grains of rice from deranged phlegm and blood.

13. *Churunā*. When the semen of the male is more copious than that of the female.

14. *Charanā*. When the male semen does not enter the uterus.

15. *Shleshmalā*. It is produced by diseased phlegm with itchiness and coldness, and the part appears as if covered with oil.

16. *Sandi*. In this variety the menses are not discharged, the breasts do not swell, and the parts are hard, and rough like a file.

17. *Palani*. When a large man has connection with a

अतिकायगृहीताया स्तरुण्ययत्वण्डुली भवेत्।
विवृता च महायोनिः सूचीवृत्तातिसंवृता।
सर्व्वलिङ्गासमुत्थाना सर्व्वदोषप्रकोपजा।
चतसृष्यपि चाद्यासु सर्व्वलिङ्गोच्छ्रयो भवेत्।
पञ्चासाध्या भवन्तीह योनयः सर्व्वदोषजाः॥

कन्दनिदानम्

दिवास्वल्पादतिक्रोधाद्व्यायामादतिमैथुनात्।
क्षताच्च नखदन्ताद्यै र्वाताद्याः कुपिता यदा॥
पूयशोणितसङ्काशं लिकुचाकृतिसन्निभम्।
उत्पद्यते यदा योनौ नाम्ना कन्दस्तु योनिजः।
रुक्षं विवर्णे स्फटितं वातिकं तत् विनिर्द्दिशेत्॥
दाहरागज्वरयुतं विद्यात् पित्तात्मकन्तु तम्।
नीलपुष्प्रतीकाशं कण्डूमन्तं कफात्मकम्॥

small, and young female he injures the parts, and produces this disease.

18. Mahatī. When the vagina is very large.

19. Suchibuktra. When the entrance is very small.

20. *Sarbalingasamutpanna*. Different varieties of pain, etc. produced by the derangement of the three humours in the part.

The five last forms of these diseases are cured with difficulty.

UTERO VEGINAL TUMORS *(Kanda)*

Theses diseases are produced by the person sleeping during the day, by an angry disposition, by great fatigue, and by too much venery. They may also like the fruit of the

मूढ़गर्भनिदानम्

भयाभिघातात्तीक्ष्णोष्णपानाशन-निशेवणात्।
गर्भे पतति रक्तस्य सशूलं दर्शनं भवेत्॥
आचतुर्थात्ततो मासात् प्रस्त्रवेद्गर्भविद्रवः।
ततः स्थिरशरीरत्य पातः पञ्चमषष्टयोः॥
गर्भोऽभिघात-विषमाशन-पीड़िताद्यैः पक्वं
द्रुमादिव फलं पतति क्षणेण।
मूढः करोति पवनं खलु मूढगर्भं
शूलञ्च योनिजठरादिषु मूत्रसङ्घम्॥
भुग्नोऽनिलेन विगुणेन ततः स गर्भः
संख्यामतीत्य बहुधा समुपैति योनिम्।
द्वारं निरुद्धशिरसा जठरेण कश्चित्
कश्चिच्छूशरीर-परिवर्त्तित-कुञ्जदेहः॥
एकेन कश्चिदपरस्तु भुजद्वयेन
तिर्य्यग्गतो भवति कश्चिदवाङ्मुखोऽन्यः।
पार्श्वापवृत्तगतिरेति तथैव कश्चिदित्यष्टधा

Lakucha tree, (a kind of Bread fruit tree, *Artocarpus lacucha, or Madar).*

When *air* produces the disease the tumor is dry, and is of a dirty or yellowish colour, and has furrows on its surface.

When diseased *bile* produces to tumor it is very hot and red, and is accompanied with fever.

When *phlegm* produces the tumor it is like the colour of the Indigo flower and is very itchy.

When air, bile and phlegm are diseased, all the separate symptoms are present. When three are so diseased in one part, it is incurable, and when produced by spirit or by phlegm, etc. it is cured with difficulty.

गतिरियं ञ्चपरा चतुर्धा।
सङ्गीलकः प्रतिखुरः परिधोऽथ वीज
स्तेषूर्द्धबाहु चरणैः शिरसा च योनिम्॥
सङ्गी चयो भवति कीलकवत् सकीलो
दृश्यैः खुरैः प्रतिखुरः स हि कायसङ्गी।
गच्छेद्धजद्वयशिराः स च वीजकाख्यो
योनौ स्थितः स परिघः परिघेन तुल्यः॥
अपविद्धशिरा या तु शीताङ्गी निरपत्रपा।
नीलोद्गतशिरा हन्ति सा गर्भ स च तां तथा॥
गर्भास्पन्दनमावीनां प्रणशः श्यावपाण्डुता।
भवेदुच्छासमूपित्वं शूनतान्तर्मृते शिशौ॥
मानसागन्तुभि र्मातु रुपतापैः प्रपीड़ित॥
गर्भो व्यापद्यते कुक्षौ व्याधिभिश्च निपीड़ितः॥
योनिसंवरणं सद्धः कुक्षौ मक्वल्ल एव च।
हन्युः स्त्रियं मूढ़गर्भां यथोक्ता व्यप्युपद्रवाः॥

सूतिकारोगनिदानम्

वायुः प्रकूपितः कूर्य्यात् संरुद्धरुधिरं स्त्रुतम्।
सूताया हृच्छिरोवस्ति शूलं मक्कल्लसंज्ञकम्॥
अङ्गमर्द्दो ज्वरः कम्पः पिपासा गुरुगात्रता॥
शोयः संक्लेशात् विषमाजीर्णभोजनात्।
सूतिकायाश्च ये रोगो जायन्ते दारुणाः स्मृताः॥
ज्वरातिसारशोथाश्च सूलानाह बलक्षयम्॥
तन्द्रारुचि प्रसेकाद्याः कफवातामयोद्भवाः।
कृच्छ्रसाध्या हि ते रोगाः क्षीणमांसबलाश्रिताः।
ते सर्व्वे सूतिकानाम्ना रोगास्ते चाप्युपद्रवाः॥

स्तनरोगनिदानम्

सक्षीरो वान्यदुग्धौ वा प्राप्य दोषस्तनौ स्त्रियाः।
प्रदूष्य मांसरुधिरं स्तनरोगाय कल्पते॥
पञ्चानामपि तेषां हि रक्तजं विद्रधिं विना॥
लक्षणानि समानानि वाह्यविद्रधिक्षणैः॥
गुरुभि र्विविधै रन्नै र्दुष्टै दोषैः प्रदूषितम्।
क्षीरं धात्र्याः कुमारस्य नानारोगाय कल्प्यते॥
कषायं सलिलप्लावि स्तन्यं मारुतदूषितम्।
कट्वम्ल-लवणं पीतराजीमत् पित्तसंयुतम्॥
कफ दुष्टं घनं तीये निमज्चति स पिच्छिलम्।
अदुष्टञ्चाम्बुनिक्षिप्तमेकीभवति पाण्डुरम्॥
मधुरञ्चाविवर्णञ्च प्रसन्नं तत् प्रशस्यते॥

बालरोगनिदानम्

वातदुष्टं शिशुः स्तन्यं पिवन् वातगदातुरः।
क्षामस्वरः मृशाङ्ग स्याद्बद्धविन्मूत्रमारुतः॥
स्विन्नो भिन्नमलो बालः कामला पित्तरोगवान्॥
तृष्ण लुरुष्णसर्व्वाङ्ग पित्तदुष्टं पयः पिवन्।

DISEASES OF INFANTS (*Bālaroga*)

The diseases of infants are supposed to be produced-

Ist. By derangement, in air, bile, and phlegm. If the child sucks the mother's milk, affected by deranged air, he becomes affected with the diseases of air. His voice is changed, his body emaciated, bowels costive, and the secretion of urine is diminished.

The diseased bile affecting the milk produces a shining appearances of the body of the infant, as if it was smeared with oil, the body is covered with perspiration, it feels hot, the child

कफदुष्टं पिवन् क्षौरं लालालुः श्लेष्मरोगवान्।।
निद्रान्वितो जड़ः शूनो रक्ताक्ष श्छर्द्दनः शिशुः।
द्वन्द्वजे द्वन्द्वजं रूपं सर्व्वजे सर्व्वलक्षणम्।
शिशो स्तीव्रामतीव्राञ्च रोदनाज्जक्षयेद्रुजम्।
कुकूणकः क्षीरदोषाच्छिशूना मक्षिवर्त्मनि।।
जायते तेन तन्नेव कण्डु रञ्च स्त्रवेन्मुहुः।
शिशुः कुर्य्याल्ललाटाक्षि कुटनासावघर्षनम।
शक्तो नार्कप्रभां द्रष्टुं न वर्त्मोन्मीलनक्षम्ः।।
मातुः कुमारो गर्भिण्यः स्तण्यं प्रायः पिवन्नपि।
कासाग्नि सादवमथु तन्द्राकर्शयरुचिभ्रमैः।।

has great thirst, with looseness, and the body becomes of a yellow colour.

When the diseased phlegm affects the milk it increases the saliva of the infant, with the symptoms produced by diseased phlegm. He is drowsy, the mouth and eyes swell, with sickness and vomiting.

When two of these diseased states act on the milk, they produce the symptoms of the combination. When three are so diseased by three classes of symptoms are present at the same time. It is only by the degree of crying of the infant, that the kind and severity of pain in known.

PURULENT OPHTHALMIA OF INFANTS (*Kukunaka*)

Bad mild produces disease of the eyelids, which, with the neighbouring parts, are very itchy; tears flow copiously, the eyes are very sensible to light, and they cannot open their eyelids.

MARASMUS (Pārigarbhika.)

When a pregnant woman continues to give suck to a child, it produces cough, bad appetite, vomiting, drowsiness, and emaciation. The child loses its vivacity, and the abdomen swells.

युज्यते कोष्ठवृद्ध्य च तमाहुः पारिगर्भिकम्।
रोगं परिभवाख्यञ्च युञ्ज्यात्तत्राग्निदीपनम्।
तालुप्रांसे कफः क्रुद्ध कुरुते तालुकण्टकम्।।
तेन तालुप्रदेशस्य निम्नता मूर्द्धि जायते।
तालुपातः स्तनद्वेषः कृच्छात् पानं शकृदद्रवम्।।
तृडक्षिकण्ठास्यरुजा ग्रीवा दुर्व्वलता वमिः।।
विसर्पस्तु शिशोः प्राणनाशनो वस्ति शीर्षजः।
पद्मवर्णो महापद्मो बाले दोष द्वयोद्भयः।
शङ्खाभ्यां हृदयं याति हृदयाद्वा गुदं व्रजेत्।।
क्षुद्ररोगे च कथिते त्वजगन्ध्यहिपूतने।
ज्वराद्या व्याधयः सर्व्वेमहतां ये पूरेरिताः।
बालदेहेऽपि ते तद्वद्विज्ञेयाः कुशलैः सदा।।
क्षणदुद्विजते बालः क्षणात्रस्यति रोदिति।
नखैद्रन्तैर्दारयति धात्री मात्मान मेव वा।।
ऊर्द्धं निरीक्षते दन्तान् खादेत् कूजति जृम्भते।
भ्रुवौ क्षिपति दन्तौष्ठ फेनां वमति चासकृत्।।
क्षामोऽति निशि जागर्त्ति शूनाक्षां भिन्नविट् स्वरः।।
मांसशोणितगन्धौ च न चाश्नाति यथा पूरा।
सामान्यग्रहदुष्टानां लक्षणं समुदाहृतम्।।

When phlegm is diseased in the soft palate small pointed elevations form there, by which the fontanell becomes depressed, the soft palate is destroyed, the child cannot suck, and there is a difficulty in swallowing, great thirst, and pain in the throat and mouth. He cannot sit up, and he vomits. This disease is called *Tālukantaka*. Children are subject to erysipelas, which is always a most dangerous disease, and requires much attention and care.

In other cases the temples swell, like the leaf of a water lily, and descends to the breast. It is produced by a disease of

एकनेत्रस्य गात्रस्य स्त्रावः स्यन्दनकम्पनम्।
ऊर्द्धदृष्ट्या निरीक्षेत वक्रास्यो रक्तगन्धिकः॥
दन्तान् खादति विस्त्रस्तः स्तन्यं नैवाभिनन्दति।
स्कन्धग्रहगृहीतानां रोदनञ्चाल्पमेव च॥
नष्टसंज्ञो वमेत् फेनं संज्ञावानतिरोदिति।
पूयशोणितगन्धित्वं स्कन्दापस्मारलक्षणम्॥
स्त्रस्ताङ्गो भयचकितो विहङ्कगन्धिः
सास्त्रवव्रण परिपीड़ितः समस्तात्।
स्फोटैश्च प्रचिततनुः सदाह पाकै
र्विज्ञेयो भवति शिशु क्षतः शकुन्या॥
व्रणैः स्फोटैश्चितं गात्रं पङ्कगन्धं स्त्रवेदसृक्।
भिन्नवर्च्चा ज्वरी दाही रेवतिग्रहलक्षणर्म
अतीसारी ज्वर स्तृष्णा तिर्य्यक् प्रेक्षणरोदनम्॥
नष्टद्रिस्तथोद्विग्नो ग्रस्तः पूतनया शिशुः।
छर्दिः कासो ज्वरस्तृष्णा वसागन्धोऽतिरोदनम्॥
स्तन्यद्वेषोऽतिसारश्च अन्धपूतनया भवेत्।
वेपते कासते क्षीणो नेत्ररोगो विगन्धिता॥
छर्द्यतीसारयुक्तश्च शीतपूतनया शिशुः।

the air, bile, and phlegm. In other cases it commences in the thorax or abdomen, and descends to the anus. Other diseases, of the class of small diseases, are produced. Fever, and other diseases of adults may occur in infants.

DISEASES PRODUCED BY DEVILS

Infants are supposed to be liable to be affected by nine kinds of spirits or devils, which may assume various forms at will. They are produced from the mother, or the nurse having committed certain improprieties, by which the devil enters their bodies, in order to amuse himself. When a devil distresses an

प्रसन्नवर्णवदनः शिराभिरभिसंवृतः।
मूत्रगन्धी च वह्वाशी मुखमुण्डतिकाग्रदी।
छर्दिस्पन्दनकण्ठस्य शोषो मूर्च्छा विगन्धिता।
ऊर्द्धं पशेच्द्दशेद्दस्तान् नैगमेयं ग्रहं वदेत्॥

विषनिदानम्

स्थावरं जङ्गमञ्चैव द्विविधं विषमुच्यते।
मूलाद्यात्मकमाद्यं स्यात् परं सर्पादिसम्भवम्॥

infant, it becomes depressed in spirits, and starts from fear. The eyes of the child swell, he cries, his fingers are contracted, and at other times he tears his body and clothes with his nails, and bites with his teeth, both himself and nurse. The child turns his face to one side, and moves about his eyes; grinds his teeth together, makes a noise like a person who cannot speak from the severity of the disease, and he frequently yawns. His eyelids and eyebrows are in continual movement, and the two foreteeth and lips remain shut and foam proceeds from the mouth. The child becomes thinner, cannot sleep, his eyes swell, has frequent motions, and an unnatural noise proceeds from the throat. The smell of the body resembles that of blood, or flesh; and the child will not take his usual food. These are the usual symptoms indicting the presence of a devil.

POISONS AND THEIR ANTIDOTES (Panata)

The origin of poison is explained in the following manner. Soon after the creation of the world, *Bramha* was displeased at the violence of *Kaitaba* one of the demons (*Asura*), and in his anger poison was generated and destroyed *Kaitaba*. The poison increased so much that the *debtās* were afraid that it would destroy the whole animated creation. They prayed to *Bramha* to relieve them, and petitioned that he would distribute the poison over the animal, vegetable, and mineral kingdoms. This was done; and when the poison is introduced into the living

निद्रां तन्द्रां क्लमं दाह मपाकं लोमहर्षणम्।
शोथञ्चैवातिसारञ्च जङ्गमं कुरुते विषम्॥
स्थावरं ज्वरं हिक्कां दन्तहर्षं गलग्रहम्।
फेनछर्द्यरुचि श्वासं मूर्च्छाञ्च कुरुते विषम्॥

body it is not digested, and produces languor,[11] and deranges all the humours of the body.

It is necessary for the practitioner to have a knowledge of the symptoms of the different poisons, and their antidotes. As the enemies of the Raja, bad women, and ungrateful servants sometimes mix poison with food. On this account the cook should be of a good family, virtuous, faithful, and not covetous, not subject to anger, pride, or laziness. He should also be cleanly, and skilful in his business. The practitioner should have like qualities with an intimate knowledge of poisons; and should examine the food to be eaten by a Raja in the cooking room. This should be large, airy, light, and surrounded with faithful servants, and no one should be allowed to enter unless he is first examined. In the *Mitākshara shāstra* there are copious directions regarding the manner of detecting a person who gives poison. He does not answer questions, or they are evasive answers; he speaks nonsense, rubs the great toe along the ground, and shivers; his face is discoloured; he rubs the roots of the hair with his fingers; and he tries by every means to leave the house. The food which is suspected should be first given to certain animals, and if they die, it is to be avoided. The authority the brāhamans assumed, and the confidence they inspired, has no doubt often had the best effect, in making the wicked shrink from perpetrating deeds, which would be detected and exposed by them.

The long account which is given of these poisons, and the means of preventing their bad effects seems to prove the frequency with which they were employed with bad intentions, at a very early period.

All poisons have the following qualities: they are drying,

इङ्गितज्ञो मनुष्यानां वाक्चेष्टामुखवैकृतैः।
जानीयाद्विषदातार मेते र्लिङ्गैः सबुद्धिमान्॥
न ददात्युत्तर पृष्टो विवक्षु मोहमेति च।
अपार्थं बहुसंकीर्णं भाषते चापि मूढ़वत्॥

heating, and stimulating; their effects, quickly extend over all the body; they destroy very quickly, are not digested, and from the rapidity with which they produce bad symptoms it is difficult to use remedies with sufficient quickness. The following stages of the effects of poisons are observed.

The tongue becomes black and rigid, the person faints, and breathes with difficulty.

Shivering, perspiration, heat, and pain in the stomach, and chest.

Severe pain in the stomach, the eye changes its colour, becomes yellow and swells, and when the poison has extended to the intestines pain of the part, hiccough, coughing, and a peculiar noise is heard in the intestines.

Heaviness of the head.

Dischage of saliva from the mouth, change of colour of the skin, and pain in the joints and belly.

Iinsensibility and purging.

Rigidity and death.

Vegetable poison *(Dushibisha)* when dried by the fire, by the air, or by the sun, may be given in solution, or in any other way in which their effects are less powerful. In this case the poison does not produce immediate death, but remains in the system for a long time; and the first effect is looseness, foetid smell of the mouth, great thirst, fainting, vomiting, and paralysis of the tongue. There are followed when taken into the stomach by diseases of phlegm and air, and in the intestines, by diseases of the bile and air. The person's hair falls off, and he becomes

हसत्यकस्मात् स्फोटदङ्गुलीर्विलिखेन्महीन्।
वेपथुश्चास्य भवति त्रस्तश्चान्योन्यमीक्षते।
विवर्णवक्त्रो ध्यामश्च नखैः किञ्चिच्छिनत्यपि।
तर्त्तते विपरीतञ्च विषदाता विचेतनम्॥

like a bird without feathers. When mixed with the hummours of the body as chyle, blood etc., the poison produces diseases of the humours, as leprosy, and various other kinds of symptoms, as languor, weakness of the joints, and pain over the body; swelling of the legs and face, dropsy, and in other cases vomiting and diarrhoea, intermittent fever, discolouration of the body, madness, impotency, and other like diseases. Alll these symptoms are aggravated in cloudy and damp weather.

Such effects may be removed by proper treatment, and a year after the person has taken the poison he will either be cured, or get worse. When weak, and the patient does not observe his diet, the poison will destroy him.

Poisons are usually arranged into two classes, the first comsisting of vegetable and mineral poisons, are named *Stābarah;* and the second animal poisons, *Jangamah*. They are not used internally, as medicines.

I. VEGETABLE AND MINERAL POISONS

The general symptoms produced by vegetable poisons are fever, hiccough, grinding of the teeth, suffocation, foaming at the mouth, vomiting,want of appetite, difficulty of breathing and fainting.

The *Mineral poisons* produce drowsiness, languor, burning of the body, indigestion, horripilation, swelling, and dysentery. The dejections of a person who has taken poison are of a black colour, large, and are discharged with wind.

Vegetable poisons are divided into nine varieties, which are derived from the roots, leaves, fruits, flowers, bark, milky juice, gum, and pith of plants.

उद्वेष्टनं मूलविषैः प्रलापो मोह एव च।
जृम्भणं वेपनं श्वासो ज्ञेयं पत्रविषेण तु।
मुष्कशोथः फलविषै र्दाहोऽन्नद्वेष एव च।
भवेत् पुष्पविषै श्छर्द्दि राध्मानं श्वास एव च॥

1. The *Roots* of the following plants are poisonous:—and when eaten they produce pain over the body, delirium, and stupidity.

   Klitaka, (Olibanum)

   Asamāsa, (Andropogon muricatum,)

   Gunja, (Abrus precatorius,)

   Sugandā, (Alpinia galanga,)

   Gargarakā, (Cissus glauca,)

   Karagāta,

   Bidyuchchikkā,

   Bijaya, (Cyperus difformis.)

2. The *Leaves* of the following vegetables produce gaping, shivering, and difficulty in breathing.

   Bisaputrikā, (Vangueria,)

   Alumbā, (Arum campanulatum,)

   Abadāruka, (Sideroxylon spinosum,)

   Karamba, (Dalbergia arborea,)

   Mahā karamba, (Antirrhinum cymbalaria,)

3. The following poisonous *Fruits* cause a loss of appetite, heat of the body, and a swelling of the testicles.

   Kamudatī, (Nelumbium speciosum,)

   Bīnākā,

   Karamba, (Dalbergia arborea,)

   Mahā karamba, (Antirrhinum cymbalaria,)

   Karakataka, (Cleome viscosa,)

त्वक्सारनिर्य्यासविषै रुपयुक्तै र्भवन्ति हि।
आस्यदौर्गन्ध्यपारुष्यशिरोरुक्कफसंस्त्रवाः।
फेनागमः क्षीरविषै र्विड्भेदो गुरुगात्रता।
हृत्पीड़नं धातु विषैर्मूर्च्छा दाहश्च तालुनि।

Ranaka,

Kadataka,

Charmara, (Viola suffruticosa,)

Ebajandā,

Sarpagata, (Hibiscus populneus,)

Nandana, (Cedrela Tuna,)

Sarapāka (Nelumbium speciosum.)

4. The following poisonous *Flowers* when eaten produce vomitting, swelling in the abdomen, and difficulty in breathing.

Betra enopdium album,)

Kadamaba, (Sinapis dichotoma,)

Ballija, (Ocymum,)

Karamba, (Dalbergia arborea,)

Mahā karamba, (Antirrhinum cymbalaria.)

5,6,7. The following poisonous *Bark, Pith, and Gums,* produce a bad smell in the mouth, a roughness of the body, head-ache, and discharge of saliva from the mouth.

Antra Pāsaka, (Aeschynomene grandiflora,)

Kutanīa, (Solanum Jacquini,)

Saurīaka, (Tetrantherea quadrifolia,)

Karagāta,

Karamba, (Dalbergia arborea,)

Nandana, (Cedrela Tuna,)

प्रायेण कालघातिनी विषान्येतानि निर्दिशेत्।
सद्यः क्षतं पच्यते यस्य जन्तोः स्त्रवेद्रक्तं पच्यते वाप्यभीक्ष्णम्।
कृष्णीभूतं क्लिन्नमत्यर्थपूति क्षतान्मांस शीर्य्यते चापि यस्य तृष्णा
मूर्च्छा ज्वरदाहौ च यस्य दिग्धाहतं तं पुरुषं व्यवस्त्येत्।

Baerātaka, (Solanum melongena.)

8. The following poisonous *Milky Juices* produce foaming from the mouth, looseness, and a swelling, and heaviness of the tongue.

Kamadugna, (Carpopogon neveum,)

Stnahu, (Euphorbia antiquorum,)

Jālakirjah,

9. The poisonous *Bulbous roots* are:

Kālakuta, (Arum colocasia,)

Batsanābha, (Sida cordifolia,)

Sarshapa, (Panicum colonum,)

Kapālaka, (Cucumis utilatissimus,)

Kardamaka,

Baerātaka, (Solanum unelongena,)

Musīaka, (Pistacena lentiscus,)

Sringībisa, (Betala,)

Prapandurika, (a small herbaceous plant,)

Mūlaka. (Tamarind,)

Halahala, (Valisneria octandra,)

Mahabisha, (a species of lily,)

Karkataka, (Cleome viscosa,)

The *Mineral poisons* are:—

Phenāshmabhasma, (white oxide of arsenic,)

Harītāla, (yellow sulphurate or arsenic: Sushruta,)

लिङ्गान्येतान्येव कुर्य्यादमित्रै र्व्रणे विषं यस्य दत्तं प्रमादात्॥
सपीतं गृहधुमाभं पुरीषं योऽतिसार्य्यते॥
फेनमुद्व मते चापि विषपीतं तमादिषेत्॥
वातपित्तकफात्मानो भोगिमण्डलिराजिला:।

Other authors have added the following poisons:—

Tuta, (Suphurate of copper,)

Tezpatra,

Deāmakā, (white oxide of arsenic.)

There are others of the same kind.

These poisons when administered to a person, produce pain in the chest and body, fainting, shivering, followed by a burning and swelling of the body, but particularly of the throat. These symptoms are succeeded by diarrhoea, languor, coma, and insensibility. When these symptoms are present, the disease will be fatal.

Poisons introduced into a wound, as by a poisoned arrow. The part quickly swells, blood flows, and from time to time pus is evacuated. The wound becomes of black colour, and dirty round it, with a bad smell and sloughing. The person is very thirsty, faintish, with fever, and the body becomes very hot. The same symptoms will be produced when poisou is placed over a sore.

II. ANIMAL POISONS

Serpents. Posion is found in all parts of the serpent, but when they are irritated the poison collects in the hood like teeth, when they snap with the head erect, they lodge the poison in the wound; but when the head is turned upside down they do not convey the poison into wound. The poison is very acid and hot.

There are some serpents *(Debya or heavenly)* which poison the air by their breathing, and by their sight. Others are

यथाक्रमं समाख्याता द्व्यन्तरा द्वन्द्वरुपिणः।
दंशो भोगिकृतः तृष्णः सर्व्ववातविकारकृत्॥
पीतो मण्डलिजः शोथो मृदुः पित्तविकारवान्॥

called *Bhauma,* which live in holes in the ground, and the poison is in their teeth.

Sushruta does not mention the symptoms, and cure of the first kind; as they kill by their breathing and sight, and the method of preventing their effects is not known. The *Bāsaki, Takhyak,* etc. belong to the first kind of serpents. Of the second class, their names, the symptoms which their bites, produce, are as follows:-

There are eighty kinds of *Bhauma* serpents, which are again divided into five classes.

1. *Dabikara, or hooded snakes.*
2. *Mantalā,* with figures of round arches on their bodies.
3. *Rajalāmanta,* with longitudinal lines.
4. *Nirbisa,* without poison.
5. *Quiranja,* or mixed class; when combine the peculiarities of several of the others.

Certain animals have poison in their teeth and nails; such as dogs, monkeys, cats, snub-nosed aligators, frogs, a kind of fish called *pāka mucha,* guanas, a shell-fish (*sambuka*), and lizards.

Others have poisonous urine and faces, as *Chipita, Phichataka, Kashāyabāsiks, Sarsapabāsika, Totaka, and Kaundilyaka.*

Musika or rats have poisonous semen. Spiders (Luta) have poisonous saliva urine, and faces, and their bites, and scratches are poisonous.

Brischika (centipede), *Bissambara, Rajibāmacha* (a fish), *Uchirangā and Samudra Brischika* have poisonous stings.

राजिलोत्थो भवेद्दंशः स्थिरः शोथश्च पिच्छिलः।
पाण्डुः स्निग्धोऽतिसान्द्रासृक् सर्व्व श्लेष्मविकारकृत्॥
अश्यत्थदेवायतनश्मशानवल्मीकसन्ध्यषु चतुष्पथेषु।
याम्ये च दष्टाः परिवर्ज्जनीया ऋक्षे च वा मर्म्मसु ये च दष्टाः।

The *Chitrasira, Surabakurdi, Satadaruka, Animadaka,* and *Sarikamukha,* convey poison by breathing, by biting, by urine, and by faces. The bones of animals killed, by poisonous arrows, and the like; the bones of serpents, and of the fish called *Barati,* produce poisonours effects when eaten.

Makkika, a kind of *flea, Kanaba,* and *Jalikā* (a kind of leech), are poisonous by biting.

The fishes called *Sākuli,* and *Raktarāji,* have poisonous bile.

General Symptoms.- There are some kinds of serpents that only produce diseases of air, others of bile, and a third kind of phlegm; accordingly diseases of air are produced by serpents of the *Baghis* (*Darbikara),* or hooded kind, the diseases of bile by those of the *Mandalā* kind, and the derangement of phlegm is produced by those of the *Rajalā* kind.

The *Baghi* leaves a black colour in the wound, with the symptoms of various air diseases. They are known by being hooded. The following symptoms are present. The skin, eyes, nails, teeth, urine, and faeces, and the part which is bitten, become black, with roughness, of the body and heaviness of the head; pain in the joints, weakness in the loins, back, and neck; gaping, shivering, alteration of voice, languor, hiccough, thirst, foaming and sluggishness of the circulation; and the secretions, and allhe external passages are closed.

The bites of the *Mandala* serpent produce in the part a yellow colour. It swells, is painful,, and soft; accompanied with the following symptoms: thirst, stupidity, fainting, fever; blood

दर्व्वी कराणां विषमाशु वाति सर्व्वाणि चोष्णे द्विगुणी भवन्ति।
अजीर्णपित्तातपपीड़ितेषु बालेषु बुद्धेषु वुभुक्षितेषु।
क्षीणक्षते मेहिनि कुष्ठयुक्ते रुक्षेऽबले गर्भतीषु चापि।।
शस्त्रक्षते यस्य न रक्तमेति राज्यो लताभिश्च न सम्भवन्ति।

is discharged from the mouth and anus, and gangrene occurs in bitten part. These serpents are shining, and are marked with different circles over the body.

The *Rajīla* serpent produces a swelling, a glistering grey-colour of the part, and blood is thick, accompanied with the various symptoms of diseased phlegm. They are distinguished by the longitudinal lines along their bodies.

There is a fourth kind of serpents called *Nirbīsa,* or serpents without poison.

Should a serpent bite a person under the sacred *pipul* tree, near a temple, where bodies are burnt, on a holy hill, on a whiteants nest, during the two hours in the evening and morning when the sun is disappearing,where four roads meet, towards the south of the house, or if the person is bit on his birthday, in the temples, or in vital parts of the body, he will not recover.

The bites are also dangerous when the food in the stomach is not digested, when the body is labouring under a bilious disease, when the person is fatigued and languid from heat, when the person is affected with a discharge from the urethra; in pregnant women, in old, weak, sickly or hungry persons; and during rainy and cloudy days. In these cases practitioners must be careful in undertaking the treatment of such patients, as they will be rarely cured. This will also be the case when no blood follows cutting the part, and when the person is senseless so that no weals are produced by the strokes of whip, or horripilation after throwing cold water on the body. The

शीताभिरद्भिश्च न रोमहर्षो विषाभिभूतश्च विवर्ज्जयेत्तु॥
कृष्णः सरक्तः स्वयथुश्च दंशे हन्वोः स्थिरत्वञ्च विवर्ज्जनीयः
वर्त्तिर्धना यस्य निरेति वक्त्वाद्रक्तं स्त्रवेदूर्द्धमधश्च यस्य॥
दंष्ट्रानि पाता श्चतुरश्च यस्य तञ्चापि वैद्यः परिवर्ज्जयेच्च।

following symptoms are likewise unfavourable: when the tongue is black, the hair falls off, the nose and mouth become changed in their shape, the voice is altered, and the bitten part becomes black and red, or tetanus supervenes; when thick mucusproceeds from the mouth, or when the blood is discharged from the mouth and anus, and there are the wounds of four teeth.

The hooded snakes are quickly fatal in their effects.

When after being bitten the person is insensible with other bad symptoms, as a stoppage of the throat, the body becoming blue, and feet and hands immoveable, the disease will be fatal.

These poisons first derange the blood, producing a blackness of the part, and a feeling as if ants are moving upon the surface of the body.

2. The poison affects the flesh, and produces a blackness and swelling of different parts of the body.
3. It next affects the fat.
4. It enters the viscera and organs.
5. The bones.
6. The marrow and lastly semen, which is followed by death.

When animals are affected by animal poisons, their bodies become swollen, they are sluggish, and saliva proceeds from their mouths, with pain in the chest. In the third stage there is pain in the head they cannot support; and fourth. The body shivers, they become insensible and die.

Birds when affected with poison first become sluggish, senseless, and die.

उन्मत्तमत्यर्थ मुप्रद्रुतं वा हीनस्वरं बाप्यथवा विवर्णम्।
सारिष्टं मत्वर्थ मवेगिनञ्च ज्ञात्वा नरं कर्म्म न तत्र कुर्य्यात्।
जीर्णं विषघ्नौषधिभिः र्हतं वा दावाग्निवातातपशोषितं वा।
स्वभावतो वा गुणविग्रहीनं विषं हि दूषीविषतासुपैति।

Posions do not affect cats, nor the mongoos,

Poisonous rats. The symptoms of different kinds of these poisons is given in the medical *shāstras*. When they discharge their semen upon any part of the body, the blood is affected, and produces, different glandular swellings, blutches, and eruptions. In other cases erysipelas accompanied with pain, fever and fainitng, followed by debility, loss of appetite, difficult breathing, and vomiting.

THE BITES OF MAD DOGS

When a dog, a jackal, a fox, a wolf, bear, or a tiger become mad they foam at the mouth, which remains open, their tails hang down, they do not hear or see well, and saliva flows from their mouths. In such a state they snap and bite each other. The part that is bitten becomes senseless, blood flows from the wound which becomes black, and the other appearances are observed; as when wounded with a poisoned arrow. The person bitten makes the same kind of noise and movements, as that of the animal which has bitten him. When such a person sees the shape of the animal which has bitten him either in water, or in a glass, it is an unfavourable symptom. It is also unfavourable when the person is afraid of water, and dreads either seeing or hearing it. This is called *Jalatrāsa* or hydrophobia, the fear of water. When the person dreams of the rabid animal, it is unfavourable. Towards the termination of the disease the person is convulsed, becomes insensible, powerless, and dies.

THE POISON OF INSECTS

These poisons are divided into four classes, one of which derange the air, another the bile, a third the phlegm, and a fourth, or a combination of the three former symptoms.

वीर्य्यल्पभावान्न निपातयेत्तु कफान्वित वर्षगणानुवन्धि।।
तेनार्द्दितो भिन्नपुरीषवर्णो वैगन्ध्या वैरस्ययुत: पिपासी।
मूर्च्छा भ्रमं गद्गदवाक् वमिञ्च विचेष्टमानोऽरतिमाप्नुयाद्वा।।
आमाशयस्थं कफवातरोगी पक्काशयख्येऽनिलपित्तरोगी।

There are 18 insects which derange air; as a kind of cricket (*Urchingarā*) the centipide (Satabāhu) etc.

There are 24 of the second class which derange bile as the wasp (*Barati*), the bee *(Bhramara)*, etc. this class produce great heat and pain in the part wounded.

There are 13 of this variety; which derange phlegm; such as the bug (*Kutuba*), and other like insects.

There are 12 varieties of this class of insects, the bites of which are very dangerous, as they affect the three humours, such as *Tungināsa*, *Bihilaka,* etc.

The bites of venomous insects thus produce a derangement of the air, bile, and phlegm of the body, and the wounds are inflamed, brown, red, yellow, or black, according to circumstances. They are sometimes followed by fever, diarrhoea, vomiting, thirst, or a burning sensation over the body. Sometimes there is a shivering, the glands proximate swell, and patches of eruptions or erysipelas appear over the body.

Different kinds of flies, gnats, mosquitoes, ants etc. produce a painful itchiness, and swelling of the part bitten.

Scorpions. There are three varieties of these bites, according as they are mild, strong, and very strong. Those which are generated in dunghills are not so poisonous as those generated in bricks and dry places. Those generated in the putrid carcases of serpents, and other venomous animals, have the most violent poisons. There are twelve kinds of the first class, three of the second, and fifteen of the third, or dangerous kind. The symptoms esemble those produced by the bites of serpents. The weak kinds produce pain, swelling, followed by

भवेत् समुद्धस्त-शिरीरुहाङ्गो विलूनपक्षस्तु यथा विहङ्गः।
स्थितं रसादिष्वथवा यथोक्तान् करोति धातुप्रभवान् विकारान्॥
कोपञ्च शीतानिलदुर्दिनेषु यात्याशु पूर्व्वं शृणु तस्य रूपम्॥
निद्रा गुरुत्वञ्च विजृम्भणञ्च विश्लेषंहर्षावथवाङ्गमर्दः।

shivering and fever, with perspiration, and stiffness of the body. The second class produce swelling of the tongue, so as to prevent swallowing, fainting, and much pain.

The third, or most dangerous class, produce delirium, fever, burning of the body, a discharge of black blood from the nose, and other parts of the body. In this case the person soon dies.

Spiders. It is stated that *Biswāmitra* made *Bashistha* anger on some occasion, and the perspiration which fell from his head fell in drops upon the grass, and in it the spiders were generated. These spiders are therefore called *Lutā*, from being generated in grass intended for the cow. There are sixteen varieties, eight are cured with difficulty, and eight are incurable. The names of the first eight are given, and they produce headache, itchiness, pain, and swelling of the part, followed by hot fever and diarrhoea, with derangement of phlegm and air. The eight other varieties produce sloughing of the part, discharge of blood, fever, burning, looseness, and diseases of the three humours. The general appearance of these eruptions over the body, are in the form of blotches or swellings. Some of them are large, others are soft or red, and others black. They pass from one part of the body to another. The first day after the bite there is no change of colour in the part, which feels itchy. The second day the part swells, and the third the characteristic symptoms of the poison develop themselves. The constitution is affected on the fourth day, and on the fifth and sixth all the severe symptoms appear. On the seventh day the person dies, when the poison is strong. If the poison remains in the upper part of the stomach it produces diseases of phlegm and air ; and if in the stomach, the diseases of air and bile, when the

ततः करोत्यन्नमदाविपाकावरोचकं मण्डलकोठजन्म॥
मांसक्षयं पादकरप्रशोथ मूर्च्छान्तथा छर्दिमथातिसारम्।
दूषीविषं श्वासतृषाज्वरांश्च कुर्य्यात् प्रवृद्धि जठरस्य चापि।
उन्मादमन्यद्धजभङ्गमन्य दानाह मन्यत् क्षपयेच्च शुक्रम्।

hair falls off. Cloudy, windy, and cold weather increase the violence of the poison. The poisons produce drowsiness, languor, and pain in different parts of the body and indigestion. Blotches appear over the body, the person loses flesh, his hands and feet swell, followed by faintness, vomiting, diarrhoea, sonorous breathing, thirst, fever, spasm, and swelling of the abdomen (*Anāha*) with delirium.

The red lizard produces a black tinge and grey colour, or mottled colour over the body. This is accompanied with delirium and diarrhoea.

Frogs if seized by a serpent and escape, and bite a person, the persons hair stands on end, severe pain is felt over the body, and the part is insensible. The part swells, and small pimples appear on the part, with vomiting and drowsiness.

Fish poison produces great heat, swelling, and severe pain.

Leeches when poisonous produce an itchiness, and swelling of the part, with fever and fainting.

When poisons have been taken and the person gets well, it is known by his feeling well, the different fluids are healthy, his appetite, urine, dejections are of the natural colour, the body has the natural appearance, as also the senses and mind, and they act properly.

Weak poisons (Apabīsha.) there are seven varieties of these poisons.

VEGETABLE POISONS

Hemp, (Gānjā or *Grinjā.)* A mixture of tobacco and the extract of hemp, (*Gānjā pitu,*) acts as a poison of a very strong

गादृगद्यमन्यज्जनयेच्च कुष्ठं तां स्तान् विकारांश्च बहुप्रकारान्।
दूषितं देशकालान्न दिवास्वल्पैरभीक्ष्णशः॥
यष्मात् संदूषयेद्घातून् तस्मात् दूषीविषं स्मृतम्।
साध्यमात्मवतः सद्यो यान्यं संवत्सरोत्थितम्॥

kind. The symptoms it produces are fever, insensibility, thirst, swelling of the abdomen, difficulty of breathing, cough, dryness of the mouth, etc.

Spirits are a kind of poison which, when taken in moderate quantities, and with food, produce good effects, being heating, pungent, subtile, light, placid, and drying. They act quickly, and increase semen. When in large quantities these qualities act unfavourably on the humours, and instead of strengthening the body they will destroy it. Spirits, like medicine, when taken in a proper manner, restore appetite and strength to the body. When taken with butter and rice, flesh, or other food, they increase the person's life beyond the period written at the individuals birth by strengthening, and increasing the person's health. When drank in large quantities it increases so much the internal heat, that it deranges the humours, and the person becomes mad. His sense becomes deranged, and whatever he fancies to do he will not desist from ; as singing, telling secrets, speaking nonsense, etc. When spirits are not drank according to rule, it produces different effects. There are three stages of drunkenness. In the first stage the person feels very happy, and strong. The energy of his body is increased, as also the acuteness of the senses, memory, appetite, and sleep. The person can apply to abstruse books, can play on instruments, and sing better than usual.

2nd. After these symptoms, the mind is obscured and memory deficient, the person speaks and works badly, and the person becomes like a fool. At his work his mind is not quiet, he is always lazy, sleepy, and is like a drunkard.

3rd. He goes after woman, or persons that are respected;

दूषीविषमसाध्यं स्यात् क्षीणस्याहितसेविनः॥
सौभाग्यार्थं स्त्रियः स्वेदं रजो नानाङ्गजान् मलान्।
शत्रुप्रयुक्तांश्च गरान् प्रयच्छन्त्यन्नमिश्रितान्॥

his father, mother, etc.; unnatural articles are eaten, and the person speaks everything, and takes no care of his body or goods.

4th. He becomes quite foolish, and falls to the earth like a piece of broken wood. He can do nothing, knows nothing, and lives like a dead man. If a good man, he can no longer perform good actions.

When cooling substances are eaten, or such food as does not increase phlegm, as oleaginous substances, the person will not become so easily drunk. Habit diminishes the susceptibility very much, but becomes liable to the attacks of the most fatal diseases, with sever pain. He also becomes passionate, fearful, thirsty, and melancholy. His body becomes covered with sores, etc. is constipated, and he is fond of eating sour things. In weak persons the body becomes hot, and the habit so bad as to produce various diseases.

When nothing is eaten with the spirit., he soon becomes drunk, accompanied with the diseases produced by great grief. When the person is very angry, and drinks spirit; as also when very fearful, severe diseases are produced; when very thirsty, or when there is a great grief, of when he is very hungry and spirits alone also taken. When violent exercise, as fencing, etc. is taken, or when fatigued with walking, spirits are very bad ; as also when the stomach, urine, etc. are constipated, or when very sour things have been taken, or what has been eaten is not digested, spirits will produce dangerous diseases. When the person is weak, when the body is very hot from the sun, etc. All these produce severe diseases of various kinds. Such as *Pānātya, Parammada, Pānārjirna* and *Pānārbibhrama,* in which the body is hot and heavy, has no taste, and there is much cough, no appetite, with a constipated state of the

तैः स्यात् पाण्डुः कृशोऽल्पाग्निर्गरश्चास्योपजायते॥
मर्म्म प्रधमनाध्यानं हस्तयोः शोथलक्षणम्।
जठरं ग्रहणीदोषो यक्ष्मा गुल्मः क्षयो ज्वरः।
एवंबिधस्य चान्यसा ब्याधेर्लिङ्गानि दर्शयेत्॥
तस्माल्लूनं तृणं प्राप्ता मुनेः प्रस्वेदविन्दवः।
तम्माल्लृतान्तु भाष्मन्ते संख्यया ताश्च षीड़श॥

dejections and urine. In *Pānārjirna* the body is hot, head-ache, thirst, pain in the joints, swelling of the abdomen, sour belching, etc.

When air is diseased by spirits, there is pain in the limbs, and the mind is deranged, hiccough, noisy breathing, head-ache, and severe pain in the side, such a person has no sleep, becoming delirious. When bile is deranged, thirst, heat of the body, fever, sweating, and *meha* are produced. When urine is deranged, *Atisar* (diarrhoea), *Abaran* (no memory), and the skin becomes of a green colour. In such cases phlegm is vomited, the person has no appetite, with nausea, and dozing. He has cold fits, and the body is heavy.

When the three are deranged, they produce all the symptoms of the separate diseases, with one named *Pānātya*. The secondary effects of ardent spirits are *Parammada* with deranged phlegm, which is discharged from the body, and the mouth. The body feels heavy, and the mouth has a bad taste with constipation, dozing, no appetite, thirst, head-ache, and the joints are pained.

Pānārjirna, or indigestion, it is a consequence of the free use of spirits. The stomach swells, with much vomiting, the body is hot, he complains of head-ache, the spirit is not digested, and *Ajirna*, in all its forms are produced.

Pānārbibhrama. Symptoms of deranged bile ; with pain of the chest and body, vomiting, fever, head-ache, and cough ;

ताभि द्रष्टे दंशकोत्थः प्रवृत्तिः क्षतजस्य च।
ज्वरो दाहोतिसारश्च गदाः स्युश्च त्रिदोषजाः॥
पिड़का विविधाकारा मण्डलानि महान्ति च॥
शोथा महान्तो मृदवो रक्ताः श्यावाश्चला स्तथा।
सामान्यं सर्व्वलूताना भेतद्दंशस्य लक्षणम्॥
दंशमध्ये तु यत् कृष्णं श्यावं वा जालकाचितम्॥
अर्द्धाकृति भृशं पाकः क्लेदशोथज्वरान्वितम्॥

mucus is discharged from the mouth and nose ; the trachea feals like smoke to the person, and the body hot. When a person in this disease appears as if drunk he will die of it. When the mouth of such a person is twisted or otherwise unnatural, the body is cold, but is supposed by the person to be hot, the mouth the colour of oil, the tongue, lips, teeth, of a dark colour, or blue, and eyes yellow or red, hiccough or fever, vomiting, or shivering, pain in the sides, cough, forgetfulness, he will not recover.

Dāha .(Inflammation), spirits producing heat, derange the blood, and bile of the skin and produce this disease. The following varieties are described:

1. The first variety affects the skin.

2. This variety affects the blood ; producing a wrinkled and dry state and copper colour of the skin with thirst. The smell of the body and mouth resembles that of blood, and the body is hot, like that produced by fever.

3. When bile is deranged it is like the fever which this produces when deranged : and the varieties are the same.

4. This resembles the last. The thirst is not gratified from the person's foolishness, the heat of the internal and external surface of the body is increased. The throat, palate and lips are dry, and the tongue is thrust out of the mouth with shivering of the body.

दूषीविषाभिर्लताभि स्तं दष्टमिति निर्दिशेत्।
शोथः श्वेतोसितारक्ता पीता वा पिड़का ज्वरः।
प्राणान्तिकाश्च जायन्ते श्वासहिक्का शिरोग्रहाः॥
आदंशाच्छोणितं पाण्डु मण्डलानि ज्वरोऽरतिः।
लोमहर्षश्च दाहश्चान्यखुदुषीविषार्द्दिते।
मूर्च्छाङ्गशोथवैवर्ण्य क्लेदशब्दा श्रुति ज्वराः।
शिरोगुरुत्वं लालासृक् छर्द्दिचासाध्य मूषिकैः॥

5. When much blood is collected in the abdomen, great heat is produced.

6. When much of the elements are discharged from the body, a form of this disease is produced. When *dāha* occurs the person swoons, is thirsty, mucus is discharged from the nose and that, and he cannot work. In other cases when severe, and a physician does not see the patient, he dies.

7. Sensible parts when wounded or bruised produce a kind of this disease, which is not cured, as blows on the temples. In all the above forms when the interior of the body is hot, and the exterior is cold, the disease is always dangerous.

IMPOTENCE (Dhajabhanga or Claiba)

There are six kinds of Impotency,

1st. It may be produced by dejection of the mind, or connection with distasteful women.

2nd. By eating too dry and pungent food, as black-peper, capsicum, etc. or too much acid, salt, or stimulating food. By such causes the secretion of semen is diminished.

3rd. Excessive venery, and eating little food.

4th. Old diseases of the organs of generation, or of injuries or diseases of the vital parts.

5th. The congenital variety ; and the

काष्ण्र्यः श्यावत्वमथवा नानावर्णत्व मेव वा।
मोहोऽथवर्च्चसो भेदो दष्टः स्यात् कृककण्टकैः॥
दहत्यग्निरिवादौ च भिनत्तीवार्द्ध माशु च।
बृश्चिकस्य विषं याति दंशे पश्चात्तु तिष्ठति।
दष्टोसाध्य्य हृद्घ्राणरसनोपहतो नरः।
मांसै पतद्भि रत्यर्थं वेदनार्त्तोजहात्यसुन्॥

6th. Variety is caused by avoiding sexual indulgences.

The fourth and fifth kinds are incurable. The other four kinds may be treated.

PROLAPSUS ANI (Gudabhrangsa)

The rectum is prolapsed during the evacuation of the faeces in weak persons ; particularly when affected with long continued diarrhoea, or much straining.

SUPERFICIAL ULCER ROUND THE ANUS, (Ahiputana)

Eruptions sometimes form round the anus, from want of cleanliness. They become itchy, are scratched, and ulcerate, producing this disease. They often occur in children.

SLIGHT DISEASES OF THE EXTREMITIES.

Painful swellings in the axilla are produced by bile, and phlegm. Deep seated swellings, which produce much heat, inflammation, and fever, like fire, kill after seven or twelve days, or after a fortnight. They are called *Agnirohīnī*.

When the nails are affected with inflammation round the edges it is called *Chipya*. It is produced by derangements of the bile, air, injuries, etc. The part which is connected to the flesh, especially at its angles swell, become very painful, and then ulcerate, particularly at its angles, when it is called *Upanaka*. When the nails become dry, rough, and discoloured, the disease is called *Kunakh* or *Kulina*.

विपर्प: श्वयथू: शूलं ज्वरश्छर्द्दि रथापि च।
लक्षणं कणभैद्रष्टे दंशश्चैवावसीदति॥
ह्रंष्टलोमोच्चिटिगेन स्तब्धलिङ्गो भृशार्त्तिमान्॥
दष्ट: शीतोदकेनेव सिक्तान्यङ्गानि मन्यते।
एकदंष्ट्रार्द्दित: शूनः सरुजः पीड़कास्तृषा॥
छर्द्दिर्निद्रा च स विषैर्मण्डूकै द्रष्टलक्षणम्।
मत्स्यास्तु स विषाः कुर्युर्दाहं शोथं रुजं तथा।
कण्डुं शोथं ज्वरं मूर्च्छा स विषास्तु जलौकसः।
विदाहं श्वयथुं तोदं स्वेदञ्च गृहगोधिका।
दंशे स्वेदं रुजं दाहं कुर्य्याच्छ्रतपदीविषम्॥
कण्डूमान मशकै र्विषं शोथस्यान्मन्दवेदनः।

When the sole of the foot is injured by some external cause, as by thorns, or the like, it produces much pain, and is called *Dari*. When the swelling is hard, indolent, and like the seed of plumbs, accompanied with much pain, and a considerable discharge, it is called *Kadara*. When the space between the toes ulcerate (*Rhagas*) the disease is called *Alasa.* The other diseases of the leg are described under *Bādobadī*.

Sometimes ulcers form near the axilla or groin, which become hard, red, and sinuous ; in such cases the deepseated parts are so affected that when opened they discharge frothy matter like a mixture of honey and ghee. The part then becomes dry, irregular, and discharges foetid matter of different colours with blood. Sometimes the hemorrhage is sudden and great. This disease is called *Sharkarārbuda, (Sarkara,* a piece of earthen pot, and *Arbuda,* tumor.) this probably an aneurismal tumor.

EMACIATION (*Kārsa*)

If a person takes dry food which does not contain much nourishment, as astringent and pungent kinds of food, much exercise, and venery, they produce emaciation ; if he indulges

असाध्यकीटसदृश मसाध्यं मशकक्षतम्।।
सद्यः प्रस्राविणी श्यावा दाहमूर्च्छा ज्वरान्विताः।
पीड़का मक्षिकादंशे तासान्तु स्थगिक्काऽसुहृत्
चतुष्पद्धि द्विपद्भिश्च नखदन्तविषञ्च यत्।।
पूयते पच्यते वापि स्रवति ज्वरवत्यपि।
प्रशान्तदोषं प्रकृतिस्थं घातुमन्नाभिकामं सममूत्रविट्कम्।
प्रसन्नवर्णेन्द्रियचित्तचेष्टं वैद्योऽवगच्छेदविषं मनुष्यम्।
दर्शन-स्पर्शनं-प्रश्नैः परीक्षा त्रिविधा मता।
वयोवर्ण शरीराणा मिन्द्रियानाञ्च दर्शनात्।।

।। इति श्रीमाधवकरप्रणीतं निदानं समाप्तम् ।।

in too much study, fer, grief, thinking, watching at night, or food in small quantities, the chyle is formed and absorbed in small quantities, does not circulate and nourish all parts of the body, and produces emaciation. In such a state the person becomes weak and cannot bear hunger or thirst, heat or cold, currents of air, or rain. Such a person is liable to the attacks of nervous diseases, or diseases of air, and will die of asthma, consumption, acitis, dyspepsia, *gulma* haematemesis, or haemopysis. Such a person has severe attacks of diseases.

UNHEALTHY (Costiveness) DISCHARGES (Amaha)

When the faeces are not properly prepared for expulsion, but are discharged in small quantities, with pain, it forms this disease. It is accompanied with great pain in the epigastric region, thirst, a discharge of mucus from the mouth and nose, accompanied with head-ache and heaviness of the body, particularly in the chest. The person has no eructations, complains of pain in the loins and back ; the urine and faeces are constipated with severe pain, and there is difficulty in breathing, fainting, and stercorous vomiting. These two last symptoms are only present when the *Pākasia* (the large intestines) are affected.

NOTES :

1. In some works the term *Ardita* is given to this discase, and others apply the term *Ardita* to Tetanus and Trismus.
2. Under this head several diseases are described; such as certain forms of rheumatism, abscesses; and such cachectic states as may terminate in true leprosy.
3. *Parinām Sul.* This variety had not been described before 1836, (see the *Indian Journal* for March, page114,) by European Physiciaus, which induced me to add the following particulars of this curious disease.

   Gastroperiodynia, or periodical pain in the stomach, often commences with symptoms of indigestion and heart-burn, succeeded by a feeling og uneasiness in the scrobiculus cordis, slight at first, and occurring at irregular intervals, and these lessening gradually white the pain increases in violence. In severer cases, the paroxyam of acute pain generally occurs rather suddenly, when the stomach is empty; sometimes early in the morning, or three or four hours after dinner; increassing slowly when the digestive process is finished, and the activity of the abdominal organs has ceased.

   The excruciating pain is confined to the pit of the stomach, particularly towards the right hypocondrium, although the neighbouring parts often participate, as the muscles of the lions, etc. The pain is of a cutting or gnawing nature; and during the paroxysm is intense, from which the patient generally obtains temporary relief from pressure. For this purpose he often turns upon his breast and places a hard ball in the pit of the stomach, on which he rests his body, and keeps rolling from side to side. A few days since I ordered an unfortunate person, in this position, to turn round for me to examine him; but such was the agony, that he could remain without the soothing influence of pressure. As a substitute, he drew from under his clothes a piece of pre-pared bamboo, an inch in diameter, and a cubit in length, round at one end. This extremity he placed to the pit of the stomach while hc rested the other on the floor; and by bending the body over it, produced such a degree of violent pressure, that at first I feared he would injure himself, and even penetrate the abdomen. He continued in this position while I gained the necessary information of his state, and then returned to his formed position, commenced rolling from side to side upon the hard ball, placed in the pit of the stomach, and low wailing proved how intense were his sufferings. This was an acute form of the disease, and until checked by remedies it occurred daily about 4 o'clock, and he continued in dreadful agony the whole night.

These paroxysms unually occur at intervals of a day or two, and remain from two hours to as many days, with occasional intervals of ease. During these accessions the state of the pulse, although full, continues slow and natural, and there is not usually more heat of body than is occasioned by a continual movement.

In the intermission the patient feels well and all the functions are pre-formed as when in perfect health. The tongue is clean, but sometimes parched, appetite good, and alvine secretions healthy and regular.

I have not been able to obtain any certain evidences of the casese which produce this disease. It appears to be the effect of a combinations, individually slight; but when occurring in a peculiar constitution, produces this distressing complaint. I have generally know it to occur in the young and robust male; to be aggravated by exposure to the weather, and by eating to occur when sleeping on the damp ground, etc. The accession seems oftener to occur when the organs are in a state of inactivity, than from causes increasing the nervous susceptiobility. I have not seen it in females, although there is no reason why they should not be also effected; and I am informed that they are sometimes atacked but in a less violent degree. Person of a nervous temperament are in general not so liable to this disease as might be supposed.

4. Under the term *Gulma* are arranged very different diseases : as tumours of the pylorus, partial enlargement of the liver, and diseases of the large intestines.

5. There is an instructive case in point. A young women became pregrant and for the uncomfortable sensation attending that state consulted a physician, who after trying various remedies, without effect, one of which was thrusting a red hot iron into the tumour, which is frequently done for spleen and sometimes with good effect by raising its activity; but in the present case the woman escaped. The physician finding that the disease did noot yield to his treatment declared the case to be one of *Gulma*, for which nothing could he done, and that it would increase, and she would

die with much pain, and violent shrinking. As this frightened very much the other females the patient was removed to a distant room, and in that state of anxiety passed some months, untill parturition commenced. That was considered as the approach of death, and not to defile the house she was put out into the compound upon a mat, and her female friends deserted her. In this state she was delivered of a female child to the astouishment of all, and to the disgrace of the medical man.

6. Form *Muta* urine, and *Krichchhra,* slow and painful.
7. See *Chikitsa Ratnasangraha,* or the jewels of treatment.
8. From *upa,* near; and *dangsha,* biting.
9. In Persian it is styled *Chechak*; in Sanskrit *Guti* and *Masūri* or *Musūrika,* resembling a pillor lentil *masūrā,* (Ervum hirsutum and Cicer lens.)
10. The translation was printed in England by Dr. Meadc, in 1747 : dee his Works, pages 297.
11. Ilence the name *Bisak.*

INDEX

H

I

J

K

L

✦✦✦